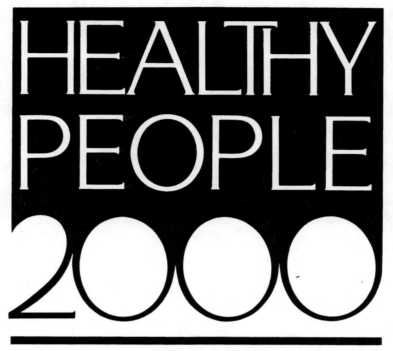

HEALTHY PEOPLE 2000

Citizens Chart the Course

Michael A. Stoto
Ruth Behrens
Connie Rosemont
Editors

Institute of Medicine

National Academy Press
Washington, D.C.
1990

NATIONAL ACADEMY PRESS • 2101 Constitution Avenue, NW • Washington, DC 20418

NOTICE: This volume was prepared as a record of the public hearings and other activities designed to gather and organize information for the United States Public Health Service in formulating national health objectives for the year 2000. The opinions expressed in this report are those of the testifiers, not the Institute of Medicine or its parent organization, the National Academy of Sciences.

The Institute of Medicine was chartered in 1970 by the National Academy of Sciences to enlist distinguished members of the appropriate professions in the examination of policy matters pertaining to the health of the public. In this, the Institute acts under both the Academy's 1863 congressional charter responsibility to be an adviser to the federal government and its own initiative in identifying issues of medical care, research, and education.

The project was supported by the Office of Disease Prevention and Health Promotion, Office of the Assistant Secretary of Health, Department of Health and Human Services under corporate agreement no. HPV-87-002-03-0.

Library of Congress Catalog Card Number 90-62772
International Standard Book Number 0-309-04340-9

Additional copies of this report are available from:

National Academy Press
2101 Constitution Avenue, NW
Washington, D.C. 20418

S224

COMMITTEE ON HEALTH OBJECTIVES FOR THE YEAR 2000

MERLIN K. DuVAL, Chairman, Committee on Health Objectives for the Year 2000, Institute of Medicine, National Academy of Sciences, Washington, D.C.

KATHARINE BAUER SOMMERS, Scholar-in-Residence, Institute of Medicine, National Academy of Sciences, Washington, D.C.

JACK ELINSON, Distinguished Visiting Professor, Institute of Health, Health Care Policy and Aging Research, Rutgers University, New Brunswick, New Jersey

ANNE HUBBARD MATTSON, Director of Adult Health Services, Jefferson County Health Department, Birmingham, Alabama

GILBERT S. OMENN, Dean, School of Public Health & Community Medicine, Professor of Medicine and of Environmental Health, University of Washington, Seattle, Washington

STAFF

GARY B. ELLIS, Director, Division of Health Promotion and Disease Prevention

MICHAEL A. STOTO, Study Director

KAY C. HARRIS, Staff Officer

CYNTHIA HOWE, Research Associate

CONNIE ROSEMONT, Research Assistant

MARTY ELLINGTON, Research Assistant

RUTH BEHRENS, Writer

RENIE SCHAPIRO, Writer

ROSEANNE McTYRE, Writer

JANE S. DURCH, Consultant

DONNA D. THOMPSON, Project Secretary

TABLE OF CONTENTS

Preface

Our nation's willingness to commit almost 12 percent of its economy to health care—from one-third to three times more than all other nations—should be rewarded with the best health outcomes in the world. Unfortunately, it isn't. On the contrary, many of our health statistics indicate poor outcomes. Some have argued that this discrepancy can be attributed to such things as our geographic size, our multiracial and ethnic diversity, and the extreme socioeconomic heterogeneity of our citizens. Others believe it is futile to seek a direct relationship between good health and what we spend in its pursuit because, as often as not, our health profiles may be an expression of the choices we make as we go through life rather than of the care we receive when we are ill.

Clearly, both views have validity. For example, some of the best health statistics in the world come from nations that are barely the size of one of our western states, and whose homogeneous populations are not even one-third as great in number. At the same time, our citizens jealously guard their right to make unconstrained personal choices about the way they wish to live. And they do, for good or for ill.

The genius of the Health Objectives for the Year 2000 project, an initiative of the U.S. Public Health Service, is that it rises above these discontinuities by acknowledging that demography, biomedical science, and personal behavior all play roles in determining our health status; therefore, all must be addressed as part of any effort to prevent diseases through the promotion of health and the reduction of risks.

To give both energy and breadth to this effort, Health Objectives for the Year 2000 solicits the active participation of America's businesses, industries, and education and professional institutions and agencies, whether for-profit or voluntary. It invites them to join hands with federal, state, and local governmental units in a common pursuit of better health for everyone. In this pursuit, the problems of particularly difficult target groups, such as those who live at the extremities of life as measured by age or circumstance, are being emphasized because of their special significance to, and impact upon, all of us.

The specific role played by the U.S. Public Health Service in orchestrating this remarkable effort deserves particular comment. For almost 200 years the PHS has served us well through its mixed missions of regulation, biomedical research, and service to specifically designated beneficiaries. Then, barely 15 years ago, our Congress added Title XVII to the Public Health Service Act authorizing the Secretary of the Department of Health, Education and Welfare (now Health and Human Services) to establish, for the first time, national goals and strategies in disease prevention and health promotion.

The Health Objectives for the Year 2000 project is the Department's principal response to that challenge. It was crafted so well that it permitted all interested parties—as exemplified by more than 800 pieces of testimony—to help define the kind of society they want for the next decade by giving form and substance to the objectives themselves. Even Marshall McLuhan might argue that, in this instance, the medium not only is the message but also may have successfully integrated the ends with the means.

Merlin K. DuVal, M.D.
Chairman
Committee on Health Objectives for the Year 2000

Acknowledgments

This volume represents the work of well over 1,000 individuals around the United States. As we explain in more detail in the introduction, the text is based on testimony presented at seven major regional hearings held in the winter of 1988 and other special hearings, and in writing to the Institute of Medicine. Much of the testimony comes from the 300 national organizations and state health departments that make up the Consortium on the Year 2000 Health Objectives, or people these organizations nominated. The individuals and organizations that submitted testimony as well as the organizers and cosponsors of the regional hearings are listed in the appendix. Although we were not able to quote every piece of testimony in the text, we are truly grateful for the efforts of the people who prepared testimony or helped to organize the hearings.

This volume was prepared under the guidance of the Institute of Medicine's Committee on Health Objectives for the Year 2000 (whose members are listed on p. iii) and the Board on Health Promotion and Disease Prevention. We have benefited from many helpful suggestions from the members of these committees, and from members of the Institute of Medicine who read and commented on early drafts. The final responsibility for the content of the report, however, rests with the editors.

The work also benefited from many Institute of Medicine staff members, only some of whom are listed with the project staff. I would especially like to note the contributions of Queta Bond, the current Executive Officer, who served as Director of the Division of Health Promotion and Disease Prevention when this project began, and Marian Osterweis, who served as Director in 1989. In addition, Connie Rosemont and Donna Thompson, the project's research assistant and secretary, respectively, worked long and hard hours revising and preparing the text for publication, checking the references, and making sure that our attributions were as accurate as possible.

Note on Authorship

The following list identifies the persons who shared the responsibility for preparing the first draft of each chapter in this volume.

Marty Ellington: Chapter 6
Kay Harris: Chapter 18
Cynthia Howe: Chapters 4, 5, and 17
Roseanne McTyre: Chapters 10 and 11
Connie Rosemont: Chapters 6, 7, 9, 15, 16, and 18
Renie Schapiro: Chapters 12, 13, 19, 20, 21, 22, 23, 24, 25, 26, and 27
Michael Stoto: Chapters 1, 2, 3, 4, 5, 6, 8, 9, and 14

The material in the chapters is drawn from testimony submitted to the Institute of Medicine. The initial drafts were submitted to the Public Health Service for use in formulating the Year 2000 Health Objectives and for review. The draft chapters also were reviewed by the testifiers cited, the Committee on Health Objectives for the Year 2000, members of the Institute of Medicine, and others. Taking these reviews into account, the editors revised and reorganized the draft chapters into what appears in this volume. *The opinions expressed in this report are those of the testifiers, not the Institute of Medicine or its parent organization, the National Academy of Sciences.* Chapter authors are listed above to give credit to individuals but not to assign final responsibility for the published text. The revision and editing of the volume were shared by Ruth Behrens, Connie Rosemont, and myself.

Michael A. Stoto, Ph.D.
Study Director
Committee on Health Objectives for the Year 2000

1. Introduction

Of the broad range of governmental responsibilities in public health, perhaps none is more fundamental than the obligation to provide perspective and direction to guide health programs along a productive course—the agenda-setting function. Its importance stems from the ability of nationally identified goals to motivate and recruit the commitment of local and private resources.[1]

Fulfilling this responsibility, the U.S. Public Health Service and other public and private organizations around the country through the Healthy People 2000 process are about to embark on a course aimed at achieving ambitious national health goals by the year 2000. This effort builds on the nation's decade-long initiative to meet a series of health promotion/disease prevention objectives established in the late 1970s aimed at making the United States a nation of healthy people, regardless of age, race, or socioeconomic status, by 1990.

These goals are national in scope, and the successes that have been achieved also must be credited to a national—not solely a federal or governmental—effort. In establishing a new set of health objectives for the year 2000, it is clear that the cooperation and commitment of every segment of the public and private sectors are needed. Only through concerted, focused efforts, made by large numbers of caring, concerned individuals and organizations, can this become a nation of truly healthy people. As a first step in this process, the views of Americans from all sectors about what the goals should be are summarized in this report.

HISTORY AND PURPOSE OF THE OBJECTIVES

Because of the fundamental public health accomplishments of earlier generations, today's national health agenda focuses increasingly on health promotion and disease prevention. This new direction was made possible by massive public health and sanitation reforms after the turn of the century that dramatically reduced infectious diseases. In the 1930s the introduction of effective vaccines and antibiotics further improved health status. More recent improvements in clinical care can be tied to revolutionary advances in medical research and medical technology.

Although disease prevention has always been a major responsibility of the Public Health Service (PHS), in the late 1970s the PHS recommitted its efforts to health promotion and disease prevention in response to Title XVII of the Public Health Service Act, which directed the Secretary of Health and Human Services to establish national goals for health promotion and disease prevention. The PHS responded in 1979 by publishing *Healthy People: The Surgeon General's Report on Health Promotion and Disease Prevention*.[2] The report presented a set of general goals for reducing preventable death and injury in different age groups by 1990.

In 1980 the PHS took the process a step further by identifying a set of 226 quantitative health promotion and disease prevention objectives for 1990 in *Promoting Health/Preventing Disease: Objectives for the Nation*.[3] The publication followed extensive reviews of the knowledge base and expert opinion in each area. The objectives were expressed as quantitative measures, for example, reducing the national rate of infant mortality to no more than 9 out of 1,000 live births by 1990. (In 1978 the infant mortality rate was 12 per 1,000 live births.) Additional objectives addressed the special needs of minorities, one stating that by 1990, no county and no racial or ethnic group should have an infant mortality rate in excess of 12 deaths per 1,000 live births. (In 1978 the rate for Blacks was 23 per 1,000 live births.) The range of endpoints encompassed by the objectives included improved health status, reduced risk factors, increased public and professional awareness, improved services and protection, and improved surveillance and evaluation systems.

During the 1980s, these objectives for improving clinical preventive services, health protection, and health promotion provided a common strategy and a frame of reference that sparked new initiatives by state and local governments and community organizations and increased interagency cooperation in the federal government. Perhaps most important, they provided a sense of unity for the disparate professional activities, both public and private, that contribute so much to the health of the country. Because the health objectives set precise numerical targets and provided baseline data for measuring progress, they have served to track improvements and to spotlight problem areas in the nation's health status. National response to the 1990 Objectives has confirmed the usefulness of the objectives approach. By 1985, the United States was on the way to meeting about half of the 1990 Objectives, and the country has seen major reductions in the amount of illness and death in specified categories for infants, children, and adults.[4]

The success of the 1990 Objectives demonstrates vividly that a well-formulated set of national health promotion and disease prevention objectives can increase interagency and intergovernmental cooperation and can provide a lasting health promotion/ disease prevention strategy that will continue to capture public interest over time. Health promotion and disease prevention deserve a massive, interdisciplinary effort from government and the private sector. In the course of developing new objectives to be achieved by the year 2000, suggestions were offered about how to make the process maximally effective.

As Jerrold Michael, Dean of the School of Public Health of the University of Hawaii, says, "Objectives are only meaningful when they reflect and are relevant to a vision that we have of the kind of society we want." The conditions necessary to achieve these objectives are important, especially

> competence in the health professions and informed supportive leadership in the community. Achievement of health objectives is not in the hands of the health professions alone. The resources of health, education, economic development, and human services must become connected to and interwoven with health objectives. (#149)

A group of state health officers, all of whom have worked to implement the 1990 Objectives within their states, summed up their view of the national objectives in this way. First, they felt that the objectives should be national, not just federal. Although the federal government is providing leadership and a process for developing the objectives, federal, state, and local government officials; industry; educational institutions; and private, nonprofit organizations must "take ownership" of the objectives and play a role in implementing them. Second, they felt that the objectives process must allow for local/regional variations in which communities can outline and address their independent needs within the national framework. Third, they said that the objectives should be tied to

a process of implementation so that states and communities can implement national goals at the local level. Finally, they felt that establishing and achieving national health objectives is a process that will require the commitment of resources from all levels of government—not just the federal government—as well as from private sources. Lawmaking bodies, from the Congress to individual city councils, must be encouraged to accept the idea of national objectives and support the objectives by appropriating funds. Resources from industry and nonprofit organizations must be identified and mobilized. (#750)

The private sector agrees. According to Paul Entmacher, who represented the Business Roundtable:

> The public sector should take the primary leadership role in establishing health objectives and providing surveillance over the nation's health, but the Business Roundtable endorses the concept of ongoing, nonpartisan, appropriate, public-private collaboration in setting and measuring the nation's health objectives. We naturally wish to contribute mainly to those objectives that could affect the employers and employees in the business community in the United States in the year 2000. There is a fundamental commonality, however, between the eventual national objectives and the nation's private sector work force because as citizens and taxpayers they either are or ought to be vitally concerned about the health of their environment. (#465)

HEARINGS AND TESTIMONY

To develop a framework for cooperation and action by the diverse groups that play important roles in improving the nation's health, the Public Health Service and the Institute of Medicine (IOM) held hearings in seven cities across the country in early 1988. The purpose of the hearings was to solicit testimony from a broad range of individuals and community organizations about appropriate and attainable national health promotion and disease prevention objectives for the year 2000.

The hearings provided a forum for groups and individuals to propose precise quantitative objectives for maintaining health and reducing death, disease, and disability; interventions to meet these objectives; and surveillance programs to assess preventive needs and efforts. The hearings also provided an opportunity to build upon the nation's earlier prevention program, the 1990 Objectives for the Nation, first presented by the Surgeon General in 1980. An outgrowth of the hearings was the promotion of widespread interest and involvement in the agenda-setting process in general, as well as a commitment on the part of virtually all testifiers to help develop and implement the Year 2000 Health Objectives specifically.

The PHS and the IOM also have convened a Year 2000 Health Objectives Consortium of more than 300 national professional and voluntary organizations and state and territorial health departments to help guide the hearing process. These organizations held their own special hearings on the objectives, submitted official written testimony, and helped review the draft objectives. Equally important, these groups (listed in the appendix) will provide leadership in all sectors and at all levels in implementing the Year 2000 Health Objectives.

The IOM and the PHS used a two-prong strategy to organize the hearings. First, local cosponsors were identified in each of the cities, including schools of public health and departments of community medicine, state health departments, and local voluntary and professional organizations. All of the local cosponsors were asked to suggest speakers from the geographical area of the hearing. Second, consortium member organizations were asked to suggest speakers for each of the regional hearings.

Day-and-a-half-long regional hearings were held in seven cities—Birmingham, Los Angeles, Houston, Seattle, Denver, Detroit, and New York—between January and March 1988. A total of almost 1,000 participants registered for the hearings, including representatives of the sponsoring organizations, representatives of consortium groups and other interested local and national organizations, public health officials, college and university faculty and students, and others. Speakers at the hearings represented the wide variety of organizations that work to promote health, including public and private health care organizations; public health agencies at federal, state, and local levels; employers; schools; insurers; community organizations; and minority groups. Almost 100 national and local organizations suggested speakers. Each hearing provided time for brief invited testimony, followed by an open session for comments from the floor. In all, 318 people testified at regional hearings. In addition, many individuals who were not able to attend the hearings submitted written testimony. In total more than 800 individuals and

organizations submitted testimony.

At each of the seven regional hearings, a panel received the testimony on behalf of the Public Health Service and questioned the speakers to help clarify their points of view and recommendations. The panels included representatives of the PHS central office (Washington or Atlanta), the PHS regional office, the Association of State and Territorial Health Officers, the IOM, and other private sector groups.

Questions for Testifiers

In preparing their testimony, testifiers were asked to address the following questions:

1. What targets for disease prevention and health promotion should be identified for achievement by the year 2000 that were not identified in the 1990 Objectives? What measures do you propose for improving health status or reducing risk factors? What measures do you propose for achieving the outcomes selected?
2. Which, if any, of the 1990 targets for prevention might be dropped in the Year 2000 Health Objectives?
3. In reviewing the 1990 Objectives in your area(s) of interest, what revisions do you suggest in the quantitative measures proposed, both in health outcomes and in prevention/promotion approaches such as professional education, information services, technology, research, and evaluation?
4. What data are available for tracking the quantitative measures you propose? What suggestions can you make for closing gaps in such data?
5. In discussing the burden of illness and the cost to society of identified target areas, what are your suggestions to improve measures of these costs?

Because their oral presentations were brief, speakers were encouraged to supplement their remarks with written testimony. They also were asked to include documentation and specific references to the literature on each subject area.

Scope of the Testimony

The testifiers addressed nearly every aspect of health promotion and disease prevention but, as might be expected, their testimony was not evenly distributed across topics, nor was it proportional to the relative magnitude of various health problems. Although most of the testimony focused on objectives themselves, many speakers addressed the needs of special populations and crosscutting areas such as implementing the objectives and financing health promotion and disease prevention programs.

Approximately one-third of the speakers testified primarily about the need to develop preventive services targeted against specific diseases and problems such as cancer, heart disease and stroke, infant mortality, unintended pregnancies (especially among adolescents), AIDS, infectious and sexually transmitted diseases, oral health problems, and other chronic conditions. Chronic diseases also were discussed frequently in testimony that focused on health promotion strategies.

More than one-fourth of those who testified stressed health promotion issues, including behavior modification and health education. Speakers asked for strengthened programs dealing with smoking and smokeless tobacco use, alcohol and drug abuse, nutrition, physical fitness, and mental health.

About one in four speakers addressed the special needs of components of the population. Some addressed the needs of racial and ethnic minorities such as Blacks, Hispanics, and Native Americans. Others focused on the needs of population age groups, especially the elderly and adolescents, as well as the disabled. Many stressed the special needs of the poor and homeless. The speakers who addressed these issues generally agreed that more objectives should be targeted specifically toward these groups than had been for 1990.

Approximately one in five witnesses testified about health problems and solutions associated with the physical and social environment. Some wrote or spoke about efforts to clean up the air, the water, and the food supply, and to improve the disposal of hazardous waste. Others addressed intentional and unintentional violence, often stemming from alcohol or drug abuse and family problems. Many speakers addressed the need for improved workplace safety and disease prevention measures.

Many witnesses identified areas in which resources were lacking, including (1) data, especially for states and smaller areas, and for minorities; (2) information about successful prevention strategies; (3) personnel resources; and above all, (4) financial resources for preventive services and health promotion programs.

Speakers also addressed technical issues, including developing and implementing national objectives at the state and local levels as well as the need to reduce the number of objectives and have them reflect national priorities.

Witnesses answered the questions given to them in advance, but most speakers did not address all of the questions. Some 450 testifiers recommended specific health promotion and disease prevention programs, and one-third of these gave some information on their efficacy. A similar number suggested objectives to be considered, at least in a generic form, and more than half of these witnesses proposed specific, quantitative values that they thought were achievable by the year 2000.

After the hearings and the submission of all written testimony, the process began that would summarize more than 800 pieces of testimony into a form that could be used by 21 PHS working groups to develop actual objectives.

First, each piece of testimony was categorized according to topic, target group, and delivery setting addressed. Then each individual piece of testimony was summarized. In addition, papers were developed synthesizing the testimony that was given on 18 individual topics, 4 target populations, and 4 implementation issues that cut across all topic areas. Finally, all of the objectives proposed by the witnesses were compiled and matched to the relevant topics. Completed summary material was then sent to the appropriate PHS working groups. Members of the working groups also had the opportunity to read the complete body of testimony or refer to it for clarification of a particular point.

PURPOSE AND STRUCTURE OF THIS REPORT

This report has two purposes:

First, it provides important information for those drafting objectives at all levels. The report does not relate every statement made in the testimony, but instead highlights major themes, puts the testimony in context, and spells out the implications of this testimony for setting objectives. All of the testimony has been distributed to the groups writing the national objectives, and this report serves as a guide to that material. Groups drafting objectives for states or local areas, or for other organizations, should also find the structure created by this report and the material summarized here useful.

Second, it serves as the record of a unique process in which over 1,000 concerned health professionals and laymen from all regions of the country contributed their knowledge and experience to the building of national objectives for health promotion and disease prevention. Those present at the regional hearings were uniformly impressed with the level of commitment that the participants exhibited to the objectives-setting process and to the activities that the objectives address. To build broader commitment to the Year 2000 Health Objectives, this report recognizes the contributions these individuals made and documents their efforts.

Although the report has been checked for factual accuracy and completeness, it is primarily the work of the individuals who submitted testimony. It does not attempt or purport to fully discuss the topics in terms of data, or of programming, evaluation, and policy issues. Rather, it is designed to document the hearings and to present highlights in a form that is useful to those attempting to adapt and implement the objectives at the state, national, or local level.

The opinions expressed in this report are those of the testifiers, not the Institute of Medicine or its parent organization, the National Academy of Sciences. Testimony cited and quoted in the text is referenced with a number in parentheses, and a list at the end of each chapter gives the name and affiliation of the testifiers (as of the date of their testimony). When testimony was received in writing from one of the consortium organizations, the statement is attributed to the organization rather than to the individual who submitted it.

This report is input to the Healthy People 2000 process, but it is not the final word. The Year 2000 Health Objectives themselves will be published by the Public Health Service in September 1990.

Structure of This Document

Because both the testifiers and the readers of this report approach health promotion and disease prevention activities from different perspectives, a number of organizing principles have been used for the report.

First, following this introduction, the report contains two chapters that address crosscutting issues relating to the development of objectives or their implementation. Chapter 2 discusses the process of developing national, state, and local objectives and is based on experience with the 1990 Objectives around the country. Chapter 3 focuses on implementing the objectives at the state and local levels, including the need for surveillance and information resources. The chapters on the structure and format of the objectives and the process of determining their content will be useful to those developing similar objectives for states, local areas, and other segments of the population. The chapter on implementation, surveillance, and information resources addresses the steps necessary to

implement the objectives at all levels.

Second, the report contains four chapters that address special health promotion and disease prevention needs and opportunities in particular components of the population. These include children and adolescents, older adults, people with disabilities, and racial or ethnic minorities. These groups deserve special attention (1) because their problems are especially severe; (2) because individualized, culturally specific approaches are sometimes required to address these problems; and (3) because the only way to make a substantial difference for the entire population is to target groups whose problems are particularly severe.

Third, the report summarizes the large amount of testimony that was received on health promotion and disease prevention in special settings, especially in the health care system, in schools, at the worksite, and in the community. Chapters address the potential for health promotion and disease prevention activities in the four settings, the barriers to these activities in medical and nonmedical settings, and the means to overcome them. Principles of health education appropriate for all settings are also discussed.

The remainder of the material is organized according to the substantive priority areas for which national objectives will be formulated. There are 18 such chapters, organized into three groups. The first group addresses behavioral risk factors and problems: tobacco use, alcohol and drug abuse, nutrition, physical fitness, and mental health issues. The second group discusses health problems related to the physical and social environment: unintentional injuries, violence and abusive behavior, environmental health, and occupational safety and health issues. The third group focuses on approaches to preventing specific diseases and health problems: human immunodeficiency virus (HIV) infection, sexually transmitted diseases, infectious diseases, maternal and infant health problems, adolescent pregnancy, heart disease and stroke, cancer, other chronic and disabling conditions, and oral health problems.

The following three groupings correspond roughly to the three categories that have come to represent health promotion and disease prevention activities and the national objectives.

1. *Health promotion* activities seek to facilitate community and individual measures to foster lifestyles that maintain and enhance the state of health and well-being.

2. *Health protection* activities target population groups and foster changes in the environment conducive to improved health and well-being. Health

protection activities include changes in the physical environment as well as changes in the social environment brought about through legislation and government regulation.

3. *Preventive health services* are targeted toward individuals to prevent the occurrence of specific diseases and disorders. These interventions are usually carried out in health care settings.

Many of the health problems addressed by the objectives, however, require a range of health promotion, health protection, and preventive service measures, and do not fall cleanly into one of these categories. Nevertheless, the categories are helpful in organizing discussion and efforts, and appear in various ways throughout this report.

REFERENCES

1. McGinnis JM: Setting nationwide objectives in disease prevention and health promotion. The United States experience. Oxford Textbook of Public Health. Edited by WW Holland, R Detels, G Knox. Oxford: Oxford University Press, 1985

2. U.S. Department of Health, Education and Welfare: Healthy People: The Surgeon General's Report on Health Promotion and Disease Prevention (DHEW Publication No. [PHS] 79-55071), 1979

3. U.S. Department of Health and Human Services: Promoting Health/Preventing Disease: Objectives for the Nation. Washington, D.C.: U.S. Government Printing Office, 1980

4. U.S. Department of Health and Human Services: The 1990 Objectives for the Nation: A Midcourse Review. Washington, D.C.: U.S. Government Printing Office, November 1986

TESTIFIERS CITED IN CHAPTER 1

149 Michael, Jerrold; University of Hawaii School of Public Health
465 Entmacher, Paul; Metropolitan Life Insurance Company
750 Richland, Jud; Association of State and Territorial Health Officials

2. Objectives Process and Structure

More than 150 witnesses focused their testimony on issues related to the process of setting objectives and to the nature of the objectives themselves. Their testimony, often based on experience in developing and implementing objectives at the state level, gave suggestions about the scope of the objectives, their organization and format, and the need to address special subpopulations. Many testifiers also addressed the need to set priorities among the objectives and suggested ways to do so.

Some of this testimony is relevant to developing national objectives, and the ideas have already been incorporated into the structure of the Year 2000 Health Objectives. The ideas in this chapter also are relevant to implementation of the national objectives. This material may, however, be most relevant for state and local governments or other organizations that are developing their own objectives, and for the future development of national objectives.

NATURE OF THE OBJECTIVES

Those who testified at the hearings and in writing had much to say about the nature of the Year 2000 Health Objectives. Their comments, for instance, addressed the need to go beyond narrow definitions of health and to include the social conditions that underlie health problems. Others addressed the basic framework for the objectives and suggested alternative frameworks for health promotion and disease prevention.

Need to Address Social Conditions

Those who addressed the issue of social conditions agreed that national objectives focusing exclusively on health matters are in danger of missing the underlying causes of illness.

"As broad as these objectives are and will be," writes Jule Sugarman, Secretary of the Washington State Department of Social and Health Services, "they are not broad enough to assure the preservation of health. The World Health Organization is asking its member nations to consider in its health policies the impact on health of education, housing, business, agriculture and the other sectors of society. We in this nation need to give more public attention to

these intersectoral impacts on health." (#337) In a similar vein, the American Public Health Association suggests that "many health problems could be ameliorated by improved social conditions, including employment, housing, nutrition, and greater access to health care." (#198)

Members of the Society for Prospective Medicine propose that the objectives address and emphasize social issues, as well as medical/technical issues, as the means to attain national health goals. (#374) Bernard Turnock, Director of the Illinois Department of Public Health, suggests that interventions be designed around models "that allow for a broad definition of health and consider such issues as transportation, ability to pay for services, and housing." (#215)

Peter Pulrang of the Washington State Bureau of Parent and Child Health illustrates this point more specifically. The 1990 Objectives, he feels, are a "one-step-at-a-time" process that is presently effective, but not enough to bring about necessary behavior changes, especially by the year 2000. Better pregnancy outcomes result not just from education, but also from emotional, economic, and environmental security, and from availability and access to appropriate medical care and support services. (#354)

Concepts of Health Promotion and Disease Prevention

Some testimony addressed the basic question of how health promotion and disease prevention activities are conceptualized and the implications for developing a structure for the objectives. Suggestions ranged from developing a more systematic and elemental approach that looks at each health problem and its causes, to developing a more holistic approach that targets basic underlying causes and requires multifactorial interventions. Another point of agreement was that the objectives should be more positive and should focus on health-enhancing factors rather than on diseases and disorders.

William Lassek, Regional Health Administrator for Public Health Service Region III in Philadelphia, calls for "a significant change in the organization of the objectives to bring them in line with accepted principles of public health epidemiology, i.e., beginning with a negative health outcome, determining its risk factors, and designing an intervention to reduce the risk factors." Lassek proposes the following:

• Define new goals by age group for reducing mortality.

• For each age group, enumerate and track the leading causes of death by race and sex.

• Within each age group, set separate goals for Whites and non-Whites, and track the rates separately.

• For each cause of death within each age group, enumerate the major risk factors.

• Set objectives for interventions known to reduce risk factors.

• Treat major causes of morbidity in the same way as major causes of death. *(#126)*

Professor Joseph Stokes of the Boston University Medical Center suggests that the Year 2000 Health Objectives be organized along the McKeown model of health and disease determinants, the model used by the Canadian Lalonde report.[1] According to Stokes, "McKeown classifies these determinants as: (1) biological factors mediated through genetic transmission; (2) factors in the physical, biological and social environment; and (3) health behaviors such as diet, exercise, cigarette smoking, alcohol and other drug use, sexual behavior, motor vehicle and other accident-risk behavior and finally health services—particularly preventive health services." *(#627)*

Others emphasize the importance of crosscutting problems and the need for multifactorial approaches. The American Academy of Family Physicians notes that the structure of the Year 2000 Health Objectives is organized on a problem-specific basis rather than a solution basis.

This is a substantial barrier to health care. In the traditional approach to medical education, the body is taken apart by various organ systems and each studied in almost complete isolation from the others. However, this is not how the body works. There are no hearts without brains, no lungs without arms and legs. The body is a highly integrated system. So too it is with medical problems. Within the practice of family medicine, no disease is an island unto itself. Most disease is multifactorial. So, too, the solutions need to be multifactorial. *(#072)*

Frank Bright of the Ohio Department of Health echoes the point.

Chronic diseases and conditions often have multiple risk factors, may be multifactorial in origin, often occur together, and may work synergistically to contribute to poor health. Chronic disease needs to be addressed in a multi-part, integrative approach that considers all of the various factors that contribute to the problem. *(#470)*

Many testifiers feel that the objectives should focus on positive states and health-enhancing factors. According to Lynn Artz of the University of Alabama at Birmingham, the 1990 Objectives are concerned with disease prevention and focus on risk factors and negative states. Positive states and health-enhancing factors should also be identified, and objectives set to achieve them. Artz gives the following examples: "Increase the proportion of Americans who consume optimal quantities of fresh fruits, vegetables and whole grains; who are physically fit; who sleep eight hours a night; who are satisfied with their interpersonal relationships; who feel good about themselves, their health, and their lives." *(#667)*

Carol Foster of the Children's Hospital of Los Angeles also feels that the overall orientation of the objectives should be more positive. "The purpose of each initiative should be to achieve some definite state (such as a positive pregnancy outcome) rather than to avoid a list of the possible negative outcomes." *(#536)* The American Society of Allied Health Professions suggests that quality of life statements be incorporated in the objectives and that the objectives not be limited to morbidity and mortality statements. It further suggests that emphasis be placed on the development and refinement of health status indicators to measure life quality characteristics. *(#631)*

Testifiers suggest that psychological, emotional, and social problems be balanced with physical problems. According to Michael Jarrett, Commissioner of the South Carolina Department of Health and Environmental Control, "Many objectives appear to be very weak regarding the influence of psychosocial issues on the health status of the nation. Greater attention needs to be paid to these issues with objectives that include intervention strategies." *(#108)*

FORMAT AND FOCUS OF THE OBJECTIVES

Many witnesses spoke about the focus and the organization of the objectives. For example, according to Mark Richards, Secretary of Health for the

Commonwealth of Pennsylvania:

One of the problems in implementing the 1990 Objectives was that there were too many different and inconsistently stated objectives. This can only dilute our effectiveness in implementing programs to address these objectives. Therefore, the Year 2000 Health Objectives should be more focused and specific, and perhaps less global than the 1990 Objectives. *(#387)*

On the other hand, numerous witnesses called for the addition of new topic areas and new target audiences which, when added together, would greatly increase the number of objectives.

Others addressed the need for more complete and accurate data, and for objectives that are grouped by or targeted to subgroups in the population.

Measurement Issues

The lack of accurate and timely data to measure progress toward the objectives, especially for local areas and minority populations, and the lack of outcome measures other than mortality have important implications for the format of the objectives. Those who testified on this issue suggested that data availability and quality be addressed directly in formulating the objectives and that attempts be made to identify potential sources for filling gaps in the information base.

According to Richards, for instance, a

major implementation problem with the 1990 Objectives was unavailability of related or proxy data to measure the status of some objectives. At the state level in Pennsylvania, we could review only 50 out of 226 objectives; at local levels, the problem of lack of data was even worse.[2] *(#387)*

Jarrett also stresses the importance of having measurable objectives and uniform or widely known data sources and advocates the Centers for Disease Control's Behavioral Risk Factor Surveillance System, or something similar. *(#108)*

The Association for Vital Records and Health Statistics (AVRHS) recommends the following:

• Objectives should be stated in quantitative terms and should be measurable.

• If data sources do not exist to measure an objective, a mechanism for obtaining adequate data should be indicated.

• Data used to measure objectives should be of high quality.

• Local and state data needs should be addressed, as well as national data needs.

• Data sources for measuring progress toward each objective should be cited.

The AVRHS adds:

Since the Year 2000 Objectives will provide a focus for many agencies working to improve the health of all citizens and are expected to be translated to state and local needs, many state and local agencies also will adopt the same objectives. Data systems should, where possible, address the needs of state and local agencies as well as those for the nation. *(#527)*

Robert Harmon, Director of the Missouri Department of Health, says that "information systems have to be built around the objectives to provide *meaningful* information about progress in achieving them. This will take an expenditure of resources." He adds, "The resources needed for this task are critical to the success of the entire objectives-setting process and should not be short-changed." *(#085)* The National Safety Council warns that requiring quantified objectives means that some important problems may be neglected. It suggests that a new format be developed for health problems such as stress and age-related disabilities, by using descriptive rather than quantitative paradigms. "It is possible, for instance, to state that situation B is better than situation A even though we cannot assign any percentage or ratio to this improvement." *(#019)*

Artz also is concerned that the objectives not be limited to easily measured outcomes. The 1990 Objectives "emphasize problems resulting in death over problems that cause relatively more morbidity and disability." The objectives stressed problems that can be measured easily such as homicide, suicide, and infant mortality. Hence, there are no objectives for sexual assault, nonfatal domestic violence, and so on. *(#667)*

Oregon's experience with using objectives at the state level suggests that the current availability of data should not be a determinant of the nature of the objectives. "Perhaps the most useful result of our project was the identification of data gaps," says Michael Skeels of the Oregon Department of Human

Resources. *(#321)*

Group Objectives by Population Subgroups

Many of the witnesses suggested that the national objectives include special objectives grouped by and targeted to various demographic, racial, ethnic, and other subpopulations. The potential groups suggested include men and women, the old and young, racial and ethnic minorities, the poor, the homeless, and various kinds of workers. The basic rationale was that separate "special population targets" are necessary to identify the groups most in need of intervention and to target programs, especially programs designed for their needs, to them.

Sheryl Ruzek of Temple University, for instance, suggests that special objectives are required for women. These would include sexual assault, problems associated with female reproductive organs and processes, and unnecessary medical interventions that are frequently applied to women such as hysterectomies, aggressive surgery for breast cancer, and cesarean sections. They would employ strategies that include providing health information; supporting community development; and promoting regulatory, legislative, and judicial measures. *(#189)*

Ronald Mazur of the University of Massachusetts at Amherst suggests a "men's health" category, focusing on violence and destructive behavior, including alcohol-related trauma. *(#530)*

Nancy Stevens of Kaiser Permanente suggests organizing the objectives by "age group (infants, children, adolescents, adults, older adults) or constituent groups (schools, worksites, municipalities), as well as diagnostic group. This type of presentation would enable providers of care, service, or employment to identify the health issues that are pertinent to specific populations, as well as diagnostic groups." *(#352)* Members of the Society for Prospective Medicine also feel that the objectives should be made for age groups, especially the elderly and children. *(#374)* Edward Wagner of the Group Health Cooperative of Puget Sound, for instance, found the 1990 Objectives useful for establishing health status goals for older Americans, but complained that specific 1990 Objectives provided little guidance in identifying specific interventions to reduce unnecessary disability among the elderly. *(#738)* According to Jerrold Michael of the University of Hawaii, representing the Association of Schools of Public Health:

[We should not] leave the differentiation of the needs of special groups as a postscript in documents that never catch up with the main body of the report. We are all special in some way. Our differences are what provides us with the spirit and creativity of our pluralistic society. These differences, in need, in aspiration, in priority, in concern, require more than a single approach. We are talking not only of groups in high risk who need special attention—although these needs must be a starting point for much of our decision making—but of the larger concept that requires us to be obligated to pattern health objectives to the needs, interests, realities, and possibilities of specific contexts. Health for all never is achieved with a standardized set of outcomes. *(#149)*

Robert Bernstein, Commissioner of the Texas Department of Health, agrees, and suggests that the objectives "target special populations such as the school-age population or a geographic area and ethnic groups like the Mexican-American populations along the U.S.-Mexico border. Attention in objective setting and initiatives developed to address the needs of these special populations will help focus attention and comprehensive action on improving the health of the high-risk and priority populations." *(#020)*

Many witnesses felt that reducing disparities in health between economic and racial groups should be an overriding goal for the year 2000. According to John Waller of Wayne State University:

The recognition of vulnerability and documented disparities in health status between White and minority populations should be sufficient justification for establishing within each of the five health status goals for age groups specific improvements in the health status of Blacks and other minorities to be achieved via targeted health promotion, health protection, and preventive service objectives that are culturally specific. The excess death methodology as defined in the *Report of the Secretary's Task Force on Black and Minority Health* should be used as the quantitative measure for tracking progress or the lack of progress toward the achievement of these Black and/or minority objectives.

Waller argues for special objectives for each of the

six causes of death identified by the task force that are the major contributors to the disparity in health status: cancer, heart disease and stroke, homicide and accidents, infant mortality, cirrhosis, and diabetes.[3] In addition, there should to be culturally specific health promotion objectives for smoking, misuse of alcohol and drugs, nutrition, physical fitness, and control of stress and violence. *(#314)*

Other testifiers suggested separate objectives for various racial and ethnic groups such as Blacks, Hispanics, Native Americans, Asian and Pacific Islanders, and Arabs. Still others felt that the objectives should target socioeconomic status instead of race, because this is the more "operative variable" in tracking health status. *(#374)* Socioeconomic groups could include the poor and the homeless, farm and migrant workers, and people who live in rural areas.

Missing Objectives

A number of witnesses testified about problem areas or approaches that were missing from the national objectives, as currently formulated. Some, for instance, addressed the infrastructure for health promotion and disease prevention. Others offered alternative approaches to health promotion and disease prevention, and mentioned particular areas that should be included in the objectives.

Joel Nitzkin, Director of the Monroe County Health Department in New York and representing the National Association of County Health Officials, points out that certain process and infrastructure issues must be addressed within a state or locality before that state or locality can effectively pursue implementation of the Year 2000 Health Objectives. He specifically suggests that an entire new section entitled "Prevention Process and Infrastructure" be added to the objectives document to provide guidance relative to assignment of responsibility for review of the national objectives, development of a local response, establishment and monitoring of needed surveillance systems, and a variety of other political, administrative, and technical issues. *(#523)*

The American Academy of Family Physicians feels that a new major category should be developed for "Systems/Programs Supporting Disease Prevention and Health Promotion." This would include (1) development of insurance or other payment systems that pay for scientifically supported disease prevention and health promotion in the doctor's office and outpatient settings; (2) development and adoption of office-based systems for health risk assessment and longitudinal

tracking for both screening examinations and health behaviors; (3) development of disease prevention and health promotion curricula within medical schools and residences on an equal par with other medical education topics; and (4) funding of research to determine appropriate assessments and interventions, as well as their frequencies and effectiveness. *(#072)*

Douglas Mack, Director of the Kent County Michigan Health Department, makes a similar suggestion.

> The Year 2000 Health Objectives should provide a category called "Administration and Support Services," with attendant measurable objectives that will provide for responsible management and design for the delivery of the more sophisticated health service delivery objectives. Without a steady improvement in the basic administrative infrastructure, the service delivery objectives run the risk of inefficient development and unequal distribution to the nation's general population. *(#137)*

The American Society of Allied Health Professions asks for "objectives to increase coverage of preventive health care services of proven efficiency and cost effectiveness." *(#631)*

According to Jarrett:

> The 1990 Objectives appear to be scant in taking into consideration the roles and importance of the family in determining and influencing health status. This was particularly evident in objectives dealing with stress, violence, substance abuse, and handicapped children. Greater attention should be paid to this area with objectives to support, maintain, and develop the strength of the family unit. *(#108)*

Carol Foster of the Children's Hospital of Los Angeles suggests that a new objective category be established, called Family Support, to include family violence, genetic services, nutritional services, and services to children including day care, school health, and early intervention. *(#536)* Foster also suggests that all substance abuse issues be incorporated into one category and that all of the health promotion activities plus family support be in a single category entitled "Maintaining Health and Quality of Life Through Health Promotion." *(#536)*

James Woodrum, President of the Wellness and Prevention Program in Houston, suggests that the objectives include a new category on the "improvement of social health" to reflect the concerns of Sugarman and others summarized earlier. Woodrum defines social health as efforts "to effect health promotion and disease prevention through the application of positive individual, group, and community social factors." *(#227)*

Other witnesses mentioned specific areas they thought were missing from the 1990 Objectives. Some of these will be addressed in the Year 2000 Health Objectives. The missing areas include adolescent health *(#125)*, aging (#125; #215; #629), chronic diseases *(#125; #215)*, mental health *(#215)*, AIDS *(#125)*, iatrogenic injury *(#191)*, smokeless tobacco *(#215)*, food-borne diseases *(#125)*, back problems *(#019)*, asbestos *(#215)*, day care *(#006; #303)*, and access to health care *(#337)*.

PRIORITY SETTING

A number of witnesses suggested that there be fewer objectives than there were for 1990 or that priorities be set among them. Some testified that priorities are required to focus efforts, allocate resources, and reduce disparities in the burden of illness. Others proposed specific analytical models or processes for setting priorities.

Need for Priorities Among the Objectives

Support for setting priorities comes from both the public and the private sector. Harmon, for instance, draws on his experience in using state objectives.

> When looking this far ahead, it helps to focus on priorities. Establishing a strategic vision or mission for the future not only helps to clarify desired achievements, it also helps eliminate those issues that may be very important but are not central to an agency's overall purpose. The nation should select priorities based on what is achievable by the year 2000, what represents a marked improvement over the status quo, what falls within the national public health mission, and what can be impacted directly or indirectly by a positive endorsement from the federal government. The collection of objectives for the nation should be limited to those objectives that are most important to the achievement of improved health status by the year 2000. *(#085)*

Based on his experience in Texas, Bernstein says:

> It is essential that priority should be given to directing resources where there is disparity between state or local morbidity or mortality rates so that interventions can be directed toward underserved or high-risk populations. This could be accomplished by utilizing the objectives as criteria in requests for funding proposals released at both the state and federal levels, as well as more closely tying block grant funds to the Year 2000 Health Objectives. *(#020)*

According to Turnock:

> Having clearly visible and repeatedly articulated priorities and broadly defining these priorities into categories is critically important. It allows all potential participants to better understand their roles in addressing a collective health problem and serves to catalyze inclusion and participation over exclusion and avoidance. It focuses our efforts on the health outcomes and on the persons affected or potentially affected by the problem, rather than on the health care delivery system as so many of our past and current so-called health priorities have done. It establishes a focal point for integration and systemization of diverse efforts—including some even outside the traditional notion of health strategies—and provides a rallying point for seeking and securing new and expanded resources. *(#215)*

Some representatives of the private sector feel the same way, for example, Charles Arnold who represents the Health Insurance Association of America.

> Regrettably, we cannot afford to specify all objectives, no matter how desirable they may be. If critical objectives are to be attained, more attention must be given to policy issues such as setting priorities, associated expenditures, managerial efficiencies, research to support the objectives, and collaboration at federal-state and public-private levels. *(#440)*

Models for Setting Priorities

Although a number of analytical and process models were proposed for determining priorities among the objectives, they all shared two factors: a concern for the burden of illness that might be alleviated, and a consideration of the possibilities (theoretical and practical) for carrying out the intervention and making it succeed.

Beverly Long, for instance, representing the National Mental Health Association, calls for a process to set national priorities, which takes into account the burden of illness (she notes the need to develop a method to assess this) and defines a role for all disciplines, public and private agencies, professional and volunteer groups. Recognizing the "distaste for saying that one sorrow is worse than another," she nevertheless calls for scientifically derived facts to help make difficult decisions. *(#270)*

A number of witnesses gave concrete suggestions about models and criteria for setting priorities. Alfred Haynes of the Charles R. Drew Postgraduate Medical School suggests that the number of objectives be drastically reduced.

My own experience in health planning in the United States and abroad convinces me that it is impossible to mobilize a nation around 226 objectives. If we want to make things happen, if we want to change the course of events by design rather than by chance, then we must sharpen the focus on items of highest priority, use the best available knowledge, and allocate appropriate resources to obtain the desired results.

Haynes suggests three criteria for setting priorities:
1. The condition or risk factor involved must be one of high priority to the nation or to a large segment of the population, based on the current or potential burden of illness and death.
2. The objective must be linked to a scientifically proven method of achieving it.
3. Resources must be available and identified to implement the objective by using a scientifically proven method. *(#276)*

Paul Entmacher of the Business Roundtable recommends the development of a "guiding conceptual framework" to bind disparate objectives together toward a common goal of improving the public's health.

The guiding framework could be based on several aggregate measures of health of the public. Candidates for objectives should be evaluated on the extent to which they are a source of preventable health loss and the extent to which strategies exist that would be effective in reducing preventable health loss. Since not all desirable objectives may be affordable, the Business Roundtable favors prioritization of the categorical goals so that resource allocation can be properly guided. The absolute and relative expenses associated with attaining each objective should be estimated. With those economic data as guidance, planners could make reasonable estimates of the national level of effort required. The ends-means-resources planning model implied here would permit an assessment of the relative value of each objective in terms of priority and cost, as well as the feasibility of having the means to reach those ends. *(#465)*

Turnock says that "in determining priorities, it is essential to focus on health outcomes and the health of the public, with a special emphasis on the disproportionate rates of excess deaths among minority populations." *(#215)* He also stresses the need to work with community organizations and local agencies to establish realistic goals. "A comprehensive process of selecting priorities, working with and through community organizations and local agencies, and setting incremental objectives specific to communities is necessary to realize objectives and establish a realistic and useful implementation process." *(#215)*

REFERENCES

1. Lalonde M: A New Perspective on the Health of Canadians: A Working Document. Ottawa: Information Canada, April 1974

2. Commonwealth of Pennsylvania, Department of Health: Pennsylvania Assessment: Health Objectives for the Nation 1990, Mid-Decade Report. Harrisburg, Pa.: 1987

3. U.S. Department of Health and Human Services: Report of the Secretary's Task Force on Black and Minority Health. Washington, D.C.: U.S. Government Printing Office, August 1985

TESTIFIERS CITED IN CHAPTER 2

006 Allensworth, Diane; American School Health Association
019 Benjamin, George; National Safety Council
020 Bernstein, Robert; Texas Department of Health
072 Graham, Robert; American Academy of Family Physicians
085 Harmon, Robert; Missouri Department of Health
108 Jarrett, Michael; South Carolina Department of Health and Environmental Control
125 Larsen, Michael; Mississippi State Department of Health
126 Lassek, William; Department of Health and Human Services, Region III
137 Mack, Douglas; Kent County Health Department (Michigan)
149 Michael, Jerrold; University of Hawaii School of Public Health
189 Ruzek, Sheryl; Temple University
191 Salive, Marcel and Wolfe, Sidney; Public Citizen Health Research Group (Washington, D.C.)
198 Sheps, Cecil; American Public Health Association
215 Turnock, Bernard; Illinois Department of Public Health
227 Woodrum, James; Wellness and Prevention Program, Inc. (Houston)
270 Long, Beverly; World Federation for Mental Health
276 Haynes, Alfred; Charles R. Drew Postgraduate Medical School
303 Grimord, Mary; Texas Woman's University
314 Waller, John; Wayne State University
321 Skeels, Michael; Oregon Department of Human Resources
337 Sugarman, Jule; Washington State Department of Social and Health Services
352 Stevens, Nancy; Kaiser Permanente, Northwest Region
354 Pulrang, Peter; Washington State Bureau of Parent and Child Health
374 Society for Prospective Medicine
387 Richards, N. Mark; Pennsylvania Department of Health
440 Arnold, Charles; Metropolitan Life Insurance Company
465 Entmacher, Paul; Metropolitan Life Insurance Company
470 Bright, Frank; Ohio Department of Health
523 Nitzkin, Joel; Monroe County Health Department (New York)
527 Freedman, Mary Anne; Association for Vital Records and Health Statistics
530 Mazur, Ronald; University of Massachusetts at Amherst
536 Foster, Carol; Children's Hospital of Los Angeles
627 Stokes, III, Joseph; Boston University
629 Kinsman, Katherine; South Dakota Department of Health
631 Freeland, Thomas; American Society of Allied Health Professions
667 Artz, Lynn; University of Alabama at Birmingham
738 Wagner, Edward; Group Health Cooperative of Puget Sound

3. Implementing the Objectives at State and Local Levels

The realization of national objectives depends, in large measure, on the extent to which national, regional, state, and local organizations—both public and private—use and adapt them to better understand and act on the health concerns of the groups and communities they serve. The testifiers made clear that translating national objectives into an action plan for the United States must involve the building blocks of the U.S. public health system—each and every state and local health department. It also must involve the efforts of the private sector, including businesses, educational institutions, community groups, and professional or voluntary organizations. "Individuals from all sectors must be encouraged to take 'ownership' of the objectives," according to the Association of State and Territorial Health Officials. (#750)

Almost 200 witnesses addressed implementation issues. Their comments summed up experience with the objectives at state and local levels, and focused especially on the relationship between the national objectives and the Model Standards for Community Preventive Health Services, an effort of a coalition of public health professional organizations.[1] Testifiers also addressed other issues that can be summed up as the need for cooperation with the general public, with communities, and with the private sector, on a state and regional basis, as well as with the federal government. Strong pleas were made for more federal funding in support of state and local health department programs aimed at achieving the objectives.

STATE AND LOCAL PUBLIC HEALTH INITIATIVES

Since the publication of the 1990 Objectives, many states, counties, and cities have developed their own objectives based on the national model, and state and local health officers testified at length about the successes and failures. Successes tend to be related to cooperation across governmental levels, with the private sector and the community, and to use of the objectives to set priorities and manage resources.

State and Local Health Department Experience

"Hawaii was one of the first states to hold a meeting addressing the 1990 Objectives," according to Julian Lipsher of the Hawaii State Department of Health. "The Governor's Conference on Health Promotion and Disease Prevention was designed, not to just establish the objectives as part of a state agenda, but as a community-based process involving organizations, agencies, and sectors of our community who would own the objectives and be, in part, responsible for their attainment." (#340)

According to Thomas Halpin and Karen Evans of the Ohio State Department of Health:

The 1990 Objectives have given Ohio strong direction in planning strategies for health promotion and disease prevention throughout the state. They have served as the primary guide in the development of the Health Promotion and Disease Prevention Component of the Ohio State Health Plan and in the preparation of the annual Preventive Health and Health Services Block Grant Plan. The objectives have strongly influenced the implementation of community-based health promotion projects and have directed attention to issues of statewide significance, such as hypertension. (#129)

The Indiana State Board of Health found the 1990 Objectives helpful in providing a framework for several activities, including developing strategic initiatives, assessing health needs, and formulating a state health plan. (#405) The Mississippi State Department of Health used the 1990 Objectives in developing an operational plan for the agency as well as a state health plan. (#125)

The Texas Department of Health also is an avid supporter of the 1990 Objectives process. It has used the process in setting and influencing state health policy and in organizing traditional and nontraditional community organizations that have the ability to influence public health within the state. Furthermore, the objectives are influencing management practice by being integrated with Model Standards language into performance contracts established with local health departments. *(#020)*

According to Dick Welch of the Minnesota Department of Health, "The 1990 Objectives had an important influence in Minnesota at both the state and local level. The 1990 goals have helped turn what were broad generalities into pragmatic goals. This pragmatism has made our job easier in developing our own statewide initiatives such as the recent Nutrition Initiative and the earlier Non-Smoking Initiative." *(#225)*

Robert Harmon, Director of the Missouri Department of Health, says that his agency "has a strong commitment to goal-directed public health management. The 1990 Objectives and the Model Standards have been acknowledged as important documents to which Missouri public health must respond. The Department of Health chose first to pursue long-range strategic planning for the year 2000, and now is in the process of addressing the 1990 Objectives in the form of a mid-range plan." *(#085)*

The West Virginia Department of Health also used the national objectives to develop health goals for the year 2000. The state health department will develop a list of the major health problems in each county that account for the most potential years of life lost. Each local health department will prioritize its major public health risk hazards and develop health promotion and disease prevention plans. *(#098)*

The national objectives have also been used at the local level. Bud Nicola, Director of the Seattle-King County Department of Public Health, states that his department

> has made good use of both the Model Standards and the 1990 Objectives in its long-range planning process and in annual program review and budget preparation. Historically, local government services are not prioritized or based on major causes of morbidity and mortality—not even on measures such as years of life lost. The use of national objectives helps us at a local level to use morbidity and mortality data to allow policy makers and the public to focus on health status outcome measures, interrelated and developed in a broad context as a basis for policy, rather than individual perceptions. *(#320)*

"The Allentown Pennsylvania Health Bureau has used the 1990 Objectives as its primary programmatic planning guide" says Gary Gurian, the bureau's director. "The Health Bureau has shifted its emphasis from what was generally an acute problem agency to a professional public health organization providing the community it serves with prevention-oriented leadership and services. Most of the Health Bureau's award-winning initiatives have their roots in the 1990 Objectives. These initiatives include home and motor vehicle injury prevention services, targeted smoking cessation and awareness activities, and cancer prevention and early detection services. Unfortunately," Gurian adds, "this nation's 1990 Objectives remain one of the best kept secrets. They have been a seldom-used tool by this nation's network of private and public sector health organizations and decision makers." *(#076)*

According to Thomas Milne, representing the Washington State Association of Local Public Health Officials, local health departments need more information and encouragement to join in the objectives. Most have not had the resources, time, or inclination to assimilate the objectives into their work plans. To increase the participation of local health departments, Milne suggests (1) seeking more active involvement of national organizations representing state and local health officers, (2) distributing the revised objectives to all local health departments and encouraging their participation, (3) promoting and providing expanded technical assistance for implementation of the Model Standards, and (4) establishing a national focus in each of the priority areas at different times during the 1990s and distributing materials to local health departments to promote their involvement. *(#328)*

Robert Spengler of the Vermont Department of Health is concerned that the 1990 Objectives lacked practical implementation suggestions, such as how to use multiple approaches, coalitions, and limited resources to achieve results at the state level. Resources, motivation, commitment, and accountability at the state level have been missing from the 1990 experience, along with valid studies about which approaches work and which do not. He has three suggestions:

1. Establish priorities. "List the top 10 achievable objectives that should be considered first as national priorities in health promotion or disease prevention. An alternative might be to identify the top priority for each of the major content areas."

2. Establish motivational efforts. "Detailed plans

are needed to translate objectives into action at the state and local levels. Motivational efforts are needed and can be fostered by more technical support and guidance from federal agencies, educational institutions and the private sector." Financial support for demonstration projects is also needed.

3. Establish evaluation efforts. "A greater emphasis must be placed on agencies/organizations with principal responsibilities being held accountable for monitoring and evaluation." These agencies should determine "efficacy, effectiveness, efficiency, cost-benefits, and transferability of program activities" and should share data and compare intervention strategies and evaluations across states. (#458)

Robert Bernstein, Texas Commissioner of Health, suggests that "as we move forward with the development of Year 2000 Health Objectives, it is essential that the roles of states are fully established in the objective-setting process." He recommends that time be provided for states to react and start a companion process to establish their own objectives while the Year 2000 Health Objectives are being drafted. Once national and state objectives are established, state and local implementation plans must be written to incorporate the appropriate strategies and actions into operational plans of appropriate organizations. (#020)

The Model Standards

The 1990 Objectives are not the only federal approach to improving health promotion and disease prevention. In particular, many state and local health officers and others make reference in their testimony to the Model Standards for Community Preventive Health Services, a collaborative effort of the Centers for Disease Control, the American Public Health Association (APHA), and a number of public health professional associations to establish local standards through planning. According to the testimony, some communities, when presented with the Model Standards and the 1990 Objectives, have had difficulty in understanding how the two are related.

This confusion results from differences between the documents. First, the 1990 Objectives are national in scope, whereas the Model Standards are oriented to local action. Although the goals of the Model Standards and the 1990 Objectives are complementary, they often are seen as two sets of policy directives for already limited resources. The Model Standards, however, can assist states and localities as an implementation tool to make the 1990 Objectives

meaningful and applicable at the local level, and as a means of gaining strong partnership and commitment to these objectives.

For instance, William Schmidt of the Wisconsin Department of Health and Social Services says, "I perceive the objectives for the nation as a statement of intent, and Model Standards as the linking mechanism between those intentions and an achievable public mission. The objectives set the direction, but Model Standards describe the organizational capacities, administrative and program processes, and by inference, the financial resources to get there. Objectives without standards are unfocused public will; standards without objectives are unfocused public resources." (#476) Richard Biery, Director of the Kansas City Health Department, adds that "setting national objectives is only an empty and futile gesture without, at the same time, promoting a practical, usable implementation plan for achieving the objectives, one that involves every unit of our public health system." (#365)

According to Susan Addiss, Director of the Quinnipiack Valley Health District in Connecticut, "The Model Standards provide the quintessential process for successful implementation of the Year 2000 Health Objectives at the state and local levels. Because the outcome objectives are set by the community itself, it is possible to establish incremental steps that are attainable and that give the community a sense of accomplishment on the way to attainment of a national objective that may by itself appear unattainable." (#460)

Nelson Frissell, Director of the City-County Health Department in Casper, Wyoming, says:

The Model Standards process is a primary and inherent ingredient in the development of any objective. It becomes a way of thinking, a way of looking at the ability to come from a common ground to diverse but specific outcomes within the overall umbrella of a national effort rather than trying to get from the diversity of local effort back into some common denominator of maximum effect. By using the Model Standards process, it is easier to see how we integrate one with another even though the ultimate objective may seem different. It's a universal tool, a common skill basis, that can highlight and emphasize the connectedness, that notices and points out the similarities, and focuses where we fit together instead of where we don't. I view the Model Standards process as the building block, as the basis for complementing efforts, the process from which the objectives for the nation can flow—an allowance and assistance of local implementation and focus, while augmenting interconnected actions in the local effort to define roles and relationships by utilizing a common process to focus on a larger national impact. *(#364)*

The fact that the Year 2000 Health Objectives are objectives for the nation is both their principal strength and their principal weakness, according to Schmidt.

The strength is in the recognition that all sections of the U.S. health care system, public and private and at all levels, need to marshal behind these objectives. The weakness is that objectives for all, conceptually, can all too easily become objectives for none in actuality. Model Standards has recognized this by stressing the concept of "A Governmental Presence At the Local Level (AGPALL)." *(#476)*

Carole Samuelson, Director of the Jefferson County Department of Health in Alabama, adds that AGPALL represents

the idea that government, either at the local or state level, is ultimately responsible for ensuring that standards are met. Not that government can or should do everything that has to be done to meet all standards, but that government must take the lead in this process (by providing necessary services or at least making sure that the necessary services are being provided). The very best objectives are unlikely to be accomplished unless a specific person or agency assumes leadership for promoting and achieving them. Likewise, it is extremely important that while one agency is responsible, objectives must be community-oriented and must promote interagency and intergovernmental cooperation. *(#260)*

The 1990 Objectives document gives specific rates and figures for objectives, whereas the Model Standards document uses an open-ended, fill-in-the-blank framework for local objectives.

Many testifiers note that in instances where the intent of the two documents is the same, incongruent terminology between them sometimes masks their agreement and complicates their relationship. Samuelson says that "one of our frustrations in using the Model Standards has been the confusion that occurs because there are two very similar documents: the Model Standards document and the 1990 Objectives document. There have been instances when the wording in the two documents is similar but different enough to cause confusion." *(#260)*

Schmidt says that the "process of using both documents works, but it takes a great deal of effort and requires patching the two together. Often, though the overall intention of the two documents is the same, the terminology differs and the relationships are difficult to ascertain. It doesn't have to be that way. It would be a tremendous service to the people using the two documents to meld them together so that they flow and complement each other." *(#476)*

Many other witnesses, such as Carol Spain of the Health Officers Association of California, suggest that the national objectives and the Model Standards be better integrated.

The Year 2000 Health Objectives need to go further by actually integrating the relevant Model Standards in the appropriate sections of the year 2000 document. This integration is critically needed in order to provide the implementation framework for achievement of process and outcome objectives that will assist each local and state health department in meeting the Year 2000 Health Objectives within their own jurisdictions. It is only through the achievement of the Year 2000 Health Objectives at the local level that the objectives will be achieved at the highest level, the nation. *(#204)*

The witnesses suggest that the merged document keep some of the philosophy (e.g., flexibility, AGPALL, community involvement) of the Model Standards for use by states and localities. The merged document "should establish national objectives but have a mechanism for local communities to convert these national objectives into attainable local objectives. The document also should stress the government's responsibility to ensure that objectives are met, but emphasize the importance of the entire community working toward a common goal." *(#260)*

The Model Standards committee and the U.S. Public Health Services (PHS) Office of Disease Prevention and Health Promotion are currently planning to develop such a document. Representatives of the Model Standards committee are working with the groups drafting the Year 2000 Health Objectives, and the Model Standards committee will produce a companion document for use by state and local health agencies that employs the Year 2000 Health Objectives as a base and focuses on the steps required to implement them on a community level.

Federal Funding

Many witnesses called for a federal leadership role in implementing as well as determining the objectives. Their suggestions ranged from providing research results and technical assistance in implementing the objectives to the financing of state and local activities.

According to William Blockstein of the University of Wisconsin-Madison, for instance, there should be a separate federal interagency work group for each health problem, and this structure should be duplicated at the state level by using a consortium of state and territorial health departments and private sector professional and voluntary organizations. These efforts should be coordinated by the PHS. The work groups should develop (1) print, radio, and television public service announcements in a variety of languages, in tune with the educational level and cultural values of the subculture being addressed; (2) help lines that will provide callers with nonthreatening, helpful, and comprehensible information on preventive measures; and (3) resource manuals that detail successful prevention programs in many languages and for various educational or cultural backgrounds. (#518)

According to Alfred Berg of the University of Washington:

The United States needs a process of identifying essential services and ensuring that they are delivered. The scientific basis underlying health promotion and disease prevention can be expected to change constantly, so that a permanent body constituted to monitor the state of the art and to advise the government should be appointed. The U.S. Preventive Services Task Force should become a permanent advisory body, and its scope of responsibilities expanded to include access and manpower issues. A mechanism for incorporating recommendations from the Task Force into national health policy should be identified; the recommendations should include a minimum core of essential im-

munizations, screening tests, and health promotion activities. All Americans should have access to the recommended core of health promotion and disease prevention services, regardless of insurance status. (#315)

Stephen Goldston of the University of California, Los Angeles suggests that federal health agencies be required to budget specific funds to implement the plans for achieving the Year 2000 Health Objectives, emphasizing primary prevention, rather than secondary or tertiary prevention. (#280) "For due consideration of the major chronic diseases, the National Institutes of Health should be involved," writes Lester Breslow of the UCLA School of Public Health.

That involvement did not occur to any great extent in setting the objectives for 1990, thereby perhaps limiting the achievement. You will recall that in the 1990 Objectives no mention of the major chronic diseases appeared. Now the Public Health Service appears to be embarking, with all of its relevant elements, on a full and appropriate health agenda. That is a highly promising development. It will tend to bring the National Institutes of Health into what many of us always thought should be included in their missions, namely, efforts to prevent the chronic diseases and promote health, especially among the elderly. (#026)

Many witnesses testified that state and local health departments lack the resources necessary to implement the national objectives. Their suggestions for addressing this problem include direct federal funding of health promotion/disease prevention activities, demonstration projects at the state or local level, and direct support through already existing funding programs. Many of these issues are discussed in more depth in Chapter 8.

The American Public Health Association's Community Health Planning Section reports that since the Midcourse Review came out in 1986,[2] there have been substantial decreases in federal funding for some health programs. If new goals are to be attained, or old ones maintained, the objectives are going to have to deal more with supporting infrastructures. Without federal funding and strong community planning, states lose focus and the ability to implement the objectives. (#756)

The Association of State and Territorial Health Officials comes to the following conclusion:

Establishing and achieving the national health objectives is a process that will require the commitment of resources from all levels of government—not just the federal government—as well as from private sources. Lawmaking bodies, from the Congress to individual city councils, must accept the idea of national health objectives and support the objectives by appropriating funds. For example, the federal government should consider funding staff for the objectives-setting process at the state level. In turn, states must work to ensure provision of technical assistance to local governments in building community support for priority health objectives.

Even when the burden is shared, resources for achieving the national health objectives will be limited. To be successful, the objectives must be realistic in terms of the expected resources available to achieve them. Existing and potential resources must be tied to the national objectives, and, in turn, the objectives must be realistic to accommodate limited resources. *(#750)*

Rhode Island's Director of Health, Denman Scott, agrees that state health departments are in a strategic position to translate the Year 2000 Health Objectives into action. To help them do this, he suggests that the federal government specifically earmark a pool of money for attainment of the Year 2000 Health Objectives at state and local levels. As a prerequisite to receiving such assistance, health departments would be required to produce a health objectives plan. "In order to give this proposed program the momentum it deserves," says Scott, "an initial funding base of $1 per person, or about $250 million per year should be allocated to the state health departments based on the size of their state populations and the quality of their national health objectives plan." Scott suggests that the Centers for Disease Control administer the process "because of its excellent track record of working collaboratively and constructively with state health departments." *(#461)*

A number of witnesses testified that some of the funding problems could be solved by tying currently existing federal funding programs to the national objectives. The preventive health and health services block grant program, funds for community health centers, and Medicare and Medicaid were all discussed.

Mark Richards, Secretary of Health for the Commonwealth of Pennsylvania, recommends "that all recipients of block and categorical grant funds should clearly demonstrate how they will help to meet the appropriate Year 2000 Health Objectives." *(#387)* Based on her experience with the 1990 Objectives in South Dakota, Katherine Kinsman suggests that one way for the federal government to consistently support the objectives is to use them as the focus and criteria for federal grants. *(#629)*

Thomas Halpin and Karen Evans report that the preventive health and health services block grants have been crucial in shaping disease prevention and health promotion plans in Ohio. "Well-prepared plans and strategies that lack resources for implementation are lofty but unobtainable ideals," they write. "The objectives must be supported with a concentrated, cooperative effort at the federal, state, and local level to continue and to increase the preventive health and health services block grant." *(#129)*

Karen Grieder, Director of Research with the Texas Association of Community Health Centers, writes that centers are federally funded and serve poor or indigent populations. In South Texas, for instance, the community health centers are primarily used by minorities, migrants, uninsured females, and border communities—people who have nowhere else to go for health care. These centers operate on limited budgets and do not have or collect very much data. They must, however, write their health plans around the 1990 Objectives when applying for grant money. This is especially difficult because the cases they are seeing—diabetes, for example—are not specifically targeted in the 1990 Objectives. Grieder asks for better coordination between state and federal agencies, improved funding, and a realistic expectation from the government of what community health centers are to monitor and implement. *(#747)*

Many testifiers also suggested that Medicare and Medicaid should more consistently cover preventive health. Richards says that "the Medicaid and Medicare programs should be restructured to encourage and allow for the reimbursement of preventive and early disease detection services." *(#387)*

INTERSECTORAL COOPERATION: ROLE OF THE PRIVATE SECTOR

Across the board, witnesses testified about the need for various sorts of intersectoral cooperation in implementing the national objectives at a local level. States and local health departments were seen as having the pivotal role in implementing national objectives locally, but testifiers repeatedly stressed the need for cooperation with other sectors. Some called for involving the general public, for community participation, and for developing partnerships with the private sector. Others stressed the need for local, state, and regional efforts, and the need for a federal role in implementation. Harmon suggests that public health institutions at each level of government take the lead in identifying other public or private participants and inviting them into the Year 2000 Health Objectives process. The objectives, he says, are "natural bridges for cooperative interagency ventures to promote public health." *(#085)*

Professional organizations also have an important role to play in formulating and implementing the national objectives. According to the American Association of Public Health Dentistry, success in meeting the objectives "is only possible through coordinated public and professional efforts, individually and collectively. Each professional association must be involved and must identify potential roles that its members may play in accomplishing the objectives and make efforts to challenge its members to do so." *(#156)*

Many of these issues are discussed in depth in Chapters 8 and 9 on health promotion and disease prevention in medical and nonmedical settings.

Community Participation

As Jerrold Michael of the University of Hawaii at Manoa says, "The achievement of health is not in the hands of the health professions alone. The resources of health, education, economic development, and human services must become connected to and interwoven with health objectives." *(#149)* Many other witnesses supported this point of view, and called for public and community participation in implementing the objectives. Some spoke about mobilizing individuals and "consumers." Others called for efforts to mobilize entire communities. Some testifiers addressed the potential role of community organizations and professional societies.

The APHA calls for strong public participation in the objectives process.

There is a need to involve the general public in health promotion and disease prevention, in order to enable individuals to determine for themselves the means to achieve optimal health. Methods should be developed to increase consumer participation and expand the roles of health consumers in achieving the objectives for the nation. The objectives should go well beyond health professionals and health agencies and develop consumer roles and outreach programs that are more conducive to achieving the objectives and reaching the population in greatest need.

The APHA testimony contains three suggestions for increasing public participation: (1) developing state implementation plans that have public service materials supporting an active role for health consumers and health professionals, (2) developing curricula material for public health professionals to promote public educational programs, and (3) building coalitions of health consumers and providers. *(#198)*

Woodrow Myers, Indiana State Health Commissioner, says that "we must do more work within our communities to revive their ability to identify and address their own health needs, to look for local solutions to local problems, and where appropriate, to link these problems to statewide solutions that affect other communities' problems and ultimately to national solutions, whether private or public, to address those needs." *(#405)*

Colorado's Governor Roy Romer agrees that communities must get involved in preventive health care. At a hearing on the Year 2000 Health Objectives in Denver, he described a successful community-based program in Colorado aimed at preventing alcohol and drug abuse. "We are talking to high school youngsters about what they can do, themselves, within their own peer groups and within their own community to begin to set the stage for mutual reinforcement of coming to terms with their own responsibility as citizens." *(#786)* Many other community-oriented programs are described in Chapter 9 of this report.

Herbert Rader of the Salvation Army uses his organization's efforts as an example of the role that community organizations can play in implementing national objectives. The Salvation Army has activities that address (1) health needs of the poor; (2) substance abuse (including intravenous drug use and

AIDS); (3) homelessness; (4) assisting young people to avoid high-risk behaviors; and (5) sexual behavior, unintentional pregnancy, and sexually transmitted diseases. Rader says that psychosocial factors and religious principles play a major role in determining the content of these programs. *(#432)*

"Our nation does not lack the epidemiological or biostatistical evidence for the benefits of disease prevention and health promotion initiatives," writes Bertram Yaffe, President of the Erna Yaffe Foundation.

> Nor do we lack the educational or primary prevention techniques for the deployment of these initiatives. What we do lack is a sustained dialogue between health professionals and the individuals who can create the political will to transform the curative model of health services into a preventive model of a health system. We need a constituency for prevention—a broad-based, advocacy process analogous to the civil rights, feminist, and environmental movements. It must be global in its concerns, but politically very local and indigenous in implementation. It is the leadership in the creation of the movement, that is the future and the real challenge of Public Health. Health status is a reflection, not of lifestyle alone, but of social, economic, political, and all other circumstances that impact on individuals. We must recognize that it is not sufficient for health status goals to be articulated by health professionals alone; they must also be delivered as messages of political commitment. All of us must be agents for the creation of a nonpartisan, but very political, movement to promote the Ecology of Health. *(#454)*

Yaffe calls for more regional consortia on health promotion and disease prevention. The New England Conference for Disease Prevention, Health Protection and Health Promotion (NECON), which Yaffe chairs, is a coalition of six New England public health departments; four schools of public health; federal health agencies in the region; various departments of the schools of medicine and allied health professions; educators; legislators; and representatives from industry, labor, and voluntary organizations. It was set up to assess the progress of the New England states toward the 1990 Objectives and to offer some strategies for further improvements in the health status of the region. It is funded by grants from the public

and private sectors.

Through a series of conferences and task force activities, NECON has developed a regional network of nearly 300 individuals "that has evolved into an effective, nonpartisan constituency to achieve healthy public policies and develop specific programs." The New England Governors' Conference has recognized the importance of NECON's goals and activities, and has established a New England Regional Health Committee to receive and consider NECON's recommendations. *(#454)*

The Colorado Trust is another group that believes that grass roots health promotion can lead to lasting improvements in health status. According to its executive director, Bruce Rockwell, the trust is a philanthropic, grant-making foundation devoted to health, medical, and human services in Colorado. One of its major programs is Colorado Action for Healthy People, which is based directly on the 1990 Objectives, funded by the Colorado Trust and the Kaiser Family Foundation, and carried out through the auspices of the Colorado Health Department. The program's strategies include (1) grants to communities that already are well organized to serve as demonstration projects for other communities; (2) technical assistance in community organization such as needs assessment, selection of interventions, and evaluation; and (3) state-level activities, including media campaigns, data collection, dissemination, and regulatory activities. *(#709)*

Corporate Partnerships

The business community, too, has a role to play in implementing the Year 2000 Health Objectives. The testimony shows that there is interest in the business world.

For instance, a survey of 48 companies about business involvement in health promotion and disease prevention, more specifically the national objectives process, conducted by the Washington Business Group on Health found the following:

> Many of the objectives are especially relevant to businesses who pay for the health care costs of not only their employees, but also their dependents and retirees. Increasingly, companies are concerned with maintaining and improving health. In addition, it is hoped that businesses will use the new objectives to help set their own health goals. Therefore, it is not only important, but necessary that America's businesses

play a key role in the process of establishing new national health objectives for the year 2000.

The survey showed that over half of the firms that responded (27) had heard of the 1990 Objectives, and almost a quarter (11) had used them in some way. Some companies used them to gain support for health promotion and disease prevention activities in general, to justify adding new programs, and as a means of comparing their company's performance to national standards. Others used them to change or reinforce existing programs, help target new programs, and set goals and objectives for long-range strategic plans. (#355)

Paul Entmacher of the Business Roundtable says that "as corporate citizens and as major taxpayers, the country's major companies have a shared interest in the health of the nation. Ceding the primary leadership role to the government, however, the Business Roundtable endorses the concept of ongoing, nonpartisan, appropriate, public-private collaboration in setting and measuring the nation's health objectives." (#465)

The New York Business Group on Health calls the worksite "a uniquely advantageous arena for programs of health education/promotion that will further help to achieve the national objectives." The work setting offers the opportunity to target individuals based on age, sex, education, and ethnic backgrounds; in addition, it offers economies of scale, ease of access, and peer pressure to increase program effectiveness. (#448)

Virtually all the objectives can be addressed through a specific workplace program, according to testimony by the American Occupational Medical Association. Health education and promotion programs developed to address problems of reproduction, childrearing, immunization, mental health, substance abuse, hazard exposure, risk taking, and self-destructive habits, can be provided efficiently and effectively at the workplace. (#071)

Carl Schramm writes that the "Health Insurance Association of America (HIAA) has encouraged coalitions by business and industry to foster a community environment" for health promotion and disease prevention. For example, the HIAA's Center for Corporate Public Involvement "sought to influence the AIDS public debate by increased public/private sector collaboration and through the expansion of industry resources to combat the epidemic." Schramm says that 21 community organizations received funds for AIDS information and education and for support programs from HIAA and the American Council of Life Insurance member companies through a challenge grant program. (#619)

SURVEILLANCE AND INFORMATION RESOURCES

The need for better data, in general, for specific health problems and special populations arose repeatedly in testimony on the Year 2000 Health Objectives. For instance, Harmon says that "data represents the single most critical element to successful planning." As part of the objectives process, the nation must identify data base weaknesses and build information systems to fill the gaps. (#085) Others discussed the need for other kinds of information, such as technical assistance in implementing the objectives and information about the effectiveness of health promotion and disease prevention interventions.

Like a number of testifiers, the American Public Health Association sees a need for an improved system of data collection and analysis in order to monitor the achievement of objectives. "The data collection and analysis system is crucial," according to the APHA, in identifying the nature and scale of problems to be faced in achieving the objectives and also in evaluating implementation activities to make sure that the most effective program is in place to achieve the objectives. (#198) Other witnesses recognized the importance of establishing baseline data in order to measure progress and evaluate outcomes.

State and Local Data Systems

Many witnesses spoke about the need for state and local data and surveillance systems to set objectives and to monitor progress toward them. Three criteria came up repeatedly: uniformity, timeliness, and quality.

The Association of State and Territorial Health Officials suggests that "data should, when feasible, be collected in standardized forms across the country, allowing for comparison of how different cities, states, and regions are faring. For data that are not collected nationally, state and local data should be utilized in lieu of establishing new data systems." (#750)

Viewing matters from the state level, Harmon calls for efforts at both national and state levels to arrive at a uniform data base with data that are no more than two years old. (#085) Mary Anne Freedman, representing the Association for Vital Records and

Health Statistics, stresses data uniformity and quality. "Data derived from systems that have multiple collection points with non-uniform collection methodologies or non-standard sampling techniques must be used with caution." Furthermore, "since the Year 2000 Health Objectives will provide a focus for many agencies working to improve the health of all citizens and are expected to be translated to state and local needs, many state and local agencies will also adopt the objectives." Therefore, says Freedman, "data systems should address the needs of state and local agencies as well as those for the nation." *(#527)*

Tom Jones, speaking for the Northwest Portland Area Indian Health Board, says that healthy communities depend on contributions from the individual and family, the health delivery system, and community government. He recommends an objective that would urge all communities to have an information system and appropriate statistical tools that could diagnose the community's health problems, assess risk factors, monitor health status progress, evaluate the effectiveness of health programs, and identify additional requirements necessary to arrive at an acceptable level of health. The Native American tribes of the Northwest, Jones reports, are currently developing such a system. *(#473)*

At the local level, "one would ideally have a local office to gather, tabulate, interpret, and disseminate those data needed to track the community's progress, or lack thereof, relative to the various objectives for the nation," according to Joel Nitzkin, Director of the Monroe County Health Department in New York. "Placing this function within the health department will facilitate access to birth and death certificate data and data on reportable communicable disease. In more realistic circumstances, one can still do pretty well with some relatively simple indicators that may indicate the presence or absence of an obvious problem." In addition, Nitzkin says, an "effective means for integrating the surveillance data and epidemiological process into the priority setting and budgeting processes" is also necessary. *(#523)*

Nitzkin suggests that "the surveillance activity not limit itself to simple totals and averages for the entire jurisdiction. The jurisdiction should be divided geographically, socioeconomically, and racially/ethnically into subpopulations representing different levels of health risk and geographic areas that might be considered for targeting of programming. By sorting both the numerator and denominator data this way, one can avoid missing small areas of high risk because they had been hidden within a larger popula-

tion at much lower risk." *(#523)*

Specific Diseases and Problems

Many witnesses call for better data and data systems on particular health issues. For example, testifiers call for the following:

• An expansion of the current nutritional data system by using registered dietitians as data gatherers. *(#572)*
• Better data on environmental issues and occupational safety and health. *(#104)*
• A "comprehensive and integrated system for periodic determination of the oral health status, dental treatment needs, and utilization of dental services of the U.S. population." *(#106)*
• A national registry to measure the incidence of fetal alcohol syndrome and fetal alcohol effects. *(#542)*
• Better data on the incidence and prevalence of AIDS and HIV (human immunodeficiency virus) infection, as well as incidence and prevalence of other retroviral illnesses. *(#698)*

Other particular data needs are discussed elsewhere in this report.

An existing data source that could be used better in setting objectives, according to Patrick O'Malley and Lloyd Johnston of the University of Michigan, is the National High School Senior Survey, "one of the country's major sources of epidemiological information on substance abuse among American adolescents and young adults." It serves as a valuable source of trends on drug and alcohol abuse, the potential for accidents, and physical fitness and nutrition, and should be used in setting and tracking objectives and teen behavior. *(#419)*

Special Needs of Minority Populations

Minority groups in the population have special data needs. First, data on minorities as groups are often lacking. Furthermore, as a number of testifiers pointed out, individual minority populations are themselves heterogeneous, which calls into question even the available data for groups such as Blacks, Hispanics, and Asians.

For example, according to Sandral Hullet, Director of West Alabama Health Services, there are no characteristics shared by all minority subgroups. Furthermore, speaking of the Black populations that she serves, Hullet says that health research policies and programs fail to differentiate among the special needs of subgroups within racial, ethnic, and social communities, which accounts for the disproportionate burden of illness among minorities. More information on the determinants of health and illness in each subgroup is necessary to account for the different susceptibilities and resistance of these groups to risk factors. *(#671)*

Similarly, David Hayes-Bautista of the University of California, Los Angeles suggests that basic data about health promotion and disease prevention are lacking for Latino populations. The problems arise from (1) lack of uniformity—some surveys are coded to names, others to national origin, others to nationality, so it is difficult to find homogenous populations for comparison purposes; (2) lack of uniform definitions and procedures; and (3) lack of data to get a baseline profile of the Latino population. Hayes-Bautista also says that a conceptual model for looking at Latino health is lacking—the Black model simply does not apply. With more than one linguistic group, more than a single cultural or economic group, and not solely an immigrant population, the Latino community has unique characteristics and structural elements that must be understood to develop appropriate interventions, he says. *(#679)*

Michael Watanabe, representing the Asian Pacific Planning Council, suggests that the Asian-Pacific community also requires special attention because it is not homogeneous. There are 17 distinct ethnic groups with different norms and problems, including a large refugee component. According to Watanabe, Asians are often represented as a model minority, but when subgroups are examined, problems with poverty, education, crime, and delinquency arise, which are not always represented in official statistics. Major health problems also emerge in subgroups: high stomach cancer rates among the Japanese and lung cancer among the Chinese. *(#683)*

Information Resources

A number of testifiers identified the need for more or better information to help implement the Year 2000 Health Objectives. This information included technical assistance about the objectives process for states and local areas, better information about the costs and benefits of disease prevention, and research to support the objectives.

Milne called for more technical assistance to help states and local areas implement the objectives.

(#328) Similarly, Kinsman suggested an addendum to the publication of the Year 2000 Health Objectives giving methods and tools needed to use objectives. *(#629)*

According to Harmon, one of Missouri's main recommendations for the Year 2000 Health Objectives is to centralize technical resources at national, state, and local levels. This requires establishing a technical resources office at the national level to provide technical assistance and training to states and local areas involved in using the national objectives and the Model Standards. This office could (1) establish a library and clearinghouse for data and technical information, (2) operate an electronic bulletin board to disseminate information and encourage communication between states and local areas, and (3) make a uniform national data set available through the clearinghouse or bulletin board. *(#085)*

Those implementing the objectives at the state or local level also require more information on the effectiveness of prevention interventions. "All too often," says Michael Eriksen of the Society for Public Health Education, "the marketplace drives the availability of effective interventions. If money can be made, programs will be marketed and sold, irrespective of need, quality, and effectiveness. Special efforts need to be made to assure that effective health promotion programs are diffused to the appropriate target groups." *(#309)*

David Lawrence of the Kaiser Foundation Health Plan of Colorado points out that employers and other purchasers of health care, as well as "bundlers" of care such as health maintenance organizations and other managed care organizations, are increasingly concerned with the quality and appropriateness of the health care they purchase. Many, however, are still not sure which preventive programs are suitable at the worksite, which are most effective, and how to evaluate success. The national objectives can be a guide for purchasers to determine how well bundlers (those who put together the pieces necessary to deliver care within systems) are doing in the areas of disease prevention and health promotion. For this to work, however, Lawrence says that data commissions or other data collection and analysis entities must be developed to evaluate the bundlers' effectiveness at health promotion and disease prevention. *(#375)*

Similarly, the Business Roundtable suggests that a public-private data consortium be organized early in the objectives-setting process to help develop baseline data and assist in the collection, retrieval, and analysis of follow-up data. The absolute and relative expenses associated with each goal should be estimated to facilitate planning and prioritizing. *(#465)*

To use the national objectives well, information about successful programs and the strategies used to implement them must be shared. According to Spengler:

> To achieve objectives and strive for improving health, it is essential that monitoring and evaluation efforts be supported throughout any project. A greater emphasis must be placed on agencies/organizations with principal responsibilities being held accountable for monitoring and evaluation. The same agencies/organizations should be held accountable for determining efficacy, effectiveness, efficiency, cost-benefits, and transferability of program activities. There also needs to be more interstate data sharing and comparison of intervention strategies and evaluations. *(#458)*

REFERENCES

1. Model Standards Work Group: Model Standards: A Guide for Community Preventive Health Services (2nd Edition). Washington, D.C.: American Public Health Association, 1985

2. U.S. Department of Health and Human Services: The 1990 Objectives for the Nation: A Midcourse Review. Washington, D.C.: U.S. Government Printing Office, November 1986

TESTIFIERS CITED IN CHAPTER 3

020 Bernstein, Robert; Texas Department of Health
026 Breslow, Lester; University of California, Los Angeles
071 Givens, Austin; American Occupational Medical Association
076 Gurian, Gary; City of Allentown Bureau of Health (Pennsylvania)
085 Harmon, Robert; Missouri Department of Health
098 Heydinger, David; West Virginia Department of Health
104 Hyslop, Thomas; Harris County Health Department (Texas)
106 Isman, Robert; The Association of State and Territorial Dental Directors
125 Larsen, Michael; Mississippi State Department of Health
129 Halpin, Thomas and Evans, Karen; Ohio Department of Health
149 Michael, Jerrold; University of Hawaii School of Public Health
156 Easley, Michael; American Association of Public Health Dentistry
198 Sheps, Cecil; American Public Health Association
204 Spain, Carol; Health Officers Association of California
225 Welch, Dick; Minnesota Department of Health
260 Samuelson, Carole; Jefferson County Department of Health (Alabama)
280 Goldston, Stephen; University of California, Los Angeles
309 Eriksen, Michael; University of Texas Health Science Center at Houston
315 Berg, Alfred; University of Washington
320 Nicola, Bud; Seattle-King County Department of Public Health
328 Milne, Thomas; Southwest Washington Health District
340 Lipsher, Julian; Hawaii State Department of Health
355 Jacobson, Miriam; Washington Business Group on Health
364 Frissell, Nelson; City-County Health Department, Casper, Wyoming
365 Biery, Richard; Kansas City Health Department
375 Lawrence, David; Kaiser Foundation Health Plan of Colorado
387 Richards, N. Mark; Pennsylvania Department of Health
405 Myers, Jr., Woodrow; Indiana State Board of Health
419 O'Malley, Patrick and Johnston, Lloyd; University of Michigan
432 Rader, Herbert; The Salvation Army in the United States

448 Warshaw, Leon; New York Business Group on Health
454 Yaffe, Bertram; New England Conference for Disease Prevention, Health Protection and Health Promotion (NECON)
458 Spengler, Robert; Vermont Department of Health
460 Addiss, Susan; Quinnipiack Valley Health District (Connecticut)
461 Scott, H. Denman; Rhode Island Department of Health
465 Entmacher, Paul; Metropolitan Life Insurance Company
473 Jones, Tom; Northwest Portland Area Indian Health Board
476 Schmidt, William; Wisconsin Division of Health
518 Blockstein, William; University of Wisconsin-Madison
523 Nitzkin, Joel; Monroe County Health Department (New York)
527 Freedman, Mary Anne; Association for Vital Records and Health Statistics
542 Weiner, Lyn and Morse, Barbara A.; Boston University
572 Williams, Corinne; California Dietetic Association
619 Schramm, Carl; Health Insurance Association of America
629 Kinsman, Katherine; South Dakota Department of Health
671 Hullet, Sandral; West Alabama Health Services
679 Hayes-Bautista, David; University of California, Los Angeles
683 Watanabe, Michael; Asian Pacific Planning Council (Los Angeles)
698 Lafferty, William; Washington State Department of Public Health
709 Rockwell, Bruce; The Colorado Trust
747 Grieder, Karen; Texas Association of Community Health Centers
750 Richland, Jud; Association of State and Territorial Health Officials
756 Reeves, Philip; American Public Health Association
786 Roemer, Milton; University of California, Los Angeles

4. Children and Adolescents

Children, as a group, constitute one of the most vulnerable segments of our society. They are subject to a wide range of health problems and are dependent on families and communities for sustenance and protection from health hazards. At the same time, childhood offers an important opportunity to set lifelong healthy behavioral patterns. Thus, the health promotion and disease prevention needs of children and adolescents need to be examined.

Almost 50 witnesses focused their testimony on issues related to the health promotion and disease prevention needs of children and adolescents. Some addressed crosscutting topics, most notably problems that children face with access to health care, but also the special needs and opportunities presented by day-care facilities, the role that the media can play in promoting child health, the necessity for coordinated services for adolescents, the special needs of children with a chronic illness or disability, and special data and information requirements for children and adolescents. Other testifiers addressed specific health problems and opportunities for health promotion, but with a special focus on children and adolescents. In health promotion, for example, testifiers addressed nutrition, substance abuse, physical fitness, and mental health with a special focus on adolescent suicide. In health protection, they addressed primarily the prevention of unintentional accidents, as well as child abuse and other forms of violence. Finally, with regard to preventive services, testifiers addressed the prevention of infectious diseases, improving oral health, and screening for chronic diseases.

Other issues of interest to children and adolescents are discussed throughout this report. Chapter 22 on maternal and infant health, for instance, deals at length with the problems of infants, so these are not discussed here. The section on the school as a setting for health promotion and disease prevention programs in Chapter 9 is clearly relevant to children and adolescents. One problem with school-based programs, however, is that not all adolescents stay in school long enough to benefit from them. Richard Eberst of the American School Health Association points out, "A large percentage of school age children are disenfranchised from the nation's schools. They are in jail, on the street, working, or on the run." Thus, health objectives regarding school children are

not enough to cover the full needs of children and, especially, adolescents. *(#055)*

CROSSCUTTING TOPICS

Some witnesses addressed issues that cut across established priority areas for the national objectives but are necessary for designing interventions to improve the health of children and adolescents. The most central issue is access to health care, which is seen as a serious impediment to improving child health. Child-care centers are seen as both a problem to be addressed and an opportunity for implementing some of the national goals. The media, too, present problems that must be addressed yet can be a powerful force in educating children about improving their health. According to a number of testifiers, many of the problems that adolescents face—substance abuse, mental health, teen pregnancy, violence, and so on—are interrelated; thus, coordinated services, not individual approaches, are required to address the complex of issues. Other testifiers addressed the problem of the growing number of children with chronic diseases and suggested programs designed to meet their needs.

Access to Care

A recurring theme in the testimony is the effect of economic and financial concerns on health, resulting in lack of both access to and availability of health care. Such concerns are of particular relevance to children because they are more likely than other age groups to be living in poverty and, thus, to be subject to the attending health problems. In 1981, 19.5 percent of children under 18 were below the poverty level, compared to 14 percent of persons of all ages.[1]

The American Academy of Pediatrics (AAP) gives access to care for all children its highest priority. "The American Academy of Pediatrics feels that the ultimate child health goal is to assure access to health care for all of America's children." The academy suggests objectives to reduce the proportion of children who are uninsured, to ensure that all Medicaid jurisdictions adopt maximum eligibility options, to reduce the proportion of uninsured chronically ill children, and to reduce the number of

U.S. counties that are underserved by child health physicians. The AAP recommends that these goals be accomplished by providing universal access to care through entitlement programs or by expanding Medicaid and private insurance coverage, encouraging states to take advantage of Medicaid services, and legislation. The academy suggests that the supply of physicians for underserved areas could be improved by making practice opportunities more attractive and available in rural areas and inner cities through such programs as the National Health Service Corps scholarship program. *(#115)*

Child-care Centers and Health

An important focus for child health mentioned by a number of testifiers is the child-care or day-care center. An increasing number of U.S. families are in need of child care, according to Thomas Hyslop and his colleagues at the Harris County Health Department in Texas. Of working mothers with children younger than three years of age, 53 percent are in the workforce.[2] *(#104)*

When parents work full time and adequate child care is unavailable, older children are often left unsupervised, according to Hyslop. He also contends that unsupervised children are at higher risk for a number of problems, including accidents leading to injury, earlier sexual involvement (potentially leading to unintended pregnancy or sexually transmitted diseases), being the victims of crimes such as sexual assault, and becoming involved in undesirable behaviors such as drug abuse or petty crime. Undue stress is another health problem experienced by children who fear being home alone and by the parents who must leave them. *(#104)*

Michael Jarrett, Commissioner of the South Carolina Department of Health and Environmental Control, says that day care should be addressed in the Year 2000 Health Objectives, especially because of the continual growth of single-parent families and employment of both parents in two-parent families. Further, he feels that day care should reflect not only the narrow perspective of care for the healthy child, but also the needs of the acutely ill child or of children with special health care problems. He recommends that the objectives address such issues as licensing, standards, staffing, availability, and accessibility of day-care facilities. *(#108)*

Improvements are needed to offer greater access to quality child care, to ensure the optimal development of children of working parents, and to ease the stress associated with working families and worries about quality child care, according to the American Academy of Pediatrics. The specific improvements suggested include making child care more affordable for low and moderate income families, increasing the number of child-care programs and qualified child-care staff, improving the quality of child care, assisting parents in locating child care that meets their needs, and coordinating child-care funding with state and local early childhood development programs—Head Start, general preschool programs, and preschool programs for handicapped children. *(#115)*

The American Academy of Pediatrics and the American Public Health Association are developing joint performance standards in health, nutrition, safety, and sanitation for out-of-home child care, and Debra Hawks, the project's director, recommends that these standards be used as the basis of new national objectives addressing child care, intervention strategies, and data collection systems. *(#089)*

Hyslop and Holly Wieland of Silver Spring, Maryland, advocate federal initiatives for child care at the national level. *(#104; #331)* Mary Grimord of Texas Woman's University wants an objective to promote affordable day care that meets minimum standards. She says that this will reduce childhood injuries and provide a more healthful environment. *(#303)* David Lurie, Commissioner of the Minneapolis Health Department, asks that all child-care facilities be required to follow proper procedures for food storage and preparation, environmental sanitation, and health and safety codes, and that health advice be available to all facilities. *(#535)*

The Media and Children's Health

According to the American Academy of Pediatrics, television has a strong, but as yet unrealized, potential for improving the health of children. The AAP mentions the adverse effects that television advertising and programming can have on the learning and behavior of children and adolescents: promoting violence; decreasing physical activity and fitness, and possibly increasing the likelihood of obesity; detracting from time spent reading; and presenting unrealistic or inappropriate messages about drugs, alcohol, tobacco, nutrition, sex roles, and sexuality. The AAP supports legislative efforts to improve the content of children's programming and promote more constructive viewing. The AAP hopes that, through improvement of the quality of children's television programming, the health of children and adolescents can be influenced positively in such areas as teenage pregnancy, alcohol or substance abuse, tobacco use, accidental injury and death, nutrition, physical fitness, suicide or homicide, and the school dropout rate. *(#115)*

The Oregon Department of Human Resources, in its own draft of objectives for the year 2000 (submitted as testimony), calls for the impact on children of violence in television and movies to be reduced through measures such as revision of the motion picture code to rate violent content separate from language and sex. The age requirement for attending "X"- and "R"- rated movies, the objectives say, should be enforced, and children should be taught to be "violence-literate" in viewing television and movies. *(#321)* Lou Large, a school nurse from La Porte, Texas, also favors regulating violence in children's television programs and educating parents and children about appropriate viewing. *(#304)*

Coordination of Adolescent Health Services

Programs for adolescents usually concentrate on a particular problem, such as drug abuse, and use a medical model of intervention, according to Claire Brindis and Phillip Lee of the University of California, San Francisco. These witnesses and many others advocate a more comprehensive, integrated approach to adolescent health, including outreach, education and counseling, and removal of financial barriers, as well as actual treatment. Coordination of services at various levels is important, as is consistent and adequate funding. *(#027)* Jarrett concurs and advocates a greater emphasis on comprehensive care centers that meet "not only health needs, but developmental needs of the adolescent" as well. After-school programs should be developed, he says, to occupy these adolescents who are often "left to fend for themselves." *(#108)*

Brindis and Lee recommend the following strategies to improve access to health care for adolescents:
• Develop comprehensive-care centers easily accessible to adolescents near the school or in the community, or expand existing facilities to meet the needs of this age group.
• Allow participation by school dropouts and the homeless as well as those who may have access to other health care services in school-based programs.
• Establish weekend and evening hours to enable a continual source of health care.
• Provide education as well as health care, and establish a networking system for referral of specific problems such as crisis counseling, family planning,

and drug abuse.
• Ensure that staff are sympathetic and qualified to deal with adolescent problems by requiring specific training in this area.
• Provide the privacy and confidentiality that is vital to participation by adolescents.
• Improve the integration of health care with social, vocational, and educational services for youth with chronic illnesses and disabilities. *(#027)*

Brindis and Lee also recommend that those who work with adolescents be proficient in adolescent health care and that this be a component of licensing and accreditation for professionals who will be treating this population. They believe that adolescent-care issues should be integrated into continuing education programs and that upgraded skills should be required of those who serve children and youth. *(#027)*

Chronic Illness and Disability in Children

According to Margaret West of the University of Washington, coping with chronic disease and disability is a way of life for an increasing number of children. Various estimates she cites suggest that 6 to 12 percent of children have chronic or disabling health conditions. In addition, one in ten chronically ill children lack any health insurance.[3] Thus, West says, objectives and programs should be developed to prepare children with chronic disease and disability for adult life. Measures of health outcomes for this population should relate to quality of, and satisfaction with, life and meaningful participation in adult roles. According to West, care for these children should focus on helping them manage their conditions and grow to their maximum potential. Programs for this group should include preparation for adult life skills; a health promotion, family-focused component; and issues of separation from families and maintaining maximum independence. Children with chronic disease or disability also need better-coordinated systems of care, says West. For example, specialty-care health clinics should expand their personnel to include nutritionists, social workers, and psychologists, and should provide continuity in the transfer from pediatric- to adult-care services; health insurance should be provided without clauses related to income or "spending down" of assets; and health care professionals who care for this population should receive training in preparing the youth for adult roles in society. *(#333)*

The use of community-based, comprehensive, coordinated care; the use of family members as care givers; and strong partnerships between families and health professionals—all are important elements in the care of chronically ill and disabled children, according to several witnesses. *(#108; #372)* Linda Henry of Children's Hospital in Denver was critical of the nation's past efforts in aiding these children.

What is America's policy toward its chronically ill children? In displacing human dignity, it resembles abandonment, neglect, and ignorance. These children deserve the same rights, protection, respect, and choices that we all would like for ourselves. They deserve choices and opportunities to see what they can become and a chance to live as independent and autonomously as possible. *(#372)*

The National Association of State Boards of Education also wants "comprehensive programs aimed at modifying behaviors that involve the broader community."

Society cannot afford to address health problems piecemeal through discrete programs aimed at reducing substance abuse, teenage pregnancy, AIDS, and other issues. Rather, they must see these problems as part of a more general at-risk syndrome that requires a comprehensive approach including school and community. *(#573)*

HEALTH PROMOTION

A number of witnesses addressed their comments to health promotion needs of children, primarily behavioral risk factors. Testimony on nutrition focused on the early formation of eating habits, as well as the special nutritional problems of children. Testimony on physical fitness stressed health-related fitness and programs to help children achieve it. Substance abuse, including the use of tobacco and alcohol, is identified as a major public health problem, and programs are proposed for dealing with it. Others testified about mental health issues, especially preventing adolescent suicide. Although the specifics differ, one underlying theme in this body of testimony is the attempt to help children and adolescents form patterns of healthy behavior that can last throughout their lives.

Many of the issues mentioned in this section are discussed more fully in the context of school-based programs in Chapter 9.

Nutrition

Those who testified on issues of childhood nutrition addressed a wide range of topics, including nutrition education and the composition of children's diets, nutritional problems such as anemia and growth retardation, and breast-feeding.

Evan Kligman, representing the Society of Teachers of Family Medicine, feels that successful educational interventions with the family can improve children's nutrition by decreasing the fat content of meals prepared at home; increasing average daily dietary fiber; increasing dietary calcium intake; decreasing salt intake; and including trace minerals, fresh fruit, and cruciferous vegetables known to have a role in the primary prevention of cancer and cardiovascular disease. *(#118)* Improving the general nutrition of children through such programs as the Special Supplemental Food Program for Women, Infants and Children (WIC) and school lunches also received support from Jarrett. *(#108)*

The American Academy of Pediatrics suggests that deaths from nutritional anemia can be prevented through education about good nutrition and, most important, through access to health care that includes correct identification of the problem and early treatment. Early recognition is needed, the AAP explains, because some anemias are recessive traits and carriers can be helped through genetic screening and counseling. *(#115)*

The AAP also believes that the number of cases of growth retardation can be reduced through better nutrition. It reports that in 1984, 7–13 percent of children had "stunted" growth, and in most cases, the cause was nutritional.[4] The AAP recommends that the situation be eased by increased use of such programs as WIC, subsidized school lunches, and Head Start, and by early recognition and treatment of the condition. *(#115)*

Breast-feeding, dealt with more fully in Chapter 22, was frequently mentioned as important to the nutrition and subsequent health of infants and children.

Physical Fitness

The Oregon health objectives sum up the primary concerns of those who testified about physical fitness in the suggested goal of increasing the proportion of children who meet health-related fitness standards and the proportion who participate regularly in a physical education and fitness program that can be carried into adulthood. *(#321)*

The American Academy of Pediatrics also believes that programs should emphasize aerobic and lifetime activities such as bicycling, swimming, tennis, and running, and decrease time spent on football, basketball, and baseball—traditional school sports that do not particularly enhance fitness. The AAP says that efforts should be made to ensure equal emphasis on sports programs for both males and females. *(#115)*

Substance Abuse

Jule Sugarman, Secretary of the Washington State Department of Social and Health Services, sees the misuse and abuse of substances as "one of the major public health menaces today." Such misuse, he feels, plays a causal or contributing role in child abuse, juvenile delinquency, adolescent pregnancy, adolescent suicide, and intentional or unintentional injury. *(#337)* Others joined Sugarman in his concern, and discussed specific problems and potential interventions. The most common substance mentioned was tobacco, including smokeless tobacco, but the problems of alcohol and addictive drugs were addressed as well.

The American Academy of Pediatrics cites a report that found that 40 percent of high school seniors did not believe there was a great health risk associated with smoking.[5] This same report says that 57 percent of high school seniors who ever smoked had their first cigarette by eighth grade or earlier.[6] Furthermore, cigarette use by high school seniors has not dropped over the last few years. The AAP attributes this to the effectiveness of advertising by the tobacco industry, which counterbalances health messages on the hazards of cigarette smoking. The AAP advocates continued education of school students and the public, as well as enhancement of legislative efforts to restrict advertisement of cigarettes. *(#115)*

The Oregon Department of Human Resources also recommends using legislation to restrict print advertising of tobacco products, especially when it is aimed at young people. Educational programs about tobacco should be targeted to children and adolescents, including the provision of smoking and health information in school and the development of incentive programs to encourage young people not to smoke. Oregon also calls for better enforcement of existing laws that prohibit the sale of tobacco to minors. *(#321)*

Kligman sees an "intergenerational" impact of smoking. He advocates programs to reduce smoking among parents of infants and young children in order to reduce the prevalence of otitis media, upper respiratory disease, and other infections associated with passive exposure to smoke. *(#118)*

According to Gabrielle Acampora of the Greater New York Association of Occupational Health Nurses, Black and low-income adolescents are more likely to begin smoking and resist quitting. She suggests that those who drop out of school and then work in small enterprises without health programs might be reached by peer group teens trained as health educators, accompanying occupational health nurses in outreach vans that travel to worksites or in community agencies. *(#002)*

Marge Reveal, testifying on behalf of the American Dental Hygienists' Association (ADHA), and others are concerned about an increase in the use of smokeless tobacco. The ADHA cites evidence that as many as 22 million people may use these products.[7] Even now, despite various health warnings, many users do not consider smokeless tobacco dangerous. The association recommends that smokeless tobacco be included in any objectives or initiatives that address the prevention and control of tobacco use. *(#575)* According to the American Public Health Association, programs to discourage the use of smokeless tobacco among youth should also be targeted toward athletes and other role models for young people. *(#198)*

Many witnesses are concerned about the use of alcohol by adolescents. Studies indicate that children and adolescents are drinking at earlier ages, and programs in the schools and the media are recommended to deal with this problem. *(#008; #675)*

Jarrett sees the need for objectives to address the abuse or misuse of commonly available substances such as cough medicine, glue, and correction fluid, and the misuse of prescribed substances such as steroids in young athletes. *(#108)* Kenneth Kaminsky of the Wayne County Intermediate School District in Michigan recommends objectives about the use of cocaine (including crack) among adolescents. *(#426)* Sugarman wants objectives to focus on all addictive and mind-altering drugs. *(#337)* The American Academy of Pediatrics spells out specific goals for reducing drug use among adolescents, including marijuana, cocaine, hallucinogens, stimulants, inhalants, sedatives, and tranquilizers, as well as tobacco and alcohol. *(#115)* These and other topics are discussed more fully in the chapters on tobacco (Chapter 10) and on alcohol and drug abuse (Chapter 11).

Mental Health and Suicide

Testimony on mental health in children focused on three issues: the promotion of mental health as a factor in general health and well-being, the prevention of severe mental illness, and the prevention of adolescent suicide. The three issues are related, of course, but the first is concerned with mental health as a contributor to other diseases, and the latter two are concerned with specific outcomes to be avoided.

Kevin Dwyer, a representative of the National Association of School Psychologists, advocates prevention of mental health problems of children through a cascade of programs composed of proven community-based preventive and treatment interventions that are interdisciplinary and dependent on interagency cooperation. Such programs would use the schools to identify risk factors in children to treat them, and to educate and involve the parents and family. A national health agenda must focus on primary and secondary prevention of mental illness in the schools, according to the association. To ensure that today's and tomorrow's diverse population of children benefit from schooling, schools must help address personal, emotional, and social development, as well as the concerns of students. (#802)

Stress is an important problem that children face. Donna Gaffney of the Columbia University School of Nursing recommends that children between 10 and 14 years of age participate in stress identification and stress reduction programs in the public schools, and that professional educational programs for mental health workers include formal course work in mental health promotion and stress reduction. (#731)

Marcia Leventhal of New York University and Nancy BrooksSchmitz of Columbia University suggest that dance can increase self-esteem and self-awareness, relieve tension, heal and strengthen the body, and provide a means of social communication. Therefore, dance should be included as a "core discipline" within the educational framework, and it should also be included in therapeutic regimens and as a common recreational activity in community organizations. (#595) Ellen Speert of Los Angeles suggests that art therapy can be used in the schools to help children deal with stresses caused by the fear of nuclear war. (#477)

Gaffney believes that too broad an age group is addressed in the current mental health objectives (15—24 year olds), which obscures the seriousness of the problem in each group and the uniqueness of cognitive, emotional, and social development during three developmental stages. She advocates looking separately at 10—14 year olds, 15—19 year olds, and 20—24 year olds. She also reports an increase in self-destructive behavior in the group age 4 to 15 years, and a concern that children under the age of 10 do not understand the finality of death. (#731)

Tom Barrett, a psychotherapist from Denver, says that there is increasing evidence that American youth are finding it difficult to cope with the stresses of growing up in a rapidly changing society. Suicide is the second leading cause of death for youth between ages 15 and 25.[8] A contributing factor, Barrett believes, is the failure to recognize suicidal behavior. Barrett cites surveys indicating that many youth agencies, including those directed at drug and alcohol use, do not fund suicide-related programs, although substance abuse accounts for many diagnoses of suicide. He recommends that the new objectives set as a goal an increase in the number of school systems with programs to identify youngsters at risk of suicide, an increase in schools with crisis intervention teams, and an increase in suicide prevention programs in colleges and universities. (#702)

Martha Medrano of the University of Texas Health Science Center at San Antonio indicates that adolescent suicide has nearly tripled over the last several decades.[9] Because of this, she proposes an objective to reduce the U.S. teen suicide rate by educating the media about what factors lead to the "contagious" effect of suicide and encouraging the media to voluntarily adopt reporting guidelines. Education about risks and warning signs for suicide in adolescents should be given to medical students, primary care physicians, emergency room attendants, teachers, parents, and students. Medrano also recommends testing professionals to assess their knowledge, as well as surveys of community-based referral sources after a suicide has occurred "to see if there has been an increase of referrals of adolescents (suicidal or not) from the victim's school." (#500)

Damien Martin of New York City reports that homosexual and bisexual young people attempt suicide at substantially higher rates than other adolescents. He recommends that questions of sexual orientation and sexual problems always be considered by those who treat or counsel adolescents who have attempted suicide. He suggests that programs about sexuality in general, including homosexuality, be offered in schools and other adolescent settings, and that such programs also be offered to adult groups such as parent-teacher associations. Research, clinical, and educational programs about teenage suicide should include sexual orientation as a possibly important factor. *(#466)*

The American Association of Child and Adolescent Psychiatry (AACAP) says that the number of children and adolescents at risk for psychiatric illness, though undocumented, is overwhelming and growing at the same time that federal resources for training in this area are shrinking. The AACAP argues that preventive programs are highly fragmented and that a systems approach is required. It cites examples of good approaches such as a new project to upgrade the visibility and services of the mental health component of Head Start, and the Child and Adolescent Service System Program, a coordinated network of children's mental health services, funded by the National Institute of Mental Health and being developed in 28 states and 11 communities. *(#009)*

Carl Hager of Seattle is concerned about the overuse of psychoactive drugs in children. He says that many children who are diagnosed as having an attention deficit disorder are put on drugs that have dangerous side effects. *(#347)*

HEALTH PROTECTION

Witnesses who addressed health protection issues focused primarily on the prevention of injuries—both accidents and intentional violence, particularly child abuse. There also was some testimony on environmental hazards for children, especially lead.

Unintentional Injury

Unintentional injury is the leading cause of death in the first decade of life,[10] and many testifiers suggested ways to prevent it in the home and especially in automobiles, where many of these injuries occur.

The Oregon health objectives suggest that special emphasis be placed on fatal injuries in children under 15 years of age, because this is the only age group in which the rate of fatal unintentional injuries is increasing. They mention specific steps that should be encouraged in the home, including installing cabinet locks, lowering water heater temperature, blocking electrical outlets, and using safety containers for potentially harmful substances. Oregon also recommends improvement of home safety through adoption and enforcement of building codes and regulations pertaining to fire alarms and smoke detectors. *(#321)*

Jarrett would also like to see emphasis placed on injury prevention for children. Parents and care givers must be educated to recognize risks and hazards that emerge as children develop, and to know what preventive measures should be taken, for example, eliminating access to guns in homes. *(#108)*

Claude Earl Fox, the Alabama State Health Officer, reports that motor vehicle accidents are the leading cause of death from birth to age 34,[11] and that increased and correct use of child safety seats can reduce loss of life and prevent serious injuries. He refers to recent studies showing that correctly used child safety seats in passenger cars are 71 percent effective in preventing fatalities, 67 percent effective in reducing the need for hospitalization, and 50 percent effective in preventing minor injury.[12] Only 44 percent of Alabama children under five, however, are fully protected by the correct use of safety seats, he reports.[13] *(#066)*

Joseph Hill of the Detroit Department of Health also recommends that the objectives seek to increase correct child safety seat use. To help promote this goal, public education should teach correct use, manufacturers should update construction of proper seats to match changes in automobile design, law enforcement agencies should clarify requirements of safety seats for children under four, and financial provisions should be made for those who cannot afford to buy seats. *(#404)*

The American Public Health Association suggests that there be a separate objective for reducing alcohol-related vehicular accidents for those under age 25, because this remains a leading cause of death in this age group. *(#198)*

The American Academy of Pediatrics focuses on several particular preventable injuries:

1. Bicycle-related head injuries could be reduced through increased use of bicycle helmets and education in proper bicycle safety procedures.

2. Drowning deaths of younger children could be reduced through increased use of secure fencing around swimming pools. Drowning accidents of older children, particularly teens, could be averted through swimming lessons, education in boat safety, proper maintenance and use of flotation devices, and enforcement of laws prohibiting consumption of alcohol with boat use.

3. Reduction in the number of deaths from accidental poisoning could be achieved through labeling poisonous products, establishing and maintaining poison control centers, maintaining and improving child-proof packaging, and increasing education and public awareness campaigns.

4. A substantial number of accidents and deaths could be avoided by banning the use of all-terrain

vehicles (ATVs) by children under the age of 16. The public should be educated about the hazards ATVs pose for children, and these vehicles should be eliminated by the year 2000. *(#115)*

Child Abuse and Family Violence

Child abuse and family violence were seen by many of the witnesses as serious problems that should be addressed in the Year 2000 Health Objectives. The American Academy of Pediatrics says that in 1987, 2.3 million cases of child abuse were reported.[14] *(#115)* According to Sugarman, intentional injuries can result in death or significant and lasting health damage to children, and such injuries should be regarded as largely preventable. "We must give up the idea that violence is something we can do nothing about except call the police after the damage has been done." *(#337)*

A representative of the Detroit Department of Health suggests a range of strategies for lowering the rate of child abuse and neglect, including support programs for new and prospective parents, parenting education, affordable and accessible child care, home visiting by health professionals, and life-skills training for children and young adults. Further recommendations are to increase public awareness of child abuse prevention; to increase the knowledge of health professionals and other service providers; to coordinate and improve the availability, accessibility, and quality of health services for families; to develop data systems for monitoring trends in incidence and prevalence; and to expand research efforts on predisposing factors and the effects of intervention and prevention activities. *(#207)* Both chronic neglect and pathological violence against children must be targeted. *(#108)*

Blanche Russ, Executive Director of Parent-Child in San Antonio, also suggests mass media awareness campaigns and more manpower in agencies that deal with child abuse and family violence. *(#748)*

A reduction in the number of cases of child abuse could be achieved through early recognition of potential abusers by social service agencies and health personnel, early intervention and treatment of abusive parents, and increased public awareness of the problem, according to the AAP. *(#115)* Oregon reports that risk factors for perpetrators of child abuse have been studied extensively. Structural factors include poverty and unemployment, too many or unplanned-for children, lack of education about childrearing, prolonged marital stress, and social isolation of the

family. Cultural factors include belief in physical punishment as a socializing agent, belief that parents have a right to do what they want with a child, and parents' unrealistic expectations of children. Psychological factors include parents having been abused as children or parents having had a violent role model. Children who are victims of violence have delayed physical, emotional, and social development; even children who witness violence may become victims, with many experiencing post-traumatic stress disorders. The Oregon objectives urge that prevention programs be developed to help parents increase their skills in raising and responding to their children; required parenting curricula should be developed for the public schools. *(#321)*

Lead Poisoning

John Strauther of the Detroit Department of Health reports that lead poisoning has been called the most common preventable pediatric disorder in the United States. It should be of concern not only in children with overt symptoms, but also in those with only moderately elevated levels. *(#412)* Ellen Mangione of the Colorado Department of Health says that since the 1990 Objectives were written, the definition of lead toxicity has changed, and lower threshold values have been established. The Year 2000 Health Objectives should strive to set a lower, scientifically feasible toxicity level or else set a population target of zero. *(#362)*

Strauther recommends a broad-based, intensive effort to reduce lead in the environment, especially in gasoline, water, street and house dust or dirt, and food. He also recommends that children ages one through five should be screened annually for lead poisoning and that the medical community should be better informed about lead hazards. *(#412)* Environmental regulations, such as establishing sanitary landfills and separating potentially contaminating materials from household garbage, also can help eliminate lead hazards. *(#108)*

PREVENTIVE SERVICES

Several testifiers addressed interventions to prevent specific diseases and health problems in children and adolescents. They focused primarily on reducing the spread of infectious diseases, preventing oral disease, and screening for chronic diseases. A large body of testimony dealt with the prevention of AIDS, sexually transmitted diseases, and teen pregnancy, all of which have an important bearing on adolescents and are discussed in Chapters 19, 20, and 23.

Infectious Diseases

The Oregon objectives point to the high levels of childhood immunization that have been achieved in many areas for most vaccine-preventable diseases and the consequent reduction in the incidence of measles, rubella, diphtheria, tetanus, whooping cough, and poliomyelitis. They recommend further improvement in the proportion of children in schools and day-care centers who are up-to-date on all their immunizations. *(#321)* One representative of the Detroit Department of Health, however, feels that it is unrealistic to expect that 95 percent of children will have up-to-date official immunization records by 1990 (the current goal), or possibly even by 2000. *(#393)*

Since the 1990 Objectives were written, new vaccines have become available, and certain populations have special needs for both new and existing vaccines, says the Oregon Department of Human Resources, which projects that immunization of all infants against *Hemophilus influenzae* during infancy could lead to at least a 90 percent reduction of *H. influenzae* invasive disease and its sequelae, including meningitis. Most such cases of meningitis are in children under five years of age; 5 percent of these children die, and 25–35 percent of those who survive sustain damage to the central nervous system. Immunization of 18-month-old children would prevent about 40 percent of the cases. A newly developed vaccine, if approved for younger infants as expected, could prevent another 50 percent of cases.[15] *(#321)*

Sugarman points out that the increased use of day-care centers suggests the need to address infectious diseases in those centers. *(#337)* George Smith of the Tennessee Department of Health and Environment says that such centers, along with schools, should educate and supervise students in proper hygiene practices (such as hand-washing techniques). *(#201)*

Oral Health

Many witnesses felt that many more opportunities exist for the prevention of oral health problems in children and adolescents than were addressed in the 1990 Objectives. Thus, they suggested interventions such as systemic fluoride, fluoride dentifrice, and pit and fissure sealants. Focusing on these three proven measures, says Stephen Moss, representing the American Academy of Pediatric Dentistry, is the most effective way to reduce caries in children. *(#154)* Others focused on special problems such as nursing bottle tooth decay, oral cancer, and the cariogenicity of foods. Jane Weintraub of the University of Michigan and others point out that the 1990 Objectives included only one objective related to the prevalence of dental caries, which focused on nine-year-old children. The new objectives, they feel, should specify additional age groups, the different types of dental caries that may develop, and the proportions of each group with decayed, unfilled teeth, indicators of unmet need. In children, much of the caries prevalence occurs among a small segment of the population;[16] therefore, mean values for a broader group may not be informative. *(#391)*

The American Dental Hygienists' Association and others raise a concern about nursing bottle tooth decay, which results from prolonged use of a nursing bottle containing milk or sugared liquid as a pacifier. The association calls for a large-scale national program directed toward educating the public about nursing bottle caries, a major contributor to decay in the primary teeth of infants that often leads to unsatisfactory oral health conditions in the permanent teeth. *(#575)*

"Oral cancers claim the lives of thousands of individuals each year, yet young persons, especially teenage females, continue their smoking habit," reports Jarrett. It is well recognized that the use of chewing tobacco and snuff, smoking, excess alcohol, and prolonged exposure to ionizing radiation significantly increase one's risk of developing oral cancer. Jarrett and other witnesses suggest development of an objective to reduce oral cancer mortality. *(#108)*

Screening for Chronic Health Problems in Children

A number of witnesses recommend more screening of children for chronic health problems, especially vision and hearing.

Lurie, for instance, recommends routine screening of young children for vision, hearing, and other health problems, with further assessment of those who do not pass a screening test and follow-up until age five of all those screened. *(#535)*

More specifically, Robert Reinecke, representing the American Academy of Ophthalmology, maintains that the screening of preschool children for visual problems is inadequate. He recommends the initiation of rigorous programs to detect visual abnormalities within six weeks of birth, with repeated testing at regular intervals as the child develops. Furthermore, whenever a child is seen by a health care worker (e.g., for immunization or routine visits), Reinecke suggests that the eyes be examined and the child referred to a pediatric ophthalmologist if necessary. He believes that testing of vision in school should be universal and carried out by properly trained individuals, and that children should be tested at least every other year throughout elementary and high school. *(#455)*

DATA NEEDS

A number of testifiers called for better data on children and adolescents, both in general and with regard to particular issues.

Ronald Feinstein of the University of Alabama at Birmingham, for instance, suggests that data be consistently reported for the age group from 8 to 22 years old to avoid grouping adolescents with children. A breakdown into several narrower ranges would be even more beneficial, he says. He also suggests that objectives be established and reported specifically for age, gender, ethnic, and racial segments of the adolescent population. Data should be collected on adolescents who have left the "system" (e.g., by dropping out

of school). *(#250)*

Brindis and Lee add to this recommendation and suggest that federal data bases on adolescent health be improved to allow for easier access, age-specific analyses, and greater comparability among data sets. They also suggest that information systems on special populations of adolescents be improved, including those for school dropouts, institutionalized youth, and chronically ill or physically disabled adolescents. *(#027)*

On more specific issues, Reveal advocates prevalence studies of nursing bottle caries because existing baseline data are limited. *(#575)* The AAP reports that data on child abuse are difficult to collect and analyze due to the lack of a uniform surveillance and reporting system. The AAP feels that development of an improved reporting procedure would yield more accurate figures on the active number of child abuse cases. *(#115)*

Patrick O'Malley and Lloyd Johnston report on the National High School Senior Survey, which is carried out each year by the Institute for Social Research of the University of Michigan. This survey of about 17,000 high school seniors, they say, is a major source of the country's reliable population data on substance abuse. It serves as a valuable source of trends in drug and alcohol abuse, the potential for accidents, and physical fitness and nutrition; it should be used to set and track objectives and teen behavior. *(#419)*

REFERENCES

1. U.S. Bureau of the Census: Statistical Abstract of the United States, 1989 (109th Edition). Washington, D.C.: U.S. Government Printing Office, 1989

2. U.S. Department of Labor: "Labor Participation Unchanged Among Mom's with Young Children." News Release. April 10, 1988

3. Hobbs N, Perrin JM, Ireys HT: Chronically Ill Children and Their Families. San Francisco: Jossey Bass Publishers, 1985

4. U.S. Department of Health and Human Services: Nutrition Monitoring in the U.S.: A Progress Report from the Joint Nutrition Monitoring Evaluation Committee (DHHS Publication No. [PHS] 86-1255), July 1986

5. Bachman JG, Johnston LD, O'Malley PM: Monitoring the Future: Questionnaire Responses from the Nation's High School Seniors, 1986. Ann Arbor: Institute for Social Research, University of Michigan, 1987

6. Ibid.

7. U.S. Department of Health and Human Services: The Health Consequences of Using Smokeless Tobacco: A Report of the Advisory Committee to the Surgeon General (DHHS Publication No. [NIH] 86-2874), 1986

8. National Center for Health Statistics: Health United States, 1987 (DHHS Publication No. [PHS] 88-1232), 1988

9. Ibid.

10. Ibid.

11. National Center for Health Statistics: Health United States, 1989 (DHHS Publication No. [PHS] 90-1232), 1990

12. U.S. Department of Transportation, National Highway Traffic Safety Administration: National Child Passenger Safety Awareness Week Idea Sampler. Washington, D.C.: U.S. Government Printing Office, 1989

13. Alabama Department of Public Health: Child and Occupant Restraint Programs: Survey Results 1988. A Report on the Child Occupant Restraint Survey Program in Alabama. Birmingham: December 1988

14. Straus MA, Gelles R, Steinmetz SK: Behind Closed Doors: Violence in the American Family. Garden City, N.Y.: Anchor Press, 1980

15. Centers for Disease Control: ACIP update: Prevention of Haemophilus Influenzae Type b disease. Morbid Mortal Wkly Rep 37(2):13−16, 1988

16. Klein SP, Bohannan HM, Bell RM, et al. The cost and effectiveness of school-based preventive dental care. Am J Pub Health 75(4):382−91, 1985

TESTIFIERS CITED IN CHAPTER 4

002 Acampora, Gabrielle; Greater New York Association of Occupational Health Nurses
008 Anderson, Dave; American Automobile Association
009 Anthony, Virginia; American Association of Child and Adolescent Psychiatry
027 Brindis, Claire and Lee, Phillip; University of California, San Francisco
055 Eberst, Richard; Adelphi University (Long Island)
066 Fox, Claude Earl; Alabama Department of Public Health
089 Hawks, Debra; American Academy of Pediatrics and American Public Health Association
104 Hyslop, Thomas; Harris County Health Department (Texas)
108 Jarrett, Michael; South Carolina Department of Health and Environmental Control
115 King, Carole; American Academy of Pediatrics
118 Kligman, Evan; Society of Teachers of Family Medicine
154 Moss, Stephen; American Academy of Pediatric Dentistry
198 Sheps, Cecil; American Public Health Association
201 Smith, George; Tennessee Department of Health and Environment
207 Gaines, George; Detroit Department of Health
250 Feinstein, Ronald; University of Alabama at Birmingham
303 Grimord, Mary; Texas Woman's University
304 Large, Lou; La Porte Independent School District (Texas)
321 Skeels, Michael; Oregon Department of Human Resources
331 Wieland, Holly; Silver Spring, Maryland
333 West, Margaret; University of Washington
337 Sugarman, Jule; Washington State Department of Social and Health Services
347 Hager, Carl; Citizens Commission on Human Rights, Seattle Chapter
362 Mangione, Ellen; Colorado Department of Health
372 Henry, Linda; Children's Hospital (Denver)

391 Weintraub, Jane; University of Michigan
393 Gaines, George; Detroit Department of Health
404 Hill, Joseph; Detroit Department of Health
412 Strauther, John; Detroit Department of Health
419 O'Malley, Patrick and Johnston, Lloyd; University of Michigan
426 Kaminsky, Kenneth; Wayne County Intermediate School District (Michigan)
455 Reinecke, Robert; Wills Eye Hospital (Philadelphia)
466 Martin, A. Damien; Hetrick-Martin Institute (New York)
467 Aguirre-Molina, Marilyn and Lubinski, Christine; National Council on Alcoholism
477 Speert, Ellen; American Art Therapy Association
500 Medrano, Martha; University of Texas Health Science Center at San Antonio
535 Lurie, David; Minneapolis Health Department
573 Wilhoit, Gene; National Association of State Boards of Education
575 Reveal, Marge; American Dental Hygienists' Association
595 Leventhal, Marcia; New York University and BrookSchmitz, Nancy; Columbia University
675 Teague, Wayne; Alabama Department of Education
702 Barrett, Tom; Center for Psychological Growth (Denver)
731 Gaffney, Donna; Columbia University
748 Russ, Blanche; Parent-Child, Inc. (San Antonio)
802 Dwyer, Kevin; National Association of School Psychologists

5. Older Adults

The need for special national objectives for older people was recognized in *Healthy People: The Surgeon General's Report on Health Promotion and Disease Prevention*, which was published in 1979.[1] Although the Surgeon General proposed mortality reduction goals for other age groups, the main goal for older adults was to improve health and quality of life, particularly to reduce the number of restricted activity days resulting from acute or chronic conditions. This priority grew out of a realization that health promotion and disease prevention activities can have profound effects on the quality of life of older Americans. The point was reemphasized in 1988 at the Surgeon General's Workshop on Health Promotion and Aging, at which almost 200 experts recommended a series of health promotion and disease prevention activities for older people in nine areas: alcohol, oral health, physical fitness and exercise, injury prevention, medication, mental health, nutrition, preventive health services, and smoking cessation. These recommendations were submitted as testimony for the Year 2000 Health Objectives.[2] (#799)

As a group, the elderly are more likely than younger people to suffer from multiple, chronic, and often disabling conditions, and they are more likely to be physically and socially dependent. However, the aging process is complex and varies substantially from one person to another. The conditions that many older people face are not inevitable: some causes of physical and mental decline can be prevented, and older people can learn to live with other conditions and still maintain high levels of physical, psychological, and social function. According to *Healthy People*, "With adequate social and health services, a greater proportion of the elderly could maintain a relatively independent lifestyle and vastly improve the quality of their lives."[3]

Some of those who testified about the special health promotion and disease prevention needs of older adults focused their comments on common and crosscutting issues, especially the quality of life. Others focused on specific health problems faced by older people and interventions for these problems. Some witnesses spoke primarily about health promotion activities for older people, including health education; modifying risk factors such as smoking and alcohol; reducing the misuse of medication; improving mental health; and increasing physical and recreational activity. Other testifiers addressed the prevention of specific diseases and health problems faced by older adults, including cancer, heart disease, osteoporosis, infectious diseases, dental problems, and hearing or communication problems. Additional testimony dealt with health protection issues such as the prevention of elder abuse and injuries. Although these topics mirror those of the general national objectives, the specific issues of concern for older adults differ substantially from those of the general population. A number of testifiers also addressed special issues that arise in the context of long-term care. Others discussed implementation issues, especially problems of access to health care and the need for better data on the health status of older people.

Although many of the issues discussed in this chapter were incorporated in the 1990 Objectives, witnesses called for even more emphasis on addressing the health concerns of those age 65 and over in the Year 2000 Health Objectives.

CROSSCUTTING ISSUES AND QUALITY OF LIFE

Many who testified about the special needs and opportunities for health promotion and disease prevention in the elderly focused their attention on measuring and improving the quality of life for older adults. Others stressed the heterogeneity among the elderly, the differences between them and the rest of the population, and the implications of these differences for setting objectives.

As Anne Somers of the University of Medicine and Dentistry of New Jersey and Victoria Weisfeld of the Robert Wood Johnson Foundation, point out:

The very concept of "old age" and all our protective policies and programs for the "aged" relate to the presumption of a sharp decline in physical and/or mental capacity, as well as life expectancy, after 65. This is now patently inaccurate—but as a nation we haven't decided how to adjust to the changed situation. (#428)

Rather than "rationing" care, Somers and Weisfeld call for "a positive national commitment to 'healthy and productive aging'."

It is no longer enough to say that older people have an equal right to good health care, including prevention and long-term care. The corollary is the obligation to take care of our own health insofar as possible, to learn to cope with various chronic conditions, and to continue working and contributing to society for as long as possible. *(#428)*

In light of this, Somers and Weisfeld propose two broad goals:

1. to improve the "health span" or "active life expectancy" of older persons, including those with some chronic impairment. In other words, increase the number of years of independent functioning and capacity for productive activity; and

2. to set the stage for upward redefinition of the concept of "old age," moving gradually from the obsolete figure of 65 toward a more realistic 75, with a target of at least 70 years of age by the year 2000. *(#428)*

Other testifiers underlined the idea that not all those referred to as "elderly" are alike. Susan Marine of Boulder, Colorado, suggests that objectives for older people should be divided into two subgroups. The subgroup for those age 65–84 should be made up of "goals for decreasing mortality from cardiovascular diseases and cancer, as well as goals for maintaining functional independence." For those 85 and older, the objectives should be "goals for maximizing functional independence and the quality of life." *(#370)* Similarly, Robert Katzman of the University of California, San Diego suggests two sets of goals for some topics: one for the "young old" (age 60–80) and another for the "old old" (over age 80). *(#794)*

Many witnesses addressed the issue of quality of life. Paul Hunter of the American Medical Student Association, quoting President John F. Kennedy, expresses it most vividly: "It is not enough for a great nation to have added new years to life. Our objective must be to add new life to those years." *(#612)*

Somers and Weisfeld suggest that the proportion of noninstitutionalized older people with self-reported health status of "excellent" to "good" should increase to 75 percent; that the labor force participation rate of those age 65 and over should be at least 20 percent (employed full-time, employed part-time, or looking for work); and that an additional 30 percent should be engaged in some form of unpaid but productive activity, including care of disabled family members. *(#428)*

Donald Patrick of the University of Washington suggests that objectives for older adults be evaluated in terms of the health-related quality of life by using the concept of quality-adjusted life years. Quality-adjusted life years measure the functional and social dependence caused by a particular disease or medical treatment, he says, thus allowing a determination of the efficacy and cost-effectiveness of a particular intervention. To improve the quality of life for older people, Patrick suggests four health promotion and disease prevention strategies for the elderly: early identification of risk factors for which there are efficacious interventions to modify the onset or course of disease, disability, and dependency; modification of physical and social environments; maintenance and improvement of desirable health habits; and enhancement of personal autonomy. *(#341)*

The Alliance for Aging Research suggests that the overall goal of health promotion/disease prevention strategies aimed at the elderly should be to decrease frailty, "a general but useful term encompassing a variety of impairments that limit functional abilities and increase vulnerability to trauma and other stresses among older persons." *(#776)* Several others recommend that overall functioning be measured in terms of the activities of daily living (ADL) scales, which assess one's ability to perform six basic functions: bathing, dressing, eating, toileting, moving from bed to chair, and independent ambulation. *(#766)* Some experts, however, find the ADL "a barely adequate measure because it relies on self-report rather than observation" *(#459),* or they criticize it because the scales are "so limited" and "skewed toward particular types of functional disability." *(#794)*

John Cornman of the Gerontological Society of America suggests four facts regarding the health of older people to guide formulation of the objectives:

1. Widespread and substantial heterogeneity of health conditions exists among older adults, even within the same age group.

2. There are physiological differences between older and younger people that should influence health care; for example, disease symptoms may vary with age, and older persons may react differently to drugs than do younger persons.

3. Because lifestyle factors at earlier ages affect health status at later ages, disease prevention and health promotion goals established for younger persons also are important to older persons.

4. Preventive measures should be applied to older

persons because modification of behavior and habits is also beneficial in older age. *(#766)*

To benefit fully from various measures aimed at improving the quality of life among older adults, they must be active participants in their own care and health promotion, rather than allowing things to be done "to" them, according to James Haviland of Seattle, Washington. *(#795)*

HEALTH PROMOTION AND HEALTH PROTECTION FOR OLDER ADULTS

Although a large number of behavior-related factors were mentioned by the witnesses, most of the testimony centered around smoking, alcohol and drug problems, mental health, physical and recreational activity, and health education. Others addressed issues that come under the heading of health protection, mainly the prevention of accidental injury and violence or abuse.

Smoking Cessation

According to Claude Earl Fox, the Alabama State Health Officer, evidence shows that people can decrease their chances of dying of a smoking-related cause even if they stop smoking at an older age. *(#066)* Rebecca Richards of the North Woods Health Careers Consortium agrees and calls for increased public and professional awareness of this fact. In particular, she recommends that smoking cessation programs aimed at the elderly be undertaken in communities and at senior centers. *(#183)*

Similarly, participants at the Surgeon General's Workshop on Health Promotion and Aging also recognized the benefits of smoking cessation and proposed a number of educational approaches aimed at opinion leaders, the media, and health professionals to convey the message that cessation can be beneficial for older people. They also proposed a range of activities to make nonsmoking the norm in environments that older people frequent and to encourage smoking cessation programs. *(#799)*

Alcohol

Richards reports estimates that one in twelve elderly men will develop a drinking problem.[4] She recommends that reimbursement be expanded for treatment of drug and alcohol problems in the elderly, citing recent research showing that older people are more likely to complete such treatment successfully and to remain free of the abused substance for longer periods of time than are young people.[5] *(#183)*

Fox says that excessive use of alcohol among the elderly can disguise certain medical problems. For example, alcohol can mask pain, leading to delay in seeking medical attention for a heart attack. Alcohol also affects blood sugar metabolism, leads to liver disease, causes digestive problems, encourages poor nutrition habits, and alters the function of the brain. Another serious problem is the dangerous interaction of alcohol and drugs. *(#066)*

In light of such problems, participants at the Surgeon General's Workshop on Health Promotion and Aging recommended professional and public education programs to inform people about the problems of alcoholism and their prevention, and service programs in the community to help older adults overcome alcohol problems. *(#799)*

Misuse of Medication

Rather than concern about the abuse of addictive substances so often expressed for adolescents and young adults, the most pressing "drug" issue for many older adults is the misuse of medication.

The American Society of Hospital Pharmacists sees a need for an objective dealing with misuse of medication by the elderly population. Some of the ways suggested to reduce misuse are heightened awareness about medication information on the part of physicians, increased cooperation among various health care professionals, and more patient education on the use of prescription and nonprescription drugs. *(#574)*

Edward Wagner of the Group Health Cooperative of Puget Sound calls for more attention to the adverse effects of prescribed medications, the use of psychoactive drugs and their relationship to injury, and the excessive or inappropriate use of commonly prescribed cardiovascular and psychoactive drugs, which may be a risk factor for falls, fractures, and hospitalization. Wagner would like to see a federal initiative to reduce the inappropriate or excessive use of antihypertensive drugs or toxic psychoactive and psychotropic drugs. *(#738)*

Mental Health

Dementia becomes a major problem over age 75, according to Katzman, and in the very elderly (over age 85) the demented constitute about one-third of the population. He recommends training "a cohort of nursing aides or other paraprofessionals" to help provide the needed optimum care and to help prevent excess disability. (#794)

Richards notes that although recent initiatives have focused attention and some resources on dementias, other mental health disorders common to older adults also require attention. A community study in North Carolina showed a prevalence rate for depression in older adults of 8.2 per 100.[6] Another study, suggesting that health care providers may not be educated to recognize mental health problems of the elderly, indicated that 90 percent of elderly men who committed suicide had visited their physicians within their last three months.[7] (#183)

John Miner of the Massachusetts Mental Health Center emphasizes that the mental health needs of the elderly, especially for emotional support and a feeling of personal caring, should be particularly stressed in the education of nurses and physicians. (#468)

James Sykes, representing the National Council on the Aging, states that "mental health is a vital goal for all Americans but especially for the large and growing population of retired persons. The insults of the psychological effects of years of purposelessness are as severe as cancer." Rather than strategies to prevent mental illness, health promotion strategies are needed that provide status, purpose, and useful roles to people whose retirement has changed their usual bases for purposeful lives. There is also a need for well-trained and appropriately compensated providers of care, as well as family members who come into daily contact with impaired older persons. (#768)

James Sugarman of the Retired Senior Volunteer Program Directors recommends volunteer work as one answer to finding productive, fulfilling roles in older age. He further comments that the exercise, regular diet, and physical and psychic benefits derived from volunteerism are important and should be emphasized in local, state, and national programs. (#769)

Physical Activity and Recreation

Scientific evidence has demonstrated that carefully planned programs of physical activity can prevent or diminish the degree of functional loss associated with some chronic diseases affecting the older population, says Fox. (#066) According to a 1987 survey, only 7.7 percent of women and 8.5 percent of men over 65 currently exercise at 60 percent of functional capacity for 20 minutes or more, three or four times a week.[8] Fox recommends as an objective that 40 percent of adults over 65 be engaging in regular, appropriate physical exercise, such as walking, swimming, or other aerobic activities, by the year 2000. (#066)

Richards points out the obstacles to exercise programs. Walking, a common form of exercise for older adults, may be difficult for those with arthritis or painful foot conditions. Walking in adverse weather can be dangerous for those with cardiovascular or balance problems. Swimming pools, particularly therapeutic pools, are not available in many communities. Richards feels that access to exercise programs for all older adults should be a priority for the new objectives and that transportation to, and reimbursement for, the cost of exercise programs at appropriate facilities must be addressed as part of this objective. (#183) Others stress the importance of building exercise' into regular daily activities rather than depending on traveling to distant facilities. (#459)

The National Recreation and Park Association (NRPA) also stresses recreational activity as crucial to the improved health and wellness of older individuals. The NRPA suggests that services be provided in settings as close to home and as consistent with usual lifestyle as possible. Each state and regional office on the aging, the NRPA says, should be required to include park and recreation programs for the aged in its referral systems to ensure greater access to recreation by the elderly. (#777)

Injury Control

Richards says that morbidity rates, not just death rates, from accidents and falls of the elderly should be examined. The cost of the morbidity (both direct medical costs and indirect costs such as subsequent institutionalization or missed work by care givers) should be compared to the cost of providing preventive services directed at known risk factors for falls. She says, for example, that vision problems are known to be a significant risk factor for falls, yet eyeglasses and examinations to prescribe, fit, or change them are not covered by Medicare.[9] (#183)

Michael Oliva of Aurora, Colorado, calls for more money to be provided from appropriate agencies for injury control programs for the elderly. All health care providers who serve the elderly, Oliva says, including Community Health Centers and those who provide health promotion and wellness programs for the elderly, should include injury control in their plans of care. (#378)

The Surgeon General's Workshop on Health Promotion and Aging calls for architects, engineers, city planners, and similar professionals to be educated about the capabilities and limitations of older persons, and recommended that they incorporate these factors into their designs. *(#799)*

Elder Abuse

Increasingly, elderly people are caring for others who are even more elderly or sick, says Richards. The added stress on older care givers, as with younger care givers, can lead to abuse. She suggests an objective to reduce elder abuse by requiring that facilities discharging Medicare patients demonstrate that comprehensive, systematic discharge planning has occurred. Elder abuse could be decreased by carrying out a systematic assessment of the older person and the potential care giver, as well as the entire family constellation.[10] *(#183)*

Melanie Hwalek, a psychologist and gerontologist in Michigan, agrees that there is a need for objectives to prevent and treat elder abuse and neglect. There also is a need for valid and reliable measurement instruments to assess both the risk of elder abuse in community populations and the substantiation of elder abuse among suspected cases from state reporting systems and human services agencies. She cites and supports the solutions advocated by the Surgeon General's Workshop on Violence and Public Health, including the development of educational programs for professionals on detection, assessment, and treatment of abuse; educational programs for the public; community outreach; research, especially national studies on incidence and prevention; and a national clearinghouse for coordinating research, training, and program development, along with services to help elder abuse victims and to help families care for older people.[11] *(#403)*

A number of people point out that many providers of long-term and chronic care are family members, usually women, and that they experience stress and often suffer from ill health and financial worries. *(#110; #451)* Olivia Maynard, Director of the Michigan Office of Services to the Aging, suggests increased awareness of the problems of family care givers through public service announcements, identification of community resources to assist in coping with family stress, and physicians providing information to family members about resources at the time of diagnosis of a serious or disabling chronic condition. More family care givers should be enrolled in support or self-help groups. In addition, more emphasis should be placed on stress identification and control

by private, voluntary, and public health organizations, as well as on the provision of education on community resources by employers. *(#145)*

PREVENTIVE SERVICES FOR OLDER ADULTS

Somers and Weisfeld report that although some of the problems older people face are beyond prevention, "a much greater proportion is amenable to preventive interventions at the primary, secondary, or tertiary levels." Many older people, however, "are still denied access to effective preventive services as a result of nonavailability, financial constraints, ignorance, or indifference—their own as well as that of many health professionals. The result is a great deal of suffering as well as unnecessary use of expensive acute care." *(#428)*

Wilda Ferguson of the Virginia Department for the Aging, representing the National Association of State Units on Aging, agrees that preventive services are not sufficiently used by older people. More creative and effective ways are required to provide older persons and their care givers with the basic information they need about the process of aging and its impact on physical and psychological health. "Myths, fatalism, or the ready acceptance of an idea that ailments among the elderly are to be borne rather than dealt with" must be overcome, says Ferguson. *(#772)*

The Preventive Health Services Working Group of the Surgeon General's Workshop on Health Promotion and Aging suggests two broad goals for preventive services: "1) to prevent physical, psychological, and iatrogenic disorders; and 2) to prolong the period of independent living with particular attention to quality of life." It recommends that preventive services be individualized according to active life expectancy; physical activity; cognitive capacity; and the presence, nature, or stage of disease, and that this individualization respect the principles of minimal disruption of lifestyle, preservation of autonomy, and minimal iatrogenic insults, and recognize that avoidance of death may not be the ultimate goal. Based on this, the working group makes a number of recommendations about the training of health professionals and others who work with the elderly, and the implementation of preventive services in programs and settings that are accessible to older people. They suggest that these programs take into account the heterogeneity in the elderly population and that they address factors that prevent disability as well as disease. More particularly, the working group is skeptical of mass screening programs for disease or risk factors outside primary care settings. *(#799)*

Other witnesses addressed a wide range of issues relevant to the prevention of specific diseases, especially those involving the provision of preventive services. The topics include cancer, heart disease, infectious diseases, oral health, hearing and communication disorders, and osteoporosis. For many of these conditions, witnesses pointed out that primary prevention in early or midlife is the most important strategy for reducing such disabilities in older people. However, primary, and especially secondary or tertiary, interventions can make a difference. Problems associated with vision loss, although still important to many older adults, have decreased in recent years due to the improved treatment of cataracts. Senile macular degeneration, however, still causes serious impairment for many. *(#794)*

Cardiovascular Disease

Somers and Weisfeld indicate that heart disease and related circulatory conditions are still the major cause of severe disability among the noninstitutionalized elderly and major risk factors are not only known but, in most cases, controllable.[12] *(#428)* Rosalie Young of Wayne State University agrees and says that, just as for other chronic diseases, the most effective strategy for controlling heart disease, postponing disability, and preventing progression of chronic conditions is risk factor reduction. *(#478)*

"The major cardiovascular risk factors (hypertension, dyslipidemia, impaired glucose tolerance, cigarette smoking, obesity, and physical deconditioning)," says Young, "are highly prevalent among elders yet all are modifiable." To do so, Young proposes health promotion objectives for older adults to increase exercise, reduce smoking, reduce serum cholesterol through diet and medication, reduce salt and total caloric intake of overweight persons and thus reduce obesity, and increase the number of physician visits to enable more preventive care. *(#478)*

Young adds that beyond primary prevention, treatment of heart disease by using the cardiologist's vast armamentarium of surgical and medical strategies offers benefits to some older patients, especially in terms of improving their quality of life. *(#478)*

Cancer

According to Ann Norman of the University of Washington, about one in ten women in the United States will develop breast cancer in any given year;[13] 75 percent of this cancer will be detected among women 50 years and older.[14] The death rate in this group is particularly high, and one reason is the low level of screening. According to Norman, the Year 2000 Health Objectives should be consistent with those of the National Cancer Institute, which recommend increasing the percentage of 50- to 70-year-old women who undergo breast examinations and mammograms, and of 40- to 70-year-old women who undergo Pap smears.[15] *(#336)* Although not as serious a problem as breast cancer is for women, prostate cancer is an important problem of aging males. *(#794)*

Osteoporosis

Osteoporosis is more common in White women over 45 than heart attacks, strokes, diabetes, and other major chronic disorders, according to Thomas Heston of the University of Washington. *(#338)* Wayne Tsuji of the Washington State Arthritis Foundation says that osteoporosis leads to vertebral compression fractures and hip fractures, which cause great pain and disability. However, measures such as calcium and estrogen supplementation, weight bearing exercise, and cutting back on alcohol or tobacco can help prevent osteoporosis and the disability it causes. Furthermore, Tsuji notes that older women at higher risk can be screened for osteoporosis so that they can be treated before the point of fracture or other damage. *(#339)* (See Chapter 27 for further discussion on this topic.) Primary prevention, however, must be started at a younger age, particularly by increasing the calcium consumption of young and middle-aged women.

Infectious Diseases

Because the elderly are at greater risk than other adults for infectious diseases, immunization is of primary importance, according to Steven Mostow of the Rose Medical Center in Denver. For example, he reports that most deaths from influenza could be prevented with a national immunization program targeted at the elderly and those with heart or lung disease; control of influenza in these groups is not only achievable but very cost-effective. "A massive annual media campaign to promote influenza vaccination among the elderly, sponsored by the Influenza Alert Committee of the American Lung Association of Colorado, has increased influenza immunization rates from 8 percent to 32 percent in the past four years (1984–1988)." *(#380)*

The impact of food-borne diarrheal illness is greater on those already physically compromised, including many elderly. The Association of Food and Drug Officials suggests that this is preventable through proper manufacturing and food handling practices. *(#384)*

Katherine Hunter, representing the American Society of Microbiology, recommends that the incidence of pneumonia in the elderly be addressed. All nursing homes should have an active, result-oriented infection control committee analogous to those in hospitals. Furthermore, all nursing homes should screen employees and patients for tuberculosis. *(#259)*

Dental Health

The American Dental Hygienists' Association (ADHA) claims that "of the entire population, older peoples' total body health is the most dependent upon their oral health. Debilitating oral conditions limit the older person's ability to eat a balanced diet, and inadequate nutritional intake results in compromised health." The ADHA recommends educational programs developed specifically to inform older people about the impact of oral health on their overall health status, and suggests that federal and private insurance programs include payment for preventive oral health services. *(#575)*

Because more people are maintaining their natural teeth as they age, caries are an increasing problem for the elderly. Ronald Ettinger of the American Society for Geriatric Dentistry suggests that caries can be reduced in the aging population by the development of techniques to identify those at risk. He also reports that dental care of the elderly in institutions is neglected and that the institutionalized have a far greater need for dental care than the noninstitutionalized elderly. *(#062)*

Hearing and Communication

According to James Lovell of the National Hearing Aid Society, it is important to recognize the high prevalence of untreated hearing impairment in older people and to include greater awareness of age-related hearing loss and its remedies in the objectives. He believes that the majority of such people can be brought back to higher functioning by the use of available technology, with a consequent improvement in the quality of life. *(#409)* Shirley Sparks of Western Michigan University also discusses communication disorders among the elderly. She suggests goals assuring that the current prevalence of significant hearing loss and speech or language problems in the elderly should not increase and that the disability of the resulting social isolation should decrease. *(#396)*

LONG-TERM HEALTH CARE NEEDS OF THE AGING

One of the issues most often addressed in testimony on older people is caring for those with permanent or chronic impairments of health and functioning. A number of witnesses suggested that the objectives should emphasize maintaining the personal independence of those with long-term dysfunctions, thus preventing their unnecessary institutionalization in nursing homes and hospitals. *(#079)* Most of the chronically ill elderly could remain at home if they were provided with the personal care services required. Physical security and appropriate living arrangements are important. Institutionalization promotes dependency and, therefore, increases disability. Deinstitutionalization (or preventing institutionalization in the first place) must, however, be accompanied by the assurance of individualized services and treatments; these are the keys to secondary prevention. *(#012)*

Violet Barkauskas of the University of Michigan reports that vulnerable elderly often are discharged from the hospital with reduced functional ability; she suggests that objectives be set to screen all over-65 hospital patients at discharge to determine the need for continuing care. *(#714)*

Patrick Griffith of Morehouse Medical School projects that the incidence of intellectual loss will escalate after the year 2000 with the growth of the elderly segment of the population. Therefore, Griffith believes it is necessary to increase the number of long-term care facilities that take Alzheimer's patients, increase the number of persons trained to treat those affected, increase the number of centers for such training, and undertake a comprehensive multidisciplinary diagnostic assessment of ways to manage this population. (#670) Several testifiers pointed to a need for coordinated and holistic home health care services for the elderly. Such care would include not only medical services, but social support; nutritionists' services; home care pharmacists; and instruction about housework, meals, and transportation. (#074)

Sharon Grigsby, President of the Visiting Nurse Foundation in Los Angeles, writes that "home care should have a bright future in the next century. It is a logical alternative to the dilemma of increasing health care demands in an era of fiscal restraints." Visiting nurses were suggested as one means of providing health care for the elderly in their own homes; prevention of further disability and dysfunction is an important part of their purview. (#074)

Kay Hollers, representing the National Association for Home Care (#686), suggests that the public be educated about the availability of home care through media, public health education, and marketing approaches. Financial disincentives to families for home care should be removed, and Medicare should provide home care benefits, says Hollers. David Lurie, Commissioner of the Minneapolis Department of Health, notes that programs to assure the quality of home health services also are necessary. (#535)

Sheldon Goldberg, President of the American Association of Homes for the Aging, has another suggestion for maintaining independence. He describes continuing care retirement communities, in which older people can live independently for as long as possible while having access to health care at whatever level is necessary. He recommends research to determine the demand for such communities; their effect on health and life expectancy; the cost and utilization of health care in such settings; and Medicare utilization rates in these communities. (#770)

Another possible answer for long-term health care needs is to provide more adult day care, reimbursable through Medicare or Medicaid. A large portion of the population served here would be those with Alzheimer's disease. (#637)

IMPLEMENTATION

Many witnesses had suggestions about implementation of the objectives for older people. Somers and Weisfeld suggest a broad range of actions at all levels. Others focus on improving access to health care and preventive service in particular, especially through Medicare and Medicaid. Still others comment about data and various information needs relevant to older people.

Somers and Weisfeld suggest a number of steps to implement the broad and specific strategies required to improve the quality of life of older Americans. At the federal level, they propose that the Public Health Service and the Health Care Financing Administration work together to determine which preventive services for the elderly are effective and to incorporate those services into Medicare or other health programs. They propose that states consider mandating clinical prevention packages in the health services they provide or regulate and that governments at all levels develop information and educational materials directed at the media and the general public. Somers and Weisfeld suggest that all health professionals devote more time and attention to prevention, and that their schools and certifying bodies move toward facilitating and ensuring this. They propose that insurance companies and employers move to adopt a full range of preventive services in the health packages they provide, and that employers implement worksite wellness programs and flexible retirement policies. Finally, they suggest that the media have an important role to play in educating the public, and they propose ways to maintain and improve the quality of its messages. (#428)

Access to Health Care

To carry out the national objectives, greater access to preventive care is necessary, according to many testifiers. (#142) Private insurance and Medicare policies about reimbursement for preventive services constitute a large part of the problem, but Marine points out that available services often are poorly coordinated. (#370)

Richards discusses barriers to cancer screening in older adults. They include transportation difficulties, lack of insurance coverage for screening and prevention, and difficulty in cancer self-detection due to physical losses (visual, musculoskeletal) and concurrent debilitating diseases. One way to overcome these problems, she says, is to conduct screening procedures at geriatric day-care centers, retirement centers, and senior centers. *(#183)*

Another way to address the access problem, according to Richards, is through Medicare versions of prepaid health plans, known as Medicare health maintenance organizations (HMOs). In addition, social health maintenance organizations (SHMOs) integrate health care with psychosocial, environmental, and informal supports to reduce dependency. The SHMO is geared to coordination of services and to maximizing the functional capacity of older adults. Richards suggests objectives to increase the availability of Medicare HMOs and SHMOs and to increase public awareness of this option. *(#183)*

Several witnesses spoke about educational efforts that should be undertaken to sensitize those who work with the aging to problems that may arise in later years and ways to deal with them. Miner feels that formal course work in geriatrics should be mandatory for those entering health care fields. In addition, primary care providers should be better educated about conditions in the elderly that suggest referral to mental health services and about their needs for emotional support and personalized caring. *(#468)* Paul Hunter and his colleagues believe that students in the health professions should have experience in facilities for the elderly. *(#612)*

Current efforts in health promotion and aging are hampered by the limited involvement of medical care providers, according to Robert Newcomer and Rena Pasick of the University of California, San Francisco. This can be improved through changes in Medicare reimbursement rules, minimum standards for professional training, and better definitions of the roles of all health providers. *(#482)*

Several testifiers stated that Medicare should reimburse a greater variety of services, especially preventive services, than it does now. *(#062; #074; #336; #612)* Richards states, "Unfortunately, a very tidy summary of the preventive services most needed in this age group can be found in a publication, *The Medicare Handbook*, under a category entitled 'What Medicare Does Not Cover'."[16] Richards suggests that the following items should be reimbursable: dental services; nutritionist's services, especially for those with multiple health problems; home care pharmacists to monitor multiple medications; mental health services; long-term care costs; periodic health and screening examinations; the costs of eyeglasses and examinations to prescribe them; breast examinations; mammography; and Pap smears. *(#183)*

Data and Information Needs

The American Association of Retired Persons (AARP) notes that the 1990 Objectives include relatively few objectives pertaining specifically to older adults. The AARP believes that this omission is due to gaps in data collection systems and measurement techniques. It recommends that the Public Health Service focus resources on expanding data collection for assessing health status and health risk in older adults. Data are needed on the use of preventive services and reimbursement for such services; accidents and injuries (especially in-home fires); misuse of alcohol or drugs (including prescription drugs); suicide; and use of mental health services by the elderly. *(#767)*

Walter Bortz of the Palo Alto Medical Foundation suggests that data are needed to show how preventive strategies work in older people and how health behavior is affected by the negative stereotype of aging. *(#508)*

Richards also believes that "while there is growing evidence that health promotion pays off in improved quality of life, we must convince policymakers that prevention also saves scarce health dollars." She recommends the researching of long-term questions: for example, do older adults with arthritis who begin a regular exercise program require institutionalization less often or at a later age than those who do not exercise? She suggests an increase in the number of projects doing follow-up to measure the long-term effects of health promotion. *(#183)*

REFERENCES

1. U.S. Department of Health, Education and Welfare: Healthy People: The Surgeon General's Report on Health Promotion and Disease Prevention (DHEW Publication No. [PHS] 79-55071), 1979

2. U.S. Department of Health and Human Services: Surgeon General's Workshop on Health Promotion and Aging, March 20–23, 1988; Proceedings. Edited by FG Abdellah, SR Moore

3. U.S. Department of Health, Education and Welfare: op. cit., reference 1

4. Atkinson R, Kofoed LL: Alcohol and drug abuse. Geriatric Medicine, Vol. II. Edited by CK Cassel, JR Walsh. New York: Springer-Verlag, 1984

5. Ibid.

6. U'Ren RC: Affective disorders. Geriatric Medicine, Vol. I. Edited by CK Cassel, JR Walsh. New York: Springer-Verlag, 1984

7. Ibid.

8. Alabama Department of Public Health: 1986 Behavioral Risk Factor Surveillance System, Alabama Statewide Survey, 1987 Weighted. February 1988

9. Health Care Financing Administration: The Medicare Handbook, 1990. Washington, D.C.: U.S. Government Printing Office, 1990

10. Kosberg J: Preventing elder abuse: Identification of high risk factors prior to placement decisions. Gerontol 28(1):43–50, 1988

11. U.S. Department of Health and Human Services: The Surgeon General's Workshop on Violence and Public Health: Report. (Publication No. [HRS-D-MC] 86-1), May 1986

12. LaPlante MP: Disability risks of chronic illnesses and impairments. Disability Statistics Report. No. 2. Institute for Health and Aging, University of California; San Francisco, November 1989

13. American Cancer Society: Cancer Facts and Figures, 1989. Atlanta, Ga.: American Cancer Society, Inc., 1989

14. National Cancer Institute: Cancer Statistics Review: 1973–1986. (NIH Publication No. 89-2789), May 1989

15. Greenwald P, Sondik E (Eds.): Cancer Control Objectives for the Nation, 1985–2000. National Cancer Institute Monographs, No. 2. (NIH Publication No. 86-2880), 1986

16. Health Care Financing Administration: op. cit., reference 9

TESTIFIERS CITED IN CHAPTER 5

012 Baker, Milton; Syracuse Developmental Services Office
062 Ettinger, Ronald; American Society for Geriatric Dentistry
066 Fox, Claude Earl; Alabama Department of Public Health
074 Grigsby, Sharon; The Visiting Nurse Foundation
079 Halamandaris, Val; National Association for Home Care
110 Angelo, Dolores; University of Colorado Health Sciences Center
142 Markstrom, Mae; Lake Superior State University, and Baker, Mary and Stanley Light, Dixie; Wellness C.A.R.E. Center (Sault Sainte Marie, Michigan)
145 Maynard, Olivia; Michigan Office of Services to the Aging
183 Richards, Rebecca; North Woods Health Careers Consortium (Wausau, Wisconsin)
259 Hunter, Katherine; Baptist Medical Center, Montclair (Alabama)

336 Norman, Ann Duecy; University of Washington
338 Heston, Thomas; University of Washington
339 Tsuji, Wayne; Washington State Arthritis Foundation
341 Patrick, Donald; University of Washington
370 Marine, Susan; Boulder, Colorado
378 Oliva, Michael; Aurora, Colorado
380 Mostow, Steven; Rose Medical Center (Denver)
384 Messenger, Tom; Association of Food and Drug Officials
396 Sparks, Shirley; Western Michigan University
403 Hwalek, Melanie; SPEC Associates (Detroit)
409 Lovell, James; National Hearing Aid Society
428 Somers, Anne; University of Medicine and Dentistry of New Jersey, and Weisfeld, Victoria; Robert Wood Johnson Foundation
451 Bennett, Ruth; Columbia University
459 Ostfeld, Adrian; Yale University
468 Miner, John; Massachusetts Mental Health Center
478 Young, Rosalie; Wayne State University
482 Newcomer, Robert and Pasick, Rena; University of California, San Francisco
508 Bortz, II, Walter; Palo Alto Medical Foundation
535 Lurie, David; Minneapolis Health Department
574 Smith, Marie; American Society of Hospital Pharmacists
575 Reveal, Marge; American Dental Hygienists' Association
612 Hunter, Paul; American Medical Student Association/Foundation
637 Adams, Gordon, Moses, Dennis and Baubman, James; Chapman College (San Diego)
670 Griffith, Patrick; Morehouse School of Medicine
686 Hollers, Kay; National Association for Home Care
714 Barkauskas, Violet; University of Michigan
738 Wagner, Edward; Group Health Cooperative of Puget Sound
766 Cornman, John; The Gerontological Society of America
767 Hurst, Victor; American Association of Retired Persons
768 Sykes, James; The National Council on the Aging
769 Sugarman, James; National Association of Retired Senior Volunteer Program Directors
770 Goldberg, Sheldon; American Association of Homes for the Aging
772 Ferguson, Wilda; Virginia Department for the Aging
776 Fainsinger, Ann; Alliance for Aging Research
777 Karlin, Steve; National Recreation and Park Association
793 Scitovsky, Anne; Palo Alto Medical Foundation
794 Katzman, Robert; University of California, San Diego
795 Haviland, James; Seattle, Washington
799 Surgeon General's Workshop on Health Promotion and Aging

6. Racial and Ethnic Minorities

An undue proportion of the disease and disability that the Year 2000 Health Objectives are intended to alleviate is concentrated in racial and ethnic minority populations, especially Blacks, Hispanics, and Native Americans. Although mortality rates for all these groups are falling, substantial differences in mortality and morbidity remain. In 1985, for instance, life expectancy was 75.3 years for Whites, but only 69.5 years for Blacks.[1] The gap between White and minority health status in the United States is so great that one testifier, Lester Breslow of the UCLA School of Public Health, labeled it "a national disgrace," and he and others called for special attention to reducing the gap in the year 2000 objectives-setting process. *(#026)*

In all, more than 125 testifiers stated the need to explicitly address minority populations in the Year 2000 Health Objectives. According to some witnesses, not only is the gap between White and minority health status so great that it must be addressed in such a forum, but targeted national objectives for such issues as infant mortality, teenage pregnancy, cancer mortality, violence and homicide reduction, and other problems will not be met unless minority rates are reduced. Furthermore, because both the conditions that lead to differentials in health status and the most effective interventions vary from group to group, the national objectives should contain specific objectives for racial and ethnic minorities, according to witnesses.

In his testimony, John Waller of Wayne State University proposes a specific way of setting minority objectives based on analyses of the differential health status of minorities documented in the Carter Center's report *Closing the Gap*[2] and the *Report of the Secretary's Task Force on Black and Minority Health*.[3] These differentials, he suggests, indicate where progress in mortality and morbidity reduction for minorities is possible, given the currently available knowledge and technology. Thus, Waller argues, these differentials should guide the selection of specific minority objectives. *(#314)*

Setting objectives that will reduce the disparity in health status between the White and non-White populations, and implementing the necessary programs and interventions to realize them, represent a formidable challenge. Providing universal access to health care is an important component of improving the health status of many ethnic groups, but it alone is not sufficient. Witnesses suggested that a broad spectrum of programs will be required to raise socioeconomic status, advance educational levels, provide social supports such as job protection and adequate housing, resolve language or cultural barriers, and clarify population-specific problems and issues.

Consistent statistics are difficult to find for minority groups. Obtaining more and better data on minority populations, especially non-Black groups, is seen as crucial. Without data, the need for health programs and health financing targeted at specific groups is neither apparent nor compelling, says Jane Delgado of the National Coalition of Hispanic Health and Human Services Organizations. *(#193)* Furthermore, as Sandral Hullet of West Alabama Health Services explains, health research and policies fail to differentiate among the sometimes very different special needs of subgroups within racial, ethnic, and social communities. She suggests that more information is necessary on the determinants of health and illness in each subgroup to account for the different susceptibilities and resistances of these groups to risk factors. Furthermore, with more specific information on the determinants, intervention strategies could be better tied to the needs of subgroups. Nutrition education, for example, would be different for a middle class home than for a home with chronic unemployment where nutritious food is not accessible. *(#671)* The need for more detailed data on minorities is discussed in Chapter 3.

Despite current limits to data on minority populations, testifiers were able to discuss specific health needs and disease patterns of Blacks, Hispanics, Native Americans, Asians, and Arab Americans in the United States. The emergent picture is that health promotion and disease prevention efforts have not yet closed the gap in health status between the majority population and racial or ethnic minorities. As in the White population, the incidence of, and mortality from, major killers such as cancer, heart disease, and diabetes, and the levels of infant mortality, teenage pregnancy, violence, and suicide in minority communities are largely associated with modifiable conditions and behaviors. Affecting behavioral changes in minority populations requires fundamental organizational changes, intensive effort, and cultural sensitivity. Though the task is difficult, witnesses say, the potential for health promotion and disease prevention activities in minority populations is great.

This chapter highlights the issues that hinder health promotion and disease prevention efforts in minority communities. These include many social, economic, and political forces, as well as communication and data gaps. It also discusses specific health problems affecting Blacks, Hispanics, and Native Americans that are amenable to prevention and the implications for establishing realistic and viable national health objectives for these disparate populations.

SOCIAL, BEHAVIORAL, AND CULTURAL FACTORS

To design better interventions to improve the health status of minorities, the social, economic, genetic, behavioral, and cultural factors that divide racial or ethnic minorities and the majority population must be understood. These groups have a disproportionate prevalence of factors known to be associated with poor health status, such as poverty, unemployment, low educational attainment, substance abuse, and poor diet. Some testifiers believe that these factors account for most, if not all, of the observed differences in health status. Others, however, believe that additional genetic and cultural components affect health status. These witnesses underline the importance of culturally appropriate interventions for minority populations.

Socioeconomic Factors

Poverty. Poverty is the single most important factor affecting the health of the non-White population, according to testimony. Harold Freeman, President of the American Cancer Society, defines poverty as "a lack of jobs, inadequate education, inadequate housing, poor nutrition, inadequate medical care, and concentration on day-to-day survival." (#443) In 1987, 31 percent of Blacks were living in poverty, whereas 28 percent of Hispanics, 39 percent of Puerto Ricans, and 28 percent of Native American families were below the poverty line. In comparison, the White poverty rate was 11 percent.[4] This calculation does not include many working poor or others who subsist just above the officially recognized standards of poverty.

Those in poverty often live in inadequate housing or have no regular housing at all. Blacks constitute more than 50 percent of the homeless, according to Ann Brunswick and David Rier of Columbia University.[5] (#031) For those who live in poor and overcrowded housing, there is greater risk of spreading and contracting communicable diseases. According to Stephen Joseph, New York City's Commissioner of Health, for example, tuberculosis is on the rise in New York City, especially in poverty-stricken communities. (#437)

Unemployment. Blacks and Hispanics, as well as other minority groups, are disproportionately unemployed. In 1987 the unemployment rates were 12 percent for Mexican-Americans, 11 percent for Puerto Ricans, 6 percent for Cubans, 13 percent for Blacks, and 5 percent for Whites, according to Brunswick and Delgado.[6,7] (#031; #193) The Black unemployment rate is 20 percent if underemployed and discouraged job seekers are included,[8] and more than 45 percent of Black youth are unemployed.[9] (#031)

Such high levels of unemployment and underemployment have devastating effects on communities and the health of their members. Unstable economic conditions are associated with high rates of crime, racism, and general despair, and these contribute to high levels of stress in many ethnic communities, according to witnesses. Reduced employment opportunity also contributes to increased levels of teenage pregnancy and to subsequent single-parent households, infant mortality, substance abuse, and violence. (#031)

Education. Educational attainment influences an individual's ability to survive and flourish in society. Many minority communities are currently affected by low levels of educational achievement. For example, high school dropout rates for Blacks in some major cities are as high as 40–50 percent.[10] Dropouts have greater rates of teenage childbearing and substance abuse, and minorities without education often get trapped in low-paying service industry jobs, many of which do not provide health insurance. (#031)

Lack of education often means limited knowledge of health matters and poor understanding of the causes and prevention of disease, according to testifiers. For example, in a study of beliefs about cardiovascular disease among Blacks and Whites, researchers found that educational level was the most important variable in being able to state the risk factors for cardiovascular disease. The impact of this conclusion on minority populations is significant.

With lower levels of educational attainment, Hispanics and Blacks are less likely to know the risk factors for cardiovascular disease. Efforts to reduce cardiovascular disease morbidity and mortality among these groups may be hampered, and interventions will have to include an attempt to improve general educational attainment in these communities.

Furthermore, medical communication or health promotion outreach frequently "requires one to have or share traditional middle class values and income in order to effect positive behavioral change," according to Waller. This tends to exclude impoverished, uneducated minority groups. *(#314)*

Behavioral Factors

As discussed in other chapters of this report, smoking, drinking heavily, using illegal drugs, or eating an improper diet can harm one's health. In many minority communities, especially where poverty and low educational achievement are found, these destructive behaviors are especially prevalent. Abuse of chemical substances is more widespread in minority populations. This abuse is harmful not only because of its immediate effect on the individual's well-being but also, as Joseph says, because substance abuse is a dynamic that is integral to all major health problems. *(#437)*

Although there has been much concern recently over the spread of AIDS through intravenous drug abuse and the onslaught of crack cocaine, the effects of tobacco and alcohol abuse cause substantially more mortality and morbidity among minority groups such as Hispanics, Blacks, and Native Americans. Smoking, for instance, leads to a variety of illnesses, among the most important of which are cancer, heart disease, stroke, and lung disease. Alcohol contributes directly to cirrhosis and cancer. Acute and chronic alcohol intoxication is also a major factor in violence, homicide, and unintentional injuries. Smoking, alcohol, and other drugs likewise lead to low birth weight, infant mortality, and other poor pregnancy outcomes.

Jose Lopez of the San Antonio Tumor and Blood Clinic and others report that Blacks and Mexican-Americans are known to have high-fat diets, which are a risk factor for cancer and cardiovascular disease. *(#488)* Dietary factors may contribute to more than one-third of all cancer deaths, says Margaret Hargreaves and the staff of the Cancer Control Research Unit of Meharry Medical College.[11] *(#615)* Obesity, a risk factor for heart disease and diabetes, is especially prevalent among Native Americans,

Mexican-Americans, and Black women. *(#255; #567)*

The Role of Culture

Testifiers generally agreed that poverty and related socioeconomic factors are the greatest source of disparity in health status between Whites and minorities. This led some witnesses to question whether poverty and other socioeconomic differences should be targeted in intervention plans, or whether race or ethnicity should underlie prevention designs.

The American Cancer Society recently studied cancer survival in the economically disadvantaged and found that ethnic differences in cancer survival are related primarily to economic status. However, according to Freeman, the study found that

> race also exerted a significant effect independently of income, but only among the low-income population. That is, at identical low-income levels for both racial groups (the same dollar amounts), non-White mortality rates were significantly higher than White, while at identical middle- and upper-income levels for both racial groups, the mortality rates for the two groups converged.[12] *(#443)*

Freeman cautions that race itself should not be construed as a health determinant. Rather, he says, race "is to be understood here as a proxy for adverse environmental and social conditions perhaps affecting non-Whites at low-income levels more strongly than they do Whites at identical income levels." *(#443)*

Others, however, say that race and ethnicity should be given greater weight in planning interventions. For instance, Michael Greenberg of Rutgers University cites studies showing that socioeconomic variables cannot explain all the differences between Blacks and Whites.[13,14,15] Because of this, interventions must contain an ethnic component and not solely a poverty component, or else the interventions will not be culturally sensitive. Furthermore, Greenberg says, programs must attack the underlying problem, which may be different for minority groups. For example, tobacco companies have been targeting Blacks in their advertising, and antismoking programs have to respond. *(#537)*

In light of these ideas, many of those who testified called for culturally appropriate interventions for minority groups. Such interventions could be as conceptually simple as providing health information in the language that the group speaks, or recruiting and training health professionals from the populations they are to serve. Mario Orlandi of the American Health Foundation in New York, for instance, lists 10 barriers that must be overcome in designing health promotion programs for racial and ethnic minorities:

- **Language:** Failure to appreciate health promotion messages when language or symbols are used that are not understandable or are misunderstood by the subgroup
- **Reading level:** Using printed materials that are too sophisticated or beyond the reading level of subgroup members
- **Models:** Using endorsements for the health promotion campaign from prominent individuals or organizations that are not well known to subgroup members
- **Inappropriate messages:** Using motivational messages that are not salient to subgroup members
- **Inappropriate target:** The belief that the health promotion campaign is worthwhile, but that program designers never really intended the subculture to participate or benefit
- **Motivational issues:** Fear that the primary motivation for the health promotion campaign is the desire to control the subculture, robbing from it the specific practices that have defined it historically
- **Welfare stigma:** A tendency to view the health promotion campaign as a "handout" and to avoid it as a matter of pride
- **Perceived responsibility:** The attitude that the campaign deals with subject areas and life choices that concern the family and the individual, not the public health establishment
- **Relevance of health promotion:** A belief that more pressing concerns such as poverty, crime, unemployment, and hunger should be addressed prior to health promotion
- **Entropy:** The tendency for subgroup members to perceive themselves as powerless or helpless when confronted with enormous economic and sociocultural barriers and to express a lack of motivation to engage in self-improvement activities *(#167)*

ACCESS TO HEALTH CARE

Another consequential element in the equation of good health is access to health care services. In general, poor and minority populations use health care services differently than the majority population. In large part, witnesses agreed, this is due to economic constraints. The problem of access is complicated, however.

Differentials between Black and White utilization of medical services have declined since the 1960s, in large part because of Medicaid and Medicare; in some cases, Blacks have higher utilization rates than Whites.[16,17] When Blacks do seek care, however, they are more likely than Whites to receive it in emergency rooms. This arrangement is obviously not conducive to preventive care, screening services, or the continuity of care needed for health promotion efforts, says Freeman. *(#443)* In general, Blacks are less likely to have a regular primary care physician.[18]

Minorities also receive fewer preventive services. Their childhood vaccination rates lag considerably behind those of Whites, as do their rates of screening for chronic diseases such as cancer, hypertension, and diabetes. In 1980, 12 percent of Hispanics, 8.8 percent of Blacks, and 4.3 percent of Whites did not receive prenatal care until the third trimester of pregnancy, or not at all, according to Peggy Smith of Baylor College of Medicine.[19,20] *(#308)* Such lack of preventive and screening services is, in large measure, the reason for the higher mortality rates. For example, 50 percent of the differences in five-year survival rates for cancer between Blacks and Whites are due to late diagnosis, according to Alvin Mauer and Mona Arreola of the University of Tennessee Memphis Cancer Center. *(#256)*

Some of the difference in access to preventive services is due to discrepancies in insurance coverage. Because minorities are more likely to be impoverished, unemployed, or employed without health benefits, they are more likely to be uninsured and unable to afford either preventive or necessary health services. *(#193)* In particular, 26 percent of Hispanics and 18 percent of Blacks have no insurance, compared to 9 percent of Whites.

Evidence suggests that Medicaid and uninsured patients receive care of inferior quality.[21] A representative from the American College of Obstetricians and Gynecologists cites a 1987 General Accounting Office report on the prenatal care of women who are on Medicaid or are uninsured, which indicates that these women are more likely to receive insufficient care.[22] *(#279)* High rates of infant mortality, heart disease, diabetes, etc., suggest a need for services from obstetricians/gynecologists, cardiologists, and other specialists. However, many physicians, particularly specialists, will not accept Medicaid, let alone treat an indigent patient, says Katherine Carr of the American College of Nurse-Midwives. *(#690)* Also, because of their lack of insurance and Medicaid status, many poor and indigent patients are often transferred from private hospitals to public facilities, according to Clyde Kay of the Louisiana Primary Care Association. (#688)

Some of the racial and ethnic differences in utilization of health services are due to cultural and geographic factors. Many ethnic groups live in areas with shortages of health providers. Inner cities and rural areas, particularly in the South, are medically underserved and have high concentrations of Blacks or Hispanics. One solution, proposed by many, is to increase the availability of minority health care providers. Studies have shown that increases in the number of physicians of a particular minority group in underserved communities of that population have raised the level of service utilization and provision within these communities.[23]

Programs to train and provide health care professionals for these communities, such as the National Health Service Corps Scholarship program and other favorable university admissions and financial aid policies, were established more than a decade ago. However, Rebecca Work of the American College of Nurse-Midwives says that in recent years, many programs have been terminated and policies reversed.[24] (#268) Thus, the increase in numbers of Black, Hispanic, and Native American physicians and the concomitant strides in cultural sensitivity and commitment to minority communities have been halted.

SPECIFIC HEALTH PROBLEMS OF MINORITY GROUPS

There are nearly 60,000 excess Black deaths yearly, according to the *Report of the Secretary's Task Force on Black and Minority Health*; that is, if Blacks had the same age- and sex-specific death rates as Whites, 60,000 fewer Blacks would die each year. These excess deaths have six principal causes: heart disease and stroke, homicide and accidents, cancer, infant mortality, cirrhosis, and diabetes. Together, these six causes represent 80 percent of the total excess deaths of Blacks. The ranking is not the same for other minority groups, but these six causes remain critical target priorities for reducing excess mortality in all minority populations.

The following section highlights health problems that are especially salient for minority groups. Witnesses frequently remarked that discussion of disease and incidence rates in these populations is limited by data gaps. In some instances, others said that the preliminary level of discussion helps shed light on how much is not yet known. (#495; #683) Although testifiers were optimistic that prevention programs could be undertaken now in all of these areas, they encouraged more research efforts.

Infant Mortality

The mortality rate during the first year of life for Blacks in 1985 was twice that of Whites (18.2 per 1,000 and 9.3 per 1,000, respectively).[25] National infant mortality rates for Hispanics are not available. George Flores of the San Antonio Metropolitan Health District says a step in the direction of reducing unacceptable rates is to set two priorities: (1) to provide prenatal care for indigent women where none exists and (2) to provide appropriate interventions to high-risk pregnant women and their infants. (#745) The first priority, if met, could likely improve the national infant mortality rate. According to Ezra Davidson of the American College of Obstetricians and Gynecologists, 76 percent of mothers across all groups began care in the first trimester of pregnancy in 1987, but only 61 percent of Hispanic women and 61 percent of Black women began care in the first trimester.[26] (#279) Those who do not receive adequate prenatal care are largely the poor and indigent. The age of the mother also plays a role in determining whether or not prenatal care is obtained. Adolescents in all populations are less likely to receive prenatal care than older women. (#279) Blacks and Hispanics both have a higher rate of adolescent pregnancy and, therefore, are at greater risk of having a low-birth-weight baby or of losing their baby.

Donald Schiff of the American Academy of Pediatrics writes that the poorly educated segments of society have the "greatest risks to the fetus and newborn infant," that a mother's self-worth "increases as dependency on welfare decreases and this is related to the availability of employment," and that "a high divorce rate, single-parent families, and early sexual activity is the milieu in which there is high infant mortality." No single professional group can resolve these social problems. Rather, they require the combined efforts and resources of different segments of society. Schiff recommends more research into the causes of low birth weight among Blacks; increased funding for outreach, prevention, and support services; greater private and public financing for insurance programs to provide coverage to all adolescents, women, and children; and increased Medicaid eligibility. (#371)

Chronic Diseases

Heart Disease and Stroke. Public education and awareness efforts to reduce heart disease and stroke in the U.S. population over the past two decades appear to have had at least some effect in reducing the mortality rates from these diseases in all population groups. However, Black mortality rates remain higher than White rates, according to testifiers. In 1987 the mortality rate for heart disease was 287 per 100,000 for Black males, compared to 226 per 100,000 for White males, and 181 per 100,000 for Black females, compared to 116 per 100,000 for White females. For Black and White males, stroke rates were 57 versus 30 per 100,000, respectively; for Black and White women, they were 46 versus 26 per 100,000, respectively.[27] Both the Hispanic and Black populations also have significant problems with obesity, high serum cholesterol levels, and high blood pressure, all of which are risk factors for cardiovascular disease. (#269; #743) To reduce obesity, high cholesterol, and hypertension in these populations, risk factors such as cigarette smoking, and compliance with treatment and diet, must be addressed, say witnesses including Eleanor Young of the University of Texas Health Science Center at San Antonio. (#261; #496)

According to Osman Ahmed of Meharry Medical College, Blacks are generally less compliant with treatment for hypertension than Whites. (#269) Michael Crawford of the University of Texas Health Science Center at San Antonio says that only 7 percent of Hispanic males in Texas with moderate to high levels of cholesterol are aware of this fact, compared to 17 percent of White males with similar cholesterol levels. Furthermore, of those Hispanic men under treatment for high cholesterol, only 40 percent are adequately controlled. (#743)

To design effective interventions for cardiovascular disease, say William Neser and John Thomas of Meharry Medical College, cultural sensitivity is necessary. In the Black community, stress, smoking, diet, and obesity, as well as compliance with treatment, should be dealt with through community interventions that include the church and schools. (#261) Similarly, Crawford encourages interventions that focus on Hispanic men and their behavior related to diet, exercise, and weight control. (#743)

Cancer. Cancer currently takes a greater share of Black life than is necessary, according to witnesses. "Scientific evidence indicates that social and environmental factors either cause the majority of cancers or promote their development," say Hargreaves and her colleagues. Bringing Blacks into treatment at earlier stages and educating them about the connection between certain cancers and behavioral risk factors, such as smoking, alcohol consumption, or dietary habits, would be effective measures. (#615)

Since 1950, Blacks have witnessed an increase in age-adjusted mortality from lung cancer, due primarily to increases in smoking two decades earlier. (#443) Blacks also suffer from the highest rate of prostate cancer in the world[28] and have among the highest rate of esophageal cancer. (#537)

"Why is there such a serious Black male cancer problem?" asks Michael Greenberg of Rutgers University. "A combination of poverty, culture, and racism has led to a greater likelihood of smoking, poor nutrition, weakened immunity, occupational exposure, and lesser chance of rapid and successful diagnosis and treatment of tumors. Heredity cannot explain the rapid increase of Black cancers, but should not be overlooked." (#537)

Blacks and Mexican-Americans show only moderate awareness of the major risk factors for cancer and are also unaware of most of the warning signs of cancer. (#488; #615) Blacks and Hispanics routinely underestimate the prevalence of cancer and overestimate its deadliness. Thus, delay in treatment and resignation to a fatal conclusion of the disease are common. (#488; #615)

Although overall cancer rates are lower for Hispanics, cultural norms can affect health outcomes for cancer in the Hispanic population, according to Lopez.

There is an evident paradox then; whereas cancer may be less frequent a problem among Hispanics, particularly for some of the most common malignancies (colon and breast cancer), Hispanics are at greater risk if one considers factors such as stage of cancer at diagnosis, nutritional habits including use of high fat products in the preparation of foods, lack of access to the health care delivery system, and certain knowledge, attitudes, and practices regarding cancer that are very peculiar to the Hispanic population. (#488)

Lopez cites a study of 800 New York Hispanics and their attitudes and knowledge about cancer. "Fifty-seven percent of Hispanic women did breast self-examination within the last year. This percentage lags behind women in general. Only 29 percent of

Hispanic women indicated that a doctor had shown them how to do breast self-examination." This study revealed some important information regarding service utilization preferences. Lopez writes, "Spanish was the language spoken at home by 63 percent of the study population. Two out of three preferred to use a doctor who was fluent in Spanish. There was clearly a strong preference that information programs be given in Spanish. Half of the study population had either been born in the United States or had lived here for more than 30 years." (#488)

Freeman suggests improving the cost-effectiveness of screening techniques and providing cancer screening to all Americans. (#443) Greenberg suggests concentrating resources on screening for prostatic carcinoma and smoking cessation programs among Black males. Cancer of the prostate and respiratory cancer cause almost 50 percent of Black male cancer deaths.[29] (#537)

Diabetes. According to testimony, one of the great differences in disease status between Hispanics and Whites is the rate of diabetes. Native Americans also have especially high rates of diabetes, according to Spero Manson of the University of Colorado Health Sciences Center. (#706) Mexican-Americans also appear to develop diabetes at an earlier age, suggesting the possibility of more complications of the disease. In fact, says Steven Haffner of the University of Texas Health Science Center at San Antonio, Mexican-Americans have a much higher rate of severe retinopathy and of end-stage renal disease. (#491) The prevalence of diabetes is 33 percent higher in the Black population than in the White population (#457), and Blacks have twice the rate of blindness secondary to diabetic retinopathy as Whites.[30]

Interventions to reduce diabetes involve improving nutrition, reducing obesity, and retraining primary physicians who treat these underserved populations in how to use the most modern techniques of diabetes detection and treatment. (#457) Young reports that "diabetes is perhaps the most significant nutrition-related health problem faced by adults in Texas, especially by Mexican-American adults," and still there is little prevention activity or funding in this area. She outlines specific nutrition objectives, which include reducing the incidence of obesity, encouraging more professional education on the fundamentals of nutrition, and establishing baseline data for all nutrition goals. (#496) However, according to Hullet, nutrition is an especially difficult area to work with in the Black population. Her recommendations that "we

involve more minorities in research in their own community" and that "we encourage more minorities to go into research" are pertinent to developing effective nutrition intervention programs for Black communities. (#671)

Common Risk Factors and Interventions

Despite the differences in these three diseases (heart disease and stroke, cancer, and diabetes), they share common behavioral risk factors. Furthermore, all three benefit from early detection and treatment. Because of these commonalities, general programs aimed at risk factor intervention and screening for chronic diseases offer some promise.

In terms of implementing prevention programs, Ahmed and Hargreaves suggest that special emphasis should be placed on diversified interventions, including (1) education and awareness programs focusing on the lay person as well as on professionals, to encourage changes in knowledge, attitudes, and practices; (2) primary prevention programs with special emphasis on smoking cessation and dietary changes; and (3) secondary prevention programs emphasizing screening practices. (#269; #615)

In a description of several community intervention programs being sponsored by a Cancer Control Consortium group made up of Meharry, Morehouse, and Drew Universities, Ahmed discusses reducing smoking among Blacks.

> Our experience suggests that to achieve a reduction in smoking rates in Blacks to about 30 percent or less by 1990 and to modify other health behaviors related to diet and nutrition, national outreach programs should be designed to reach Blacks. These programs should address Black needs and contain culturally-sensitive curricula. In this respect, the expertise and resources of a coalition of interested community organizations should be fully explored and properly utilized. (#269)

HIV Infection and AIDS

According to witnesses, AIDS has levied a disproportionate toll on both Blacks and Hispanics in this country. Although considered by many to be a gay White male's disease, increasing numbers of minority heterosexuals have been infected. Alvin Thompson of the Washington State Association of Black Professionals in Health Care writes, "We recommend urgent implementation of improved outreach campaigns of public education and particularly of health education, devising effective techniques for changing the behavior of the noncompliant IV [intravenous] drug-using population." (#358)

Of all the 1989 AIDS cases reported to the Centers for Disease Control (CDC), Blacks made up 29 percent and Hispanics 16 percent, compared to their proportions of 12 percent and 6 percent, respectively, in the overall population.[31] The cumulative risk of AIDS then was almost three times higher in Blacks and Hispanics than in Whites. For men, the relative risks of AIDS were 2.8 and 2.7 for Blacks and Hispanics, respectively; for women, the relative risks were 13.2 for Blacks and 8.1 for Hispanics. For children, the relative risks were 11.6 for Blacks and 6.6 for Hispanics. Much of the difference between the minority and White populations is due to a higher prevalence of intravenous drug use among Blacks and Hispanics. According to CDC researchers, however, Blacks and Hispanics also have been more likely than Whites to contract AIDS through most of the important routes, especially bisexuality in men, suggesting that other AIDS risk factors also may be more prevalent in Blacks and Hispanics.[32]

Ignorance of AIDS and its risk factors is a special area of concern for minority youth. Ralph DiClemente of the University of California, San Francisco says that Black, Asian, and Hispanic adolescents are less knowledgeable than Whites about AIDS, its risk behaviors, and preventive measures.[33] (#273)

Homicide, Suicide, and Violence

Homicide and interpersonal violence are significant problems in the Black community. Indeed, homicide is the leading cause of death for Black men between the ages of 15 and 44 and for Black women age 15 to 24. The lifetime risk for homicide is 1 in 21 for Black men and 1 in 104 for Black women. In comparison, the risk for White men is 1 in 131 and for White women, 1 in 369.[34]

"As a Black psychiatrist practicing community psychiatry in a predominantly Black community on the south side of Chicago," says Carl Bell, Executive Director of the Community Mental Health Council, "I have seen the lethal and nonlethal effects of interpersonal violence firsthand." For example, based on a survey of his clinic population, Bell says that one out of three women has been raped, 40 percent of the male and female patients have been physically assaulted, and one in four people reports personally

knowing someone who has been murdered. Other studies that he and others have conducted indicate that most violence in Black communities stems from conflict in interpersonal relations, and not from a desire to acquire resources from another person. (#018)

Bell also argues that homicide prevention strategies are hampered by myths, ethnic tensions, and ignorance of homicide dynamics, which vary according to local culture and circumstance. He points out that the lack of clarity on homicide dynamics prevents suitable solutions from being adopted. For example, reducing drug-related homicides would require different strategies than reducing domestic violence. Similarly, designing a prevention program for reducing Hispanic violence does not mean copying an existing intervention targeted at a different population, according to Bell. (#018)

Still, Bell says that many interventions can be undertaken immediately, within the existing social structures. First, a major media effort can be made to encourage handgun owners to keep their guns unloaded. This reduces the immediate availability of a deadly weapon. Second, primary physicians, especially in high-risk communities, can screen patients for victimization and perpetration of violence and at least provide them with a list of follow-up services. Third, antiviolence curricula should be introduced in the schools. Fourth, the community can provide emotional and medical services to the victims of violence and their families. (#018)

Hispanics also have homicide rates that exceed those of White Americans. Age-adjusted homicide rates for Hispanic men in five southwestern states from 1976 to 1980 were 2.5 times those of Whites, whereas those of Hispanic women were approximately the same as those of White women, according to Delgado.[35] (#193) John Bruhn, representing the American Society of Allied Health Professions, writes that mortality due to violent deaths is fairly high among Cuban-, Mexican-, and Puerto Rican-born adolescents and young adults, particularly males. He states that a specific objective "to reduce these deaths by one-half of their current prevalence, through education and prevention programs, should be of high priority." (#235)

According to David Besaw of the Wisconsin Tribal Health Directors, the higher incidence of alcohol and drug abuse problems, coupled with a younger, more impoverished population, puts Native Americans at greater risk for both intentional and unintentional injuries. Alcohol is involved in many Native

American suicides and is related to the high number of unintentional injuries among Native Americans. (#514)

Native Americans also have suicide rates that are much higher than those of the general population. Although rates vary among tribes, most suicides are in the 15–39 age group and peak rates are reached in the 20–24 age range. "Unlike in the general population, it's basically a youth and young adult problem as opposed to an older adult problem, which is more common in the mainstream population," according to Manson. A recent series of suicide epidemics has prompted tribal leaders and other community members to research the causes of such despair and to devise interventions for the young population. In one study of over 300 Native Americans in the Pacific Northwest, "only 16 percent knew of agencies or other types of resources for coping with stressful life experiences." (#706)

To combat suicide among Native Americans, testifiers suggested several intervention strategies. Among them, for example, are programs to develop stress-coping skills among young people, drug education and peer counseling programs, and crisis hotlines to provide immediate access to counseling.

Tobacco, Alcohol, and Substance Abuse

The prevalence of cigarette smoking in the Black community is a distressing sign of the gap between White and Black health behaviors. Smoking rates are 39 percent for Black men age 18 or older and 27 percent for Black women, whereas the rates are 30 percent for White males and 27 percent for White females.[36] Although Black men tend to be lighter smokers than White men, successful interventions to reduce the smoking rate in this population are not widespread, according to Hargreaves. (#615) Thompson says that as the White community decreases its consumption of tobacco, the tobacco industry has begun to direct its advertising and promotional efforts increasingly toward the Black community. (#358) He calls the Black community to action: "In addition to the present admirable activities of the Public Health Service, the Black community and the Black media must resolve this competition of vital communication to the Black community and the health of Black people by discouraging tobacco advertising and smoking among

Blacks." (#358)

Jacqueline Morrison, representing the National Black Alcoholism Council, considers alcoholism the number one public health problem in the Black community. In addition to high rates of liver cirrhosis and esophageal cancer, alcohol consumption is linked to auto accidents, domestic violence, and homicide. Morrison calls for government and private agencies to coordinate their efforts to develop alcohol prevention and treatment services that are sensitive to Black culture. She also argues that the Year 2000 Health Objectives should address the problems of children of alcoholics. One such program, called "B Co-Adapt," developed by the council, includes establishing groups to repair children's self-esteem, training qualified professionals, and improving public and professional awareness. (#723)

James Sall of the Detroit Department of Health also focuses on community interventions for substance abuse prevention. He offers three strategies: (1) vigorous enforcement of drug laws; (2) strengthening the value systems in public schools; and (3) supporting a community movement toward parenting education by developing a culturally specific curriculum without literacy barriers that addresses issues of achievement, as well as the prevention of violence, teenage pregnancy, and drug use. (#389)

Although alcohol abuse varies tremendously among Native American tribes, it remains the major health problem of that population. Manson notes that Native American youth "use alcohol and marijuana, earlier, more frequently, and with significantly greater consequences than any other minority youth." According to Jerome West of the Five Sandoval Pueblo Villages, the Albuquerque Area Tribal Coordinating Committee in conjunction with the Bureau of Indian Affairs and the Indian Health Service has established a regional alcohol treatment center and is training 175 alcohol and drug counselors to provide counseling in New Mexico. (#565)

High rates of inhalant abuse are reported among Mexican-American and Native American youth. Studies performed in San Antonio suggest that "barrio" children and adolescents are 14 times more likely than a national sample to abuse inhalants and also more likely to use other substances.[37] (#494) To reduce inhalant abuse, Ricardo Jasso of Nosotros Human Services Development urges a comprehensive continuum of interventions at the individual, community, and national levels. (#494)

Teenage Pregnancy

Edna Batiste of the Detroit Department of Health feels that adolescent childbearing in an impoverished Black community is only one part of a syndrome that makes the Black teenager an "endangered species." The cycle, as she sees it, is as follows: have a baby; drop out of school; get a low-paying job (if she can get one at all); not marry the child's father because he does not have a job, is on drugs, doesn't care, or disappears; go on welfare; develop low self-esteem; and so on. Batiste concludes that "no community, especially the Black community, can afford to keep losing one-fifth of each generation because of failure to complete their high school education, because of an unplanned pregnancy or for any of the reasons of the syndrome." Batiste's solution to adolescent pregnancy, as well as many other health problems of poor communities, is a "resurgence of the public health model" where teams of professional community workers would provide care in primary care health centers. (#016)

Louis Bernard, Dean of Meharry Medical College, supports Batiste's view and reports that unwanted childbearing in the Black community is especially high among teenagers and is exacerbated by "lack of income and job protection, limited access to essential services, and the indifference of society to their aspirations." (#253)

Smith discusses the problems of adolescent pregnancy in the Hispanic population in Texas. Like others, she mentions social factors that help determine fertility rates, age of pregnancy, attitudes toward seeking family planning services, marital status, and attitudes toward childbearing among Hispanics. She also outlines some childbearing patterns that are unique. One-half of all Hispanic women migrating to Texas are 18 years of age or younger, and in 1980, the fertility rate for Hispanic women age 15 to 44 was 95 births per 1,000 women. This rate is 33 percent higher than the rate for White women (62 per 1,000).[38] (#308) Finally, Smith says, "estimates suggest that from 22 to 63 percent of Hispanic adolescents stated their pregnancies were planned and that for them the negative consequences associated with the out-of-wedlock conception status of the infant were negligible."[39] (#308)

Smith emphasizes the need to develop intervention models appropriate to the community and to improve data collection for this population. Reluctance to use services because of the citizenship, employment, or residency status of family members affects the utilization of services by Hispanic immigrants.

The effect of acculturation and its impact on health care practices should be determined. If the degree of acculturation turns out to be one of the independent variables in effective contraceptive utilization and health care, providers must be prepared to assess the patient's sociocultural status as well as her contraceptive and maternity needs. (#308)

REFERENCES

1. National Center for Health Statistics: Health United States, 1987 (DHHS Publication No. [PHS] 88-1232), 1988

2. Amler RW, Dull HB (Eds.): Closing the Gap: The Burden of Unnecessary Illness. New York: Oxford University Press, 1987

3. U.S. Department of Health and Human Services: Report of the Secretary's Task Force on Black and Minority Health. Washington, D.C.: U.S. Government Printing Office, 1987

4. U.S. Bureau of the Census: Statistical Abstract of the United States, 1989 (109th Edition). Washington, D.C.: U.S. Government Printing Office, 1989

5. Brown LP: Crime in the black community. The State of Black America, 1988. Edited by J Dewart. New York: National Urban League, Inc., 1988

6. U.S. Bureau of the Census: Current Population Reports. The Hispanic Population in the United States, 1986 and 1987. March (Advance Report). Series P-20, No. 416, August 1987

7. U.S. Bureau of the Census: op. cit., reference 4

8. Jacob JE: Black America, 1987: An overview. The State of Black America, 1988. Edited by J Dewart. New York: National Urban League, Inc., 1988

9. Hare BR: Black youth at risk. The State of Black America, 1988. Edited by J Dewart. New York: National Urban League, Inc., 1988

10. Chavez L: "Crisis over dropouts: A look at two youths," New York Times, 2/16/88, p.B1.

11. Doll R, Peto R: The causes of cancer: Qualitative estimates of avoidable risks of cancer in the United States today. J Natl Cancer Inst 66(6):1191–1308, 1981

12. American Cancer Society: Cancer in the Economically Disadvantaged: A Special Report. The Subcommittee on Cancer in the Economically Disadvantaged. American Cancer Society, June 1986

13. U.S. Department of Health and Human Services: op. cit., reference 3

14. Levin D: Cancer Rates and Risks (NIH Publication No. 75-691), 1975

15. Haan M, Kaplan G, Camacho T: Poverty and health: Prospective evidence from the Alameda County study. Amer J Epid 125:989–998, 1987

16. Davis K, Lillie-Blanton M, Lyons B, et al.: Health care for Black Americans: The public sector role. Milbank Q 65(Suppl. 1):213–47, 1987

17. Manton KG, Patrick CH, Johnson KW: Health differentials between Blacks and Whites: Recent trends in mortality and morbidity. Milbank Q 65(Suppl. 1):129–99, 1987

18. Davis, et al.: op. cit., reference 16

19. National Center for Health Statistics: Health United States, 1989 (DHHS Publication No. [PHS] 90-1232), 1990

20. Ventura SJ: Births of Hispanic parentage, 1980. Hyattsville, Md.: U.S. National Center for Health Statistics 32:6, 1983

21. Manton, et al.: op. cit., reference 17

22. U.S. General Accounting Office: Prenatal care: Medicaid recipients and uninsured women obtain insufficient care. Report to the Chairman, Subcommittee on Human Resources and Intergovernmental Relations, Committee on Government Operations, House of Representatives. GAO/HRD 87-137, September 1987

23. Davis, et al.: op. cit., reference 16

24. Ibid.

25. National Center for Health Statistics: op. cit., reference 1

26. National Center for Health Statistics: op. cit., reference 19

27. Ibid.

28. U.S. Department of Health and Human Services: op. cit., reference 3

29. National Center for Health Statistics: op. cit., reference 19

30. U.S. Department of Health and Human Services: op. cit., reference 3

31. Centers for Disease Control: HIV/AIDS Surveillance. Atlanta, Ga., January 1990

32. Selik RM, Castro KG, Pappaioanou M: Racial/ethnic differences in the risk of AIDS in the United States. Am J Pub Health 78:1539−1545, 1988

33. Diclemente RJ, Zorn J, Temoshok L: Adolescents's knowledge of AIDS near an AIDS epicenter. Am J Pub Health 77:876-877, 1987

34. U.S. Department of Health and Human Services: op. cit., reference 3

35. Ibid.

36. National Center for Health Statistics: op. cit., reference 19

37. Padilla AM, Trimble JE, Bell CS: Drug Abuse Among Ethnic Minorities. National Institute on Drug Abuse (DHHS Publication No. [ADM] 87-1474), 1987

38. Smith, PB, Wait RB: Adolescent fertility and childbearing trends among Hispanics in Texas. Texas Medicine 82:29−32, 1986

39. Smith PB: Sociologic aspects of adolescent fertility and childbearing among Hispanics. J Dev Behav Ped 7(6):346−349, 1986

TESTIFIERS CITED IN CHAPTER 6

016 Batiste, Edna; Detroit Department of Health
018 Bell, Carl; Community Mental Health Council (Chicago)
026 Breslow, Lester; University of California, Los Angeles
031 Brunswick, Ann and Rier, David; Columbia University
167 Orlandi, Mario; American Health Foundation
193 Delgado, Jane; The National Coalition of Hispanic Health and Human Services Organizations (COSSMHO)
235 Bruhn, John; University of Texas Medical Branch at Galveston
253 Bernard, Louis; Meharry Medical College
255 Blumenthal, Daniel; Morehouse School of Medicine
256 Mauer, Alvin and Arreola, Mona; University of Tennessee, Memphis
261 Thomas, John and Neser, William; Meharry Medical College
268 Work, Rebecca; University of Alabama at Birmingham
269 Ahmed, Osman; Meharry Medical College
273 DiClemente, Ralph; University of California, San Francisco
279 Davidson, Ezra; King-Drew Medical Center (Los Angeles)
308 Smith, Peggy B.; Baylor College of Medicine
314 Waller, John; Wayne State University
358 Thompson, Alvin; University of Washington
371 Schiff, Donald; American Academy of Pediatrics
389 Sall, James; Detroit Department of Health
437 Joseph, Stephen; New York City Department of Health

443 Freeman, Harold; State University of New York at Buffalo
457 Altschuler, Alan; Prudential-Bache Securities, Inc.
488 Lopez, Jose; San Antonio Tumor and Blood Clinic
491 Haffner, Steven; University of Texas Health Science Center at San Antonio
494 Jasso, Ricardo; Nosotros Human Services Development (San Antonio)
495 Andrew, Sylvia; Our Lady of the Lake University (San Antonio)
496 Young, Eleanor; University of Texas Health Science Center at San Antonio
514 Besaw, David; Wisconsin Tribal Health Directors
537 Greenberg, Michael; Rutgers University
565 West, Jerome; Five Sandoval Indian Pueblos, Inc. (Bernalillo, New Mexico)
567 Diehl, Andrew and Stern, Michael; University of Texas Health Science Center at San Antonio
615 Hargreaves, Margaret et al.; Meharry Medical College
671 Hullet, Sandral; West Alabama Health Services
683 Watanabe, Michael; Asian Pacific Planning Council (Los Angeles)
688 Kay, Clyde; Louisiana Primary Care Association
690 Carr, Katherine; American College of Nurse-Midwives
706 Manson, Spero; University of Colorado Health Sciences Center
723 Morrison, Jacqueline; Wayne State University
743 Crawford, Michael; University of Texas Health Science Center at San Antonio
745 Flores, George; Metropolitan Health District, San Antonio

7. People with Disabilities

Between 20 and 40 million Americans live with physical disabilities. Figures vary depending on whether disabilities are classified by health condition, which means any condition or limitation impairing the normal functioning of an individual, or by work disability, which looks at conditions preventing an individual from taking, finding, or maintaining employment.[1] *(#223)* In either case, the number of individuals directly affected by disabilities and those indirectly affected, such as family members, is significant enough that many testifiers find it meaningful to discuss a manifold of conditions and issues in terms of a single, aggregate population.

For people concerned about disabilities, the year 2000 objectives-setting process offers two opportunities. First, it provides a forum for those most directly concerned to discuss the implementation of goals to prevent disabilities in the first place. Michael Marge of Syracuse University says that "the 1990 Health Objectives for the Nation provided a blueprint for prevention that focused primarily on premature death with little attention to premature disability." *(#433)* In the Year 2000 Health Objectives, Marge and others hope to see an expanded focus on the prevention of disabilities.

In total, 50 testifiers commented on prevention of disabilities, and their specific suggestions covered many of the priority objective areas, including maternal and infant health, alcohol and drug abuse, infectious diseases, unintentional injuries, violent and abusive behavior, nutrition, sexually transmitted diseases and AIDS, environmental health, occupational health, mental health, and chronic diseases. The prevention of disabilities is addressed in this report primarily in the context of specific objective areas.

Second, the Year 2000 Health Objectives process provides an opportunity to discuss health promotion and disease prevention activities, and barriers to the same, for those currently disabled. Health promotion and disease prevention mean something different to a population already affected by an "unhealthy" condition. As a result, several testifiers, including Jeffrey Brandon of the University of New Orleans, feel it is necessary to redefine health promotion to include activities and attitudes that aid an individual and family in achieving or maintaining optimal functional capability and self-dependence, regardless of whether or not they are "healthy." *(#568)* Defined this way, it becomes possible to talk about health promotion for people with disabilities.

This chapter addresses the special health promotion and disease prevention needs of people with disabilities and the problems they face in gaining access to programs to meet those needs. Most of the testimony addresses prevention of secondary consequences due to disabling conditions, plus general health promotion and disease prevention activities for other conditions.

HEALTH PROMOTION FOR PEOPLE WITH DISABILITIES

A number of witnesses made the case that people with disabilities can benefit from health promotion as much as, or more than, others. A health promotion approach, they argued, can help people with disabilities improve the quality of their lives despite the physical problems they face. Health promotion, also is consistent with established rehabilitation practices.

Robert Guthrie of the State University of New York at Buffalo points out that mental retardation and developmental disabilities are "life-long, non-lethal handicaps" for people affected by them. *(#529)* Spinal cord injuries, chronic diseases, sensory impairments, and brain injuries can periodically or permanently disable individuals, while still allowing them to live long lives. Because these disabling conditions cannot be "cured," argues Margaret West of the University of Washington, it is necessary to look at measures of health promotion and disease prevention that "relate to quality and satisfaction with life, ability to participate meaningfully in adult roles such as work, and accessibility, availability, and affordability of care." *(#333)* For example, the provision of occupational, physical, and speech or language services to infants in the first two years of life substantially influences developmental outcomes and can prevent further deteriorating conditions.

Others underscore the significance of secondary prevention programs for those with disabilities, not only to enable the disabled to overcome social and environmental barriers to full social participation, but also to provide training and support in maximizing their potential for independent living and reducing the chance of secondary disability. These needs, argues Brandon, are quite suited to health promotion activities. In fact, he says, rehabilitation parallels wellness programming in many respects. Health promotion, he argues, takes a holistic approach to health that encompasses more than just physical wellness. Similarly, rehabilitation provides patients with physical, emotional, and social support activities.

Since traditional rehabilitation includes an emphasis on self-responsibility, health promotion could be incorporated as an additional component within this area. Depending upon the needs of the client, specific health promotion activities also may be incorporated into his or her rehabilitation plan. Stress management, for instance, may be recommended for chronic pain sufferers, while exercise may be recommended to increase muscle strength or to help relieve anxiety or depression.[2] *(#568)*

Health promotion programs in areas such as nutritional awareness, exercise and fitness, stress management, and alcohol and drug abuse prevention, "are of much, if not even greater, relevance" to the disabled population, Brandon argues, precisely because of their mental or physical disabilities. *(#568)*

ACCESS TO HEALTH SERVICES

Despite their need for health promotion and disease prevention, people with disabilities face numerous problems gaining access to health promotion programs and preventive services. The barriers, the testifiers point out, are financial, social, physical, and logistical.

Linda Henry, representing the National Association for Home Care, points out that advances in medical technology over the past century have not been matched by similar advances in health policy. Whereas technology now allows many ill children to live into adulthood, there are significant barriers to enabling these children to live and grow in a family and community environment. Quoting Val Halamandaris of the National Association for Home Care, Henry writes:

Ten million fragile and disabled children and their families struggle to find a quality of life that maximizes their potential, supports independence and self-care, and promotes family attachment and integrity. Unfortunately, they often struggle in isolation, remaining in hospitals or institutions because changes in policy have not kept up with changes in technology. *(#372)*

The largest barrier that Henry sees to community health care for chronically ill children is financial reimbursement. Others express similar difficulties for other disabled groups. Examples include (1) insurance policies with riders that exclude coverage of preexisting conditions and their resulting medical problems; (2) drugs, wheelchairs, special appliances, special foods, and formulas that are not covered if used on an outpatient basis; and (3) services such as home nursing, social work services, and physical or occupational therapy that either are not reimbursed or are covered only on a short-term or intermittent basis. *(#372)*

Alfred Tallia, Debbie Spitalnik, and Robert Like of the University of Medicine and Dentistry of New Jersey say that the

inadequacy of the level of Medicaid reimbursement, or the complete absence of reimbursement for medical services is extensively cited as a major, if not the major, disincentive in providing preventive health care to the chronically disabled population. The inadequate Medicaid reimbursement limits accessibility of services to clients as few providers can deliver services and products under this type of system. *(#209)*

The picture of health care coverage for those with disabilities is especially grim, notes Ann Zuzich of Wayne State University. In the United States, one out of five disabled adults has no health insurance and is ineligible for Medicaid or Medicare, she says. Many are denied insurance because they are not poor enough for public programs or because preexisting conditions prevent them from using private programs. When coverage is available, it is difficult to know what services are covered. Zuzich says that delays in processing papers for Medicaid recipients often deny essential equipment for long periods. For children, these delays can increase the disability. Home care services are more difficult to obtain than the same services in an institution. *(#727)*

In addition to financial barriers to adequate preventive services, the disabled population also faces additional difficulties in obtaining quality health care. Institutional living, argues the Association for Retarded Citizens of the United States, compounds health problems for the retarded largely due to lack of qualified medical and support staff trained to apply appropriate health promotion and disease prevention approaches for people who have multiple severe disabilities. *(#048)* In the community, disabilities can impede individuals from gaining access to existing services. People with disabilities have special problems with inconvenient locations and communication with providers, according to Tallia and his colleagues. *(#209)*

Tallia, Spitalnik, and Like say that to provide adequate health care to a community's disabled population, a systematic and comprehensive network of health care services must be established. They cite Allen Crocker of Children's Hospital Medical Center in Boston, who offers the following criteria for comprehensive service to this community:

1. A medical home where an individual's records, needs, and idiosyncrasies are known by a provider population that is responsive to his or her needs

2. A primary health care provider who takes longitudinal responsibility for individual needs, including prevention

These elements, they say, "must occur in the context of a comprehensive network of other health care elements." Such a community-oriented, primary care model also should include access to trauma centers, regional rehabilitation centers, follow-up programs, clinics that include interdisciplinary professional coordination, (e.g., nutritionists and physical therapists), and so on. One trial program built on this model is now being implemented with help from the Robert Wood Johnson Foundation at the University of Medicine and Dentistry of New Jersey. In addition to providing primary care services to a disabled population, this program is undertaking some measurement and evaluation activities. According to Tallia, Spitalnik, and Like, "This project will use health status program measures and volume measures to evaluate wellness, morbidity, reliance on polypharmacy, and the need for hospitalizations, as well as measure cost effectiveness, quality of life, and level of adoptive functioning in this patient population." *(#209)*

IMPLEMENTATION

In all areas of disability—mental retardation, congenital birth defects, developmental disabilities, sensory impairments, chronic illness, and so on—testifiers encourage increased research into the unknown causes of disabilities and continued focus on the prevention of disabilities. They also propose better injury and disability reporting mechanisms, better financial access to preventive services, and improved physician education about serving persons with disabilities so as to improve the delivery of health care services to them. Finally, they call upon the nondisabled population to recognize that many disabilities would not be disabling for individuals in the context of a supportive and accessible social and economic environment.

According to some testifiers, once there is broad-based recognition that the problems of disability are not essentially medical, the necessary community-wide endorsement of disability prevention activities and programs for persons with disabilities will be possible. Allen Crocker points out 15 to 20 states that now have developmental disabilities prevention plans "of some maturity" and argues that through such plans the prevention of developmental disabilities "can be expedited within the policy resolves of individual states." Most plans, he observes, start with a "common public constituency" that works to develop a statewide conference on prevention and eventually results in an implementation process involving commitments from a wide range of public and private groups. Crocker argues that with a state prevention plan the chances of funding prevention research projects and understanding the causes of developmental disabilities will improve. *(#326)*

Irving Zola of Brandeis University makes perhaps the most fundamental recommendation for health policy directed toward those with disabilities. He contends that the development of effective health policies for the disabled requires reexamination of many basic values by which every member of society lives. Instead of building systems of employment, transportation, and health care that "break the rules of order for a few," and thus undermine human interdependence, policies must begin to look at designing a "flexible world for the many," where interdependence and independence are not in conflict. *(#798)*

REFERENCES

1. National Council on the Handicapped: Toward Independence: An Assessment of Federal Laws and Programs Affecting Persons with Disabilities. Washington, D.C.: U.S. Government Printing Office, February 1986

2. Brandon JE: Health promotion and wellness in rehabilitation services. J Rehab 51(4):54–58, 1985

TESTIFIERS CITED IN CHAPTER 7

048 Davis, Sharon; Association for Retarded Citizens of the United States
209 Tallia, Alfred, Spitalnik, Debbie, and Like, Robert; University of Medicine and Dentistry of New Jersey
223 Waldrep, Kent; Kent Waldrep National Paralysis Foundation (Dallas)
326 Crocker, Allen; Children's Hospital (Boston)
333 West, Margaret; University of Washington
372 Henry, Linda; Children's Hospital (Denver)
433 Marge, Michael; Syracuse University
529 Guthrie, Robert; State University of New York at Buffalo
568 Brandon, Jeffrey; University of New Orleans
727 Zuzich, Ann; Wayne State University
798 Zola, Irving; Brandeis University

8. Health Promotion and Disease Prevention in the Health Care System

Because of the important role it plays in detecting, treating, and preventing diseases and injuries, the health care system is critical to implementation of the Year 2000 Health Objectives. However, according to the nearly 100 people who addressed this in their testimony, there are severe problems with access to preventive services and an unfulfilled potential role for health professionals in preventing disease and promoting the health of the U.S. population. Some witnesses digressed from the narrow focus of the objectives to the broader problems of access to health and medical care in general.

Milton Roemer of the University of California, Los Angeles gets directly to the essence of the problem.

Many, if not all, of the priorities of positive health activity on the national agenda can be substantially influenced by access to professional health care. To cite just a few examples, the detection of and intervention against hypertension and cancer, immunization against preventable infectious diseases, control of obesity, or the preventive management of depression require the services of physicians or other skilled health personnel. Yet some 35 to 40 million Americans do not have economic access to doctors through voluntary health insurance, Medicare, or Medicaid. A larger number lack economic and physical access to primary health care, although they may have insurance for hospitalization.

Access to professional care may have very broad impacts on health promotion. Education and advice from a doctor can affect lifestyle—smoking, alcohol use, contraception, exercise, diet, stress—more effectively than the most skillful messages of mass media. We have long ago learned that almost any person is more receptive to advice on changed behavior, if this advice is offered by a health care provider who is giving treatment for a specific symptom. Prevention is more effective if it is integrated with the delivery of medical care. *(#277)*

The Medical Care Section of the American Public Health Association (APHA) agrees with this assessment: "The goals for the year 2000 will not be attained unless all Americans have access to high quality health care." This is true across the broad range of national objectives—whether the health problem being addressed is heart disease and stroke through the control of hypertension; cancer through screening and early detection; or infant mortality through the provision of prenatal care. Consequently, the APHA Medical Care Section suggests that the Public Health Service add an additional goal for the year 2000 that "all Americans will be assured adequate access to quality health care." *(#755)*

Senator Chet Brooks, Dean of the Texas State Senate, sums up the political view.

From my perspective as a state legislator, our success in achieving the national health objectives for the year 2000 will depend to a large extent on improving access to programs and services we already have in place and on increasing the availability of information regarding disease prevention. For example, perhaps the greatest success in a preventive health effort with significant effect on the nation's health status was the discovery and uniform administration of vaccines. The diseases we faced were so frightening and widespread, we took immediate and definitive action. Every child had access to immunizations to prevent these diseases. The results: almost a virtual elimination of debilitating and life-threatening diseases such as polio, diphtheria, and smallpox. The undisputed key to this success was access. As we begin to formulate our goals for the year 2000 and beyond, we must determine why certain objectives for 1990 were not achieved. I suggest we look closely at our policies and programs to see whether they are accessible to the persons for whom they are intended. *(#234)*

Clearly, the Year 2000 Health Objectives can not be achieved without full participation of health professionals and the organizations in which they work. This chapter summarizes testimony on two interrelated issues: the great potential value of providing health promotion and disease prevention services through the health care system, and the serious problems faced by many in gaining access to that system. Access to health care in general, and to preventive services in particular, is primarily a problem of specific populations, especially the poor and minorities, so the problems confronting these groups are discussed first. Testimony on potential contributions of the various health professionals and the settings in which they work is next, along with suggestions on strengthening their roles as providers of health education and preventive services. The next section discusses problems and solutions in the financing of health promotion and disease prevention programs, including changes in existing federal funding programs and in the insurance system. The last section discusses four issues in the implementation of health promotion and disease prevention in health care settings: coordination of services, training health professionals, underserved areas, and the need for minority practitioners.

PROBLEMS WITH ACCESS TO HEALTH CARE

Access to health care is very unevenly distributed in the United States. As discussed in Chapter 6, the poor, the homeless, and many racial and ethnic minorities have severe problems gaining access to preventive services and even basic health care. People with disabilities have access problems of a different sort (Chapter 7). To set the stage for the interventions and changes called for in the latter part of this chapter, testimony on the problems faced by the poor, minorities, and the disabled is presented first.

Poor and Homeless

According to many who testified, today's poor and homeless represent special populations that both are large enough and include enough of America's most vulnerable citizens to warrant particular concern in the Year 2000 Health Objectives. The difficulties these people face in maintaining their health and attaining access to the medical system go beyond the obvious economic ones and include the horrendous physical and social conditions in which they must live. For these disadvantaged, issues of preventing disease and promoting good health often are secondary to the problems associated with everyday survival.

According to Mary Sapp of the San Antonio Health Care for the Homeless Coalition, the number of homeless people is growing, and their ranks include families and people at the highest risk for health problems. Their needs are exacerbated by special health risks inherent in their lifestyles: exposure to the elements, poor nutrition, inadequate sanitation, lack of a place to recuperate from minor illnesses, vulnerability to violent acts, psychological stress, and alcohol or substance abuse. This group needs access to every preventive measure available to the general population and would benefit more from them than the average person. (#507)

According to Harold Shoults, the Salvation Army works with the most "down-and-out," the working poor and those who "fall through the cracks" in public welfare programs. Their experience, revealed in reports from Salvation Army officers around the country, is enlightening. The "barriers to health care for our clients might be summed up in three words: access, understanding, and conditions," says Shoults. The Memphis and Dallas offices discuss access:

One of our biggest problems is lack of medical insurance among the unemployed, temporarily employed, and those working for temporary labor providers. These people would have to apply for Medicaid if they got into a crisis. There is nothing for minor problems. They must present themselves to an emergency room and take what they can get there.

Preventive health service is only able to take life-threatening cases. As an example, this past winter our local public hospital had to refuse inpatient care unless an individual had pneumonia in both lungs.

Others deal with understanding:

Barriers to access include a fragmented system and not understanding the treatment or instructions.

There is no continuity of service, they probably see a different physician every time, never develop a relationship with a doctor or nurse and get little in the way of health education.

Finally, there is the question of condition:

The socioeconomic condition of clients creates, perpetuates, and exacerbates major health problems.

Particularly in the case of a homeless family, there are multiple needs that must be addressed. Stress related problems of the families we see today may be due to (1) unemployment or underemployment, (2) inadequate public assistance programs, (3) substandard housing, (4) exorbitant utility costs, (5) poor health care, (6) lack of transportation, (7) inadequate support systems, and (8) lack of experience and education about good parenting.

Many children are being raised in a state of sheer survival. As a result, they are faced with some serious malaise: malnutrition, long-term sleep deprivation, depression, developmental lags, educational deprivation, dental and other chronic health problems; these can only bring perpetuation of the homeless syndrome. *(#579)*

Stephen Joseph, New York City Commissioner of Health, writes that "the health problems of New York inevitably reflect the conditions of poverty in which too many families live. Confronting these environments means confronting the failures of our formal and informal education systems, chronic unemployability, the too-frequent drift into a lifetime of crime and drugs, the collapse of the nuclear family, and a worsening housing crisis." *(#437)*

As an example of what needs to be done to prevent disease and promote the health of the homeless, consider the situation of New York City. In 1987 the city provided room for over 27,000 homeless people, including more than 5,000 families, in shelters, temporary apartments, and hotels. For homeless families living in hotels the infant mortality rate is twice the city average. According to Joseph, the Homeless Health Initiative is being expanded to provide essential health screening and referral services to homeless individuals and families. New York City has 25 public health nurses working in 37 hotels that house approximately 90 percent of the city's homeless; these nurses refer residents to medical or social service agencies, and teach them about proper nutrition and prenatal or pediatric care. To reduce the infant mortality rate and reach women who traditionally have not sought prenatal or pediatric care, the Department of Health is implementing a plan in which 30 public health nurses and 35 public health advisers will work with community groups to refer pregnant women and infants to local providers of medical and social services. *(#437)*

Racial and Ethnic Minorities

The problems that minorities face in attaining access to health care are severe and complex (see Chapter 6). They are caused not only by socioeconomic factors, but also by different cultural attitudes and beliefs about health and medicine.

According to Daniel Blumenthal of the Morehouse School of Medicine, millions of Americans—especially Blacks—lack adequate access to quality health services. The reasons for this include (1) lack of insurance (even "adequate" insurance does not cover preventive services); (2) living in rural or inner-city areas that are poorly served by physicians; and (3) the shortage of Black physicians. Although 12 percent of the U.S. population is Black, fewer than 3 percent of U.S. physicians are Black.[1] *(#255)* The APHA Medical Care Section reports that a substantial portion of the disparities in Black and minority health "may be attributed to differences in access to health care, both preventive and curative between the two population groups." *(#755)*

Osman Ahmed of Meharry Medical College writes that "Blacks are known to delay seeking health care within the traditional health care system, preferring to rely upon family, friends, and even spiritualists and healers, during periods of economic and emotional stress." Unique value systems, together with medical care expenses, may prevent Blacks from utilizing the health care system. Since different "loci of control are operating in Blacks, different health promotion strategies should be used to reach them. Eliminating barriers to care seeking and behavior change will require new, culturally sensitive approaches to information dissemination, health planning and resources management, and may even require the institutionalization of new health policies." *(#269)*

As an example of what should be done to improve access to preventive services, Ahmed cites Meharry Medical College's "Community Coalition on Minority Health." This coalition, led by Meharry, consists of local governmental, professional, voluntary, community, and religious organizations and tries to "bring together the knowledge, expertise, and resources to provide solutions." The coalition's objective is to decrease diet- and nutrition-related cancer and cardiovascular disease risk factors and hypertension in the Black community. *(#269)*

Other minority groups have similar difficulties with access to health care. The National Coalition of Hispanic Health and Human Services Organizations says that Hispanics are more than twice as likely to be without either public or private health insurance than non-Hispanic Whites or Blacks.[2] Hispanic mothers are more likely than non-Hispanic Whites or Blacks to begin prenatal care in the third trimester or not at all; Hispanics are less likely to have a regular source of health care; 30 percent of Hispanics lack this, compared to 20 percent of Blacks and 16 percent of Whites. Hispanics are also less likely to receive public health messages. *(#193)*

"Hispanics, in particular Puerto Ricans, continue to have poorer health status, and excess morbidity and mortality compared to the majority population," according to Eric Munoz of the Long Island Jewish Medical Center in New York. Munoz suggests that this disparity is due in part to less access to health care and preventive services in particular. For example, fewer Puerto Rican women undergo breast exams and mammography, or Pap smears and gynecological exams. Puerto Ricans also have inadequate detection and treatment of hypertension. *(#431)*

People with Disabilities

"Adults with chronic disabilities," write Alfred Tallia, Debbie Spitalnik, and Robert Like of the University of Medicine and Dentistry of New Jersey, "either those who have developmental disabilities or chronic mental illness, individually and as a collective group, have a history of inadequate health care and a lack of access to quality medical services, including preventive health services." They say that deinstitutionalization of the chronically disabled from large, congregate institutions assumes the availability and accessibility of health services in the community, but services are not being delivered adequately to this population. Chronic disabilities are accompanied by complex needs for an array of preventive health, social, educational, vocational, and other supportive services; health services for the chronically disabled, however, tend to be targeted to specific problems, and general preventive health needs tend to go unattended or are poorly "coordinated." Furthermore, Tallia, Spitalnik, and Like say that the nature of chronic disabilities may create barriers to participation in a primary care setting with preventive health measures; problems include economic disadvantages due to difficulty in sustaining employment, physical access issues, difficulties in obtaining adequate health histories, and negative prejudicial attitudes from health care workers. *(#209)*

HEALTH PROMOTION AND DISEASE PREVENTION IN THE HEALTH CARE SYSTEM

Implementation of the national objectives for health promotion and disease prevention in medical and health care settings depends on the participation of physicians, other health professionals, and the organizations in which they work. Those who testified had many recommendations about how to make better use of health professionals in disease prevention and health promotion programs. The suggestions generally included changes in training programs, compensation and reimbursement systems, and recruitment.

Physicians

Many who testified felt that physicians can play a much larger role in health promotion and disease prevention than they currently do. The evidence of their effectiveness is strong, according to witnesses. Testimony, therefore, called for enhanced training opportunities and changes in insurance payment policies to allow physicians to become more active.

According to the American Academy of Family Physicians:

> Physicians in primary care can have a positive effect on health behaviors in very cost effective ways. For example, the simple offering by a general practitioner of advice to stop smoking to patients who come to the doctor for some reason other than smoking, results in a 5 percent quit rate at the end of one year.[3]

To take advantage of the opportunities presented by physicians, the American Academy of Family Physicians makes four recommendations:

1. Insurance should cover scientifically supported disease prevention and health promotion interventions in the doctor's office and other outpatient settings.

2. Office-based systems for health risk assessment and longitudinal tracking for both screening examinations and health behaviors should be developed and adopted.

3. Disease prevention and health promotion curricula must be developed in medical schools and residencies and put on a par with other medical education topics.

4. Research to determine appropriate assessments and interventions, as well as their frequencies and

effectiveness, needs to be funded. (#072)

Donald Logsdon reports on a series of studies funded by the insurance industry under the banner of Project INSURE, which he directs. These studies have shown that (1) physicians are interested in clinical prevention; they will effectively provide preventive services, including patient education in their practices, if they receive practice-based training and if the financial barriers to preventive care are removed; (2) such interventions can be effective in changing risk behaviors; and (3) their costs can be controlled. Therefore, Logsdon suggests that the Year 2000 Health Objectives include clinical preventive services provided by physicians. He also sees a need for continuing medical education programs and incentives for physicians to become more effective at preventive health services and health promotion. (#463)

According to Michael Eriksen, Director of Behavioral Research at the University of Texas M.D. Anderson Hospital:

The potential impact of health professionals, especially physicians, in furthering our disease prevention and health promotion goals is vast. However, they were rarely included in the 1990 Objectives. The Year 2000 Health Objectives should stipulate specific health promotion objectives for each patient encounter, consistent with the guidelines being developed by the U.S. Preventive Services Task Force.

Eriksen offers this example: "Smoking patients should be counseled by their physician to stop smoking during 75 percent of routine office visits." (#309)

Other Health Professionals

Witnesses discussed the roles that a wide range of health professionals can play in implementing health promotion and disease prevention objectives. The professional groups include pharmacists, nurses, midwives, public health professionals, and allied health professionals. In many cases, these groups are oriented to disease prevention and health promotion and are reportedly effective at it, so that minimum changes in training and funding patterns can have important effects.

The American Pharmaceutical Association (APhA), for instance, urges recognition of the important role pharmacists play in health promotion and disease prevention. Their testimony addresses the following matters:

1. The pharmacists' role as health educators and medication counselors: Pharmacists provide education and information to patients regarding the control of high blood pressure, family planning, sexually transmitted diseases, poison prevention, smoking and health, nutrition and weight control, and the control of stress.

2. The role of pharmacists in promoting rational prescription drug therapy: The 1990 Objectives focus on adverse drug reactions, but counseling should be much broader and should emphasize the correct use of all medication to avoid complications. Pharmacists also play a role in assuring the quality of drug therapies on the regulatory level.

3. The need to pay all health care providers for counseling that fosters health promotion and disease prevention: Unless there are economic incentives for pharmacists (like other care providers) to provide health education, the APhA feels that their maximum effort will not be brought to bear on the problem. (#564)

Many witnesses testified about the contributions that nurses already make to health promotion and disease prevention efforts and stressed the role that they can play in implementing the Year 2000 Health Objectives. Patty Hawken, Dean of the School of Nursing at the University of Texas Health Science Center at San Antonio, says that because nurses have traditionally been the constant care giver in the community and in the home, they are well prepared to assist with health promotion and disease prevention. (#501)

Sharon Grigsby, President of the Visiting Nurse Foundation in Los Angeles, reports that the initial efforts of visiting nurses a century ago concentrated on the prevention of disease through education on the rudiments of good hygiene and helped reduce maternal and infant mortality, as well as the spread of infectious diseases. Visiting nurses have kept up with technological advances in medicine, she reports, but their historical commitment to community-based care has not lessened. Grigsby still sees a role for visiting nurses in preventing illness and disability through education. Their efforts would be most effective for vulnerable populations such as the elderly, pregnant women, and infants. (#074)

Sapp reports on her coalition's goal of promoting the utilization of nurse practitioners to the fullest extent of their training and skills in all programs targeting the homeless. (#507)

However, according to Hawken the number of new

nurses is declining. The current shortage of professional nurses has a critical impact on health care in the country. *(#501)* As the population ages, the shortage of nurses to care for the elderly will become particularly acute, says Anita Beckerman of the College of New Rochelle in New York. She suggests that federal and state governments develop programs to facilitate the entrance of prospective nursing students into the profession, perhaps through full tuition payments with service payback provisions, scholarships, grants, or capitation payments to nursing schools. *(#436)* Hawken suggests that encouraging groups in health care to highlight the importance of nurses in meeting national health care objectives would help ease the shortage. *(#501)*

Mary Mundinger, Dean of the Columbia University School of Nursing, says that the major reasons for the unavailability of nurses are their low status within the medical system, low salaries, and shift work. To prevent a nursing shortage and restore nursing to a viable and useful profession, funding changes must be initiated at the federal level. These would include transferring federal resources for training physicians (who are in oversupply) to nurse training programs; using National Health Service Corps funds to bring nurses into underserved areas; finding ways to bring nonworking nurses back into the work force; and changing credentialing practices to recognize and reward nurses at the highest levels of education and practice. *(#589)*

A number of testifiers discussed the preventive services that midwives can provide, especially high-quality prenatal care and obstetrical services. Representatives of the American College of Nurse-Midwives believe that nurse midwives can deliver quality services at low cost and would be particularly effective for low-income populations. Thus, they urge the removal of barriers to practice, such as noncompetitive salaries, restraint of trade by physicians, and the malpractice crisis. *(#268; #292; #690)*

Allan Rosenfield, Dean of the Columbia University School of Public Health, reports on a shortage of well-trained public health professionals. "Only a small percentage of the people working in city, county, and state departments of health and in other parts of the public health infrastructure have been formally trained in public health." *(#633)* Bernard Goldstein of the University of Medicine and Dentistry of New Jersey notes that one impediment to reaching the important goal of a sufficient number of trained public health professionals is the "poor geographical distribution and relative lack of outreach of our existing accredited

graduate training facilities in public health." He suggests the development of easily accessible, rigorous graduate education programs. *(#625)*

According to Keith Blayney, Dean of the School of Health-Related Professions at the University of Alabama at Birmingham, allied health professionals engage in millions of patient interactions each week and thus represent a tremendous potential for disease prevention and health promotion efforts. *(#258)* According to John Bruhn, Dean of the School of Allied Health Sciences at the University of Texas Medical Branch at Galveston, physician's assistants, physical and occupational therapists, dental hygienists, and other allied health professionals are in positions to provide one-on-one patient education regarding lifestyles and habits that can prevent illness. 'Teachable moments' are not limited to the physician-patient dyad." *(#235)*

To make them a potent force for implementing the Year 2000 Health Objectives, Blayney feels that every allied health professional in the country should be cross-trained to provide patient and public education and services in the area of health promotion and disease prevention. *(#258)*

Lisa Fleming, President of the Alabama Dental Hygienists' Association, wants to "emphasize the role that dental auxiliaries can play in the Year 2000 Health Objectives. As education and prevention professionals, dental hygienists can have a significant role in meeting these objectives. With proper education, hygienists can actively participate in educational and preventive programs to reduce dental caries, apply preventive procedures to periodontal patients, and educate the public about the prevention of accidents and oral cancer." *(#262)*

Health Care Settings and Organizations

Health professionals, especially nonphysicians, generally work in organizations, and the policies and structure of these organizations have an important effect on access to preventive services. Along these lines, witnesses discussed health promotion and disease prevention activities in hospitals, community health centers, health maintenance organizations, group practices, and long-term care facilities. The general feeling is that these facilities are interested in providing more preventive services and health promotion programs, but funding patterns inhibit their ability to do so.

For instance, the American Hospital Association (AHA) reports:

As chronic disease has replaced acute infectious disease as the major cause of morbidity and mortality, as the locus of care has shifted to the outpatient setting, and as the research base for broadly defined health promotion/disease prevention services has solidified, hospitals have expanded the range of services they offer. During the 1980s, hospitals across the United States became major providers of health promotion services and active partners with other local organizations in addressing community health problems. Historically, patient education has been the primary focus of hospital health promotion services as a complement to acute medical services. A 1979 policy statement recognized hospitals' responsibility "to take a leadership role in helping to insure the good health of their communities."

According to the AHA, hospitals now have a wide variety of health promotion activities such as cardiac rehabilitation, care giver education, wellness programming, and occupational health services. Increasingly, hospitals are recognizing the limits of their acute inpatient and outpatient services in meeting the needs of patients with chronic conditions, and are establishing linkages with self-help/mutual aid groups. (#576)

However, AHA reports that changes in hospital care—more outpatient services, shorter inpatient stays, and more care of chronic than acute illness—mean that hospitals have less opportunity to offer prevention or health promotion education to patients. Also, work force shortages, especially in nursing, and inadequate resources or reimbursement may prevent health care professionals from offering the range of educational efforts called for in the 1990 Objectives, such as counseling in safety belt use, nutrition education, physical fitness regimens, and stress-coping skills. Given the lack of progress toward some key objectives such as infant mortality among minorities and the lack of access to private health insurance, "it is perhaps time to elevate financing for preventive services to the status of an objective if risk reduction and health status objectives are to be achieved for all populations." (#576)

The National Association of Community Health Centers reports that these centers present a good opportunity for implementing the objectives in poor and minority communities. Clients of these centers are largely poor, minorities, women, and children, and the illnesses reported are preventable if diagnosed early. For example, among the top 10 diagnoses reported at community health centers around the country were hypertension, upper respiratory infections, pregnancy, and diabetes. (#635)

Health maintenance organizations (HMOs) have "several distinct advantages" that enable them to efficiently deliver preventive and health promotion services, according to David Sobel of the Permanente Medical Group in Oakland, California. (#780)

1. Their financial incentives are such that the organization benefits from the implementation of efficient, cost-effective preventive services.
2. Large HMOs and group practice models can achieve economies of scale and efficiency in delivering these services through such mechanisms as health education centers, group classes, and telephone tapes or advice nurses.
3. Centralized medical records and patient profiles provide outstanding opportunities for evaluation of health promotion initiatives.

But, Sobel cautions that even the physicians who work in HMOs may not be skilled or comfortable in providing health education and counseling. Thus, to be successful, HMOs must
• define and specify a basic benefit package of prenatal, immunization, and age-related periodic health evaluation services to assure consistency;
• use nonphysician health professionals, such as nurses, nurse practitioners, dietitians, and pharmacists, to provide health education and prevention services; and
• include self-care education to help people understand when to seek medical and preventive care, and when or how to use self-treatment safely. (#780)

FINANCING HEALTH PROMOTION AND DISEASE PREVENTION PROGRAMS IN THE HEALTH CARE SYSTEM

Many testifiers identified problems with financing health promotion and disease prevention programs as an obstacle to implementing the national objectives. Robert Black of Monterey, California, states, "Health promotion and disease prevention have been the stepchild of the American health care system and there is no incentive or reward for keeping people healthy. The financial structure needs complete revision and arrangement differently than it is presently conceived." (#796)

Some saw the problem in the context of a larger

concern about overall health expenditures in the United States, and proposed changes in Medicare and Medicaid or in already existing federal grant programs. Most of those who testified on these issues, however, proposed major changes in the financing of health care, including a national health insurance policy.

According to the APHA Medical Care Section, "Access to health care for those most in need of care has actually been reduced since the Surgeon General's goals were first published. This is because of cutbacks in the several programs that have been established to increase access for the underprivileged and because of increasing corporatization of health care." (#755)

William Hagens, a senior research analyst for the Washington State Legislature, said that the number one health problem facing Olympia and all other state capitals is the question of financing. At a time when access to health care for low-income people is declining and costs are rising, there is the feeling that all the money spent is not contributing to happier, healthier people. Therefore, it is important that no new program be added, but that those already on the books be implemented more aggressively. Hagens feels that people must to be taught to be more responsible for their own health, and that prevention activities by businesses should be expanded. (#694)

Federal Funding Programs

Many witnesses suggested that already existing federal funding programs could do more to finance health promotion and disease prevention, and to improve the access to health care generally. In particular, testifiers addressed the possibilities of changing Medicare reimbursement policies for preventive services; increasing the coverage of Medicaid to include more poor people and more services, especially maternal health services; and better coordinating block and categorical grant programs with the national objectives.

Medicare. A number of speakers suggested that Medicare should cover more health promotion and disease prevention services. Paul Hunter of the American Medical Student Association/Foundation, for instance, says that Medicare should reimburse at least 50 percent of the costs of the following preventive services: "health screenings, health-risk appraisals, immunizations, nutrition counseling, stress reduction, injury prevention, alcohol and drug abuse

counseling, smoking cessation, and medication use." (#612)

Medicaid. A number of witnesses suggested changes in the Medicaid system to improve access to preventive services for the poor. These proposals ranged from changes for specific services, especially prenatal care, to an overall expansion of the number of people insured and the services covered.

Milton Arnold of the American Academy of Pediatrics, for example, says that adequate prenatal care is the single most important factor in reducing infant morbidity and mortality, and he calls for more complete Medicaid reimbursement for it. With better prenatal care, he says, many of the 40,000 deaths that occur annually to babies in their first year of life can be prevented.[4] However, he cites a General Accounting Office (GAO) report that found insufficient prenatal care for women of all races, ages, and economic groups, but especially for low-income minorities.[5] According to the GAO report, 81 percent of privately insured women surveyed received adequate prenatal care compared to 36 percent of those who qualify for Medicaid and 32 percent of uninsured women.[6] The American Academy of Pediatrics would like to see prenatal care made available to all pregnant women early in pregnancy; Medicaid can help meet this goal by providing a regularly updated list of approved and reimbursable services and procedures and by improving reimbursement and paying claims promptly. (#678)

Other witnesses complained that Medicaid is not realizing its potential. The APHA Medical Care Section says that "the Medicaid program still does nothing to improve access to health care for the majority of low-income Americans. The program actually covers less than half of all persons living in poverty; even those who are technically covered are often unable to find a physician who will accept Medicaid patients." (#755)

Judith Glazner of the Denver Department of Health and Hospitals says that federal and state cutbacks in the early 1980s resulted in some of the poor becoming ineligible for Medicaid; she recommends that all states be required to use the same Medicaid eligibility standards. (#377) The Health Policy Agenda for the American People, a collaborative effort of nearly 200 health, health-related, business, government, and consumer groups to promote health sector change, recommends that

1. Medicaid be revised to establish national standards that result in uniform eligibility, benefits,

and adequate payment mechanisms for services across jurisdictions; and

2. Medicaid eligibility standards be expanded to include the medically indigent and payments be related to their ability to pay. *(#583)*

Block Grants. A number of state and local health officers suggest that federal block grant funds should be an important tool in financing prevention activities called for in the objectives. Mark Richards, Secretary of Health for the Commonwealth of Pennsylvania, says that all recipients of block and categorical grant funds should demonstrate clearly how they will help meet the appropriate objectives. *(#387)*

Thomas Halpin and Karen Evans of the Ohio Department of Health say that federal preventive health and health services block grants were crucial to the success of the objectives in Ohio and should continue with the Year 2000 Health Objectives. *(#129)* Diana Bonta suggests using Title X family planning grants to implement family planning objectives. *(#024)* Maternal and child health block grants and the Special Supplemental Food Program for Women, Infants, and Children (WIC) can help improve access to early prenatal care and other services for pregnant women, infants, and children. *(#044)*

Health Insurance

Many witnesses called for some form of national health insurance system that would pay for preventive services, saying that without major changes in the current system, from which many are disenfranchised and which provides little preventive care for those who are covered, it will be difficult to make progress in the Year 2000 Health Objectives. Although some witnesses felt that a national health system or at least a national health insurance system is the only answer, others proposed changes in the existing private insurance system.

According to Rosenfield:

There should be a much greater emphasis on disease prevention/health promotion as a number one national health priority with adequate funding at federal, state, and local levels. Health care financing in this country remains a tragic problem for an unacceptably large percentage of the population. As the only Western nation without some form of national health insurance or health service, a sizable percentage

of our population is either unserved or underserved. The problem is greatest for the uninsured working poor, the homeless, and the poor generally. A national health insurance program remains an urgent, if misunderstood, national priority. *(#633)*

Derrick Jelliffe of the University of California, Los Angeles goes further:

Until the country has some form of national health insurance coverage or other national health system enabling preventive and curative health services to be available to all economic levels in the country, the rest of the deliberations on the objectives border on the farcical. Unless one is careful, a potpourri of fragmented programs of limited extent and coverage may emerge in the usual sort of way. There is no way that the country can move from being a second-class nation as far as health services are concerned until a national health coverage has been achieved. *(#271)*

"Millions of people are going without needed medical care, both therapeutic and preventive, because of financial barriers," writes Marjorie Wilson of Olympia, Washington.

It is time for us to stop Band-Aiding a sick medical system. It is time now to start implementing a comprehensive national health plan. In addition to preventing serious conditions caused by neglect of early diagnosis and treatment, the national health plan should provide other preventive services such as: (1) primary prevention of mental conditions, early screening, and tertiary prevention for symptom control; (2) age-related health screening for all citizens with emphasis on the very young and the very old; (3) mammograms, Pap smears, and cholesterol and diabetic screening, as risk related; (4) health education in the community, the workplace, and the schools for healthy living; and (5) environmental and personal changes for injury prevention. *(#346)*

Members of the Society of Teachers of Family Medicine at a hearing on the national objectives suggested the following objective: "The number of Americans not covered by health insurance, currently 37 million, should be reduced by at least half—and preferably more; alternatively, more than 95 percent of Americans should have health insurance that covers 90 percent of hospital and 80 percent of outpatient costs, including primary and secondary prevention, as recommended by the U.S. Preventive Services Task Force." *(#143)*

According to Glazner, insurance coverage is a key factor in gaining access to preventive health care, and lack of insurance particularly affects the young, the old, and the poor.

> Without health insurance, low-income families must rely on a frequently fragmented and difficult-to-use public system of health care. Regular preventive care, including prenatal care, immunization, and well-child care, is sometimes difficult to get, and its availability may not be well understood. Only when families do not have to make a choice between food on the table and a visit to the doctor or clinic will adequate care for those most at risk be provided.

Because health insurance in the United States is largely employment based, "the practical focus of increasing insurance coverage at this time must primarily be on employers that don't provide health insurance and on the insurers themselves." *(#377)*

Thus, Glazner suggests adding a new category to the objectives, "Improvement of Economic Access to Health Care." Its aim would be to reduce the number of Americans not covered by public or private insurance programs, including Medicare and Medicaid, to less than 7.5 percent (a reduction of 50 percent), and she suggests a number of specific changes in legislation and regulation to achieve this goal. *(#377)*

The Health Policy Agenda for the American People also is addressing the current insurance system, especially its coverage. The Health Policy Agenda has developed a "basic benefits package" to serve as the foundation for private health insurance plans and for public programs that finance health care. The package includes the following prevention and health promotion activities: maternal and child care, dental examination and teeth cleaning, immunizations, and periodic medical examinations. *(#583)*

IMPLEMENTATION WITHIN THE HEALTH CARE SYSTEM

Witnesses also identified four interrelated implementation issues especially relevant to assuring access to preventive services: coordination of services, training of health professionals, underserved areas, and the lack of minority practitioners.

Coordination of Services

Helen Farabee, representing the March of Dimes Birth Defects Foundation, suggests as an objective that "by 2000, all pregnant women and infants should have access to and at least 95 percent shall receive quality care and case management from a coordinated and comprehensive system of public and private health-care providers." According to Farabee, recent efforts in Texas have (1) expanded services, to make prenatal care available in every county; (2) instituted a comprehensive managed care program for pregnant women with high-risk conditions; and (3) tried to better coordinate services that should be targeted toward the poor, such as the WIC program, family planning programs, infant care programs, and early childhood intervention programs. *(#289)*

George Silver of Yale University writes of the need "to focus on the inadequacies, inefficiencies, uncontrollable inflation of cost, and evidence of poor quality plaguing the U.S. medical care system" in order to meet the Year 2000 Health Objectives. However, in implementing programs, he emphasizes the need to start with a state, rather than a full-scale national, program because the "national tradition in connection with social policy has always been to start with a state model." *(#510)*

Training of Health Professionals

Many testifiers identified training issues as key in realizing the potential of health professionals, especially physicians, in implementing the objectives. One issue is the necessity for more specialists in preventive medicine. Other witnesses called for better integration of the knowledge and skills needed for health promotion and disease prevention in the basic education of all health professionals.

William Scheckler of the University of Wisconsin,

for instance, notes a decline in choice of primary care careers by medical students, despite an increasing need for such specialists. He suggests that training grants in these areas be increased, residency programs in primary care be promoted, and medical schools be encouraged to emphasize primary care. (#194)

The American Occupational Medicine Association (AOMA) makes a similar suggestion about training more specialists in occupational medicine. (#071) The Society of Teachers of Family Medicine (STFM) calls for a 25 percent increase in the number of residency graduates in family medicine and general preventive medicine who plan to emphasize clinical preventive medicine in their practice, as well as development of a clinical preventive medicine fellowship to meet this objective. (#118)

The Association of Preventive Medicine Residents agrees with this approach and recommends creation of a specific objective dealing with the training of health professionals in disease prevention and health promotion, with emphasis on training physicians in preventive medicine. Although shortages of preventive medicine specialists are predicted, the federal government has cut funding for preventive medicine residencies in recent years; thus, the association recommends that this funding be restored at least to the earlier level. (#560)

The other approach suggested in testimony is incorporation of health promotion and disease prevention material into the general medical curriculum. Sue Lurie of the Texas College of Osteopathic Medicine points to the importance of prevention in the training of physicians and physician's assistants. She feels that integration of specific topics into the existing curriculum is the most effective approach and that increasing the clinical training of physicians in outpatient settings would increase their focus on preventive health care. (#136) The AOMA recommends that broad-based orientation courses in occupational medicine be established in the curriculum of all schools of medicine and osteopathy. (#071) The STFM calls for a 25 percent increase in the curriculum time spent in medical schools and primary care residency programs on health promotion and disease prevention. (#118) The National Board of Medical Examiners sets certification standards for practicing physicians and develops tests to evaluate current medical education and practice. It reports that the major priority areas of the 1990 Objectives are covered in the examination and that the "educational imperative" of the Year 2000 Health Objectives will be reflected in new examinations.

Thus, setting appropriate objectives will have some impact on medical practice. (#221)

The National Council for the Education of Health Professionals in Health Promotion (NCEHPHP) suggests that

> students of medicine, nursing, dentistry, and the allied health professions be adequately prepared to intervene effectively with those patients at risk and to organize health promotion/disease prevention services. Therefore, those responsible for the education, training, and certification of health professionals must develop goals and objectives to assure that health promotion and disease prevention becomes an integral part of the repertoire of skills of those charged with the responsibility of providing health care.

The NCEHPHP also addresses specific recommendations for the health professions curriculum, academic institutions and faculty, accreditation, certification and licensure, and continuing education. (#169)

Underserved Areas

According to some witnesses, the problem is not a shortage of health professionals but rather their distribution. Many inner cities and rural areas have few physicians or other health professionals; furthermore, according to witnesses, the primary federal program for addressing this problem, the National Health Service Corps, is insufficient. The solutions proposed involve the medical education system, reimbursement, and substituting one kind of professional for another.

According to the APHA's Medical Care Section, "Millions of Americans who live in rural or inner-city areas lack access by reason of living in these areas. The National Health Service Corps, which offered one approach to this problem, has been all but phased out over the last several years." (#755)

Donna Denno, representing the American Medical Student Association, says that the health objectives cannot be attained without a consistent health care work force available to implement them, particularly to serve the indigent in health manpower shortage areas. Despite reports of a physician surplus, the manpower shortage is increasing, particularly of primary care physicians in underserved regions. The steps Denno lists to address the problems include funding the National Health Service Corps, exposing medical students to health manpower shortage areas during their training period, and recruiting minority medical students. *(#717)*

In a more specific case, according to Lisa Kane Low and colleagues from the Michigan chapter of the American College of Nurse-Midwives:

> The distribution of health care providers is a main contributor to the problem of patient access to maternity services. While major urban and resort areas have long had ample numbers of physicians, there are many areas of Michigan that have far fewer physicians than necessary, and despite the ample number of providers, all women are not provided equal access to these resources. Many of the underserved areas are rural, geographically removed from the social and professional benefits of large urban areas. However, a number of urban areas in Michigan contain "pockets" of underserved populations.

They offer three recommendations for dealing with these problems:

1. Reestablish the National Health Service Corps or provide incentives for states to develop their own programs.

2. Reimburse certified nurse midwives and other nurses in advanced practice for services they are qualified to deliver.

3. Improve reimbursement rates for services provided to Medicaid recipients and provide parity in reimbursement for the same services provided by various health care professionals, including nurse midwives. *(#628)*

Minority Practitioners

The problems of underserved areas often intersect with the lack of access for minority populations. A number of testifiers suggested that one solution to this joint problem could be found in training more minority health professionals at all levels.

One testifier who calls himself "a state health commissioner with a vision toward the new millennium," says that "ultimately, achievement of the nation's health objectives will depend not only on clearly articulated measures, but also on the availability of appropriately trained personnel who are representative of the communities served, and who recognize the fact that health is the outcome of many complex factors, involving individual, institutional, and community behavior patterns." Objectives for the year 2000 should include training health professionals in culturally appropriate interventions and recruiting health personnel from the communities most in need of interventions. *(#599)*

More specifically, the APHA Medical Care Section says that "the continued shortage of Black physicians exacerbates access problems for Black Americans. *(#755)* Denno adds that minority physicians tend to work in health manpower shortage areas more often than their White counterparts; thus, recruiting minority medical students through specific grant and loan programs would help underserved areas. *(#717)*

James Young, Dean of the School of Allied Health Sciences at the University of Texas Health Science Center at San Antonio, says that allied health professionals have an important potential role in promoting and achieving the nation's health goals, specifically as they concern minorities. Young's recommendations include (1) increasing minority representation in the allied health professions, and assessing the incentives that exist to encourage student, faculty, and clinician entry into needed areas; (2) aggressively recruiting students from underserved communities; and (3) developing strategies and incentives to attract allied health professionals to enter practice in underserved areas and to increase the number of minority students who practice in these settings. *(#497)*

REFERENCES

1. U.S. Bureau of the Census: Statistical Abstract of the United States, 1987 (107th Edition). Washington, D.C.: U.S. Government Printing Office, 1986

2. National Center for Health Statistics: Health United States, 1984 (DHHS Publication No. [PHS] 85-1232), 1985

3. Russell MAH, Wilson C, Taylor C, et al.: Effect of general practitioners' advice against smoking. Brit Med J 2:231–235, 1979

4. Hughes D, Johnson K, Rosenbaum S, et al.: The Health of America's Children: Maternal and Child Health Data Book. Washington, D.C.: Children's Defense Fund, 1988

5. U.S. General Accounting Office: Prenatal care: Medicaid recipients and uninsured women obtain insufficient care. Report to the Chairman, Subcommittee on Human Resources and Intergovernmental Relations, Committee on Government Operations, House of Representatives. GAO/HRD 87-137, September 1987

6. Ibid.

TESTIFIERS CITED IN CHAPTER 8

024 Bonta, Diana; Los Angeles Regional Family Planning Council
044 Corry, Maureen; March of Dimes Birth Defects Foundation
071 Givens, Austin; American Occupational Medical Association
072 Graham, Robert; American Academy of Family Physicians
074 Grigsby, Sharon; The Visiting Nurse Foundation
118 Kligman, Evan; Society of Teachers of Family Medicine
129 Halpin, Thomas and Evans, Karen; Ohio Department of Health
136 Lurie, Sue; Texas College of Osteopathic Medicine
143 Martin, Robert; Society of Teachers of Family Medicine
169 Osterbusch, Suzanne; National Council for the Education of Health Professionals in Health Promotion
193 Delgado, Jane; The National Coalition of Hispanic Health and Human Services Organizations (COSSMHO)
194 Scheckler, William; University of Wisconsin
209 Tallia, Alfred, Spitalnik, Debbie, and Like, Robert; University of Medicine and Dentistry of New Jersey
221 Volle, Robert; National Board of Medical Examiners
234 Brooks, Chet; Texas State Senate
235 Bruhn, John; University of Texas Medical Branch at Galveston
255 Blumenthal, Daniel; Morehouse School of Medicine
258 Blayney, Keith; University of Alabama at Birmingham
262 Fleming, Lisa; Alabama Dental Hygienists' Association
268 Work, Rebecca; University of Alabama at Birmingham
269 Ahmed, Osman; Meharry Medical College
271 Jelliffe, Derrick; University of California, Los Angeles
277 Roemer, Milton; University of California, Los Angeles
289 Farabee, Helen; Benedictine Health Promotion Center (Austin)
292 Wente, Susan; Jefferson Davis Hospital (Houston)
309 Eriksen, Michael; University of Texas Health Science Center at Houston
346 Wilson, Marjorie; Olympia, Washington
377 Glazner, Judith; Denver Department of Health and Hospitals
387 Richards, N. Mark; Pennsylvania Department of Health
431 Munoz, Eric; Long Island Jewish Medical Center
436 Beckerman, Anita; College of New Rochelle (New York)
437 Joseph, Stephen; New York City Department of Health
463 Logsdon, Donald; INSURE Project (New York)
497 Young, James; University of Texas Health Science Center at San Antonio
501 Hawken, Patty; University of Texas Health Science Center at San Antonio
507 Sapp, Mary; Benedictine Health Resource Center (San Antonio)
510 Silver, George; Yale University
560 Salive, Marcel and Parkinson, Michael; Association of Preventive Medicine Residents
564 Schlegel, John; American Pharmaceutical Association
576 Owen, Jack; American Hospital Association
579 Shoults, Harold; The Salvation Army

583 McCarthy, Diane; Health Policy Agenda for the American People (Chicago)
589 Mundinger, Mary; Columbia University
599 Adams, Frederick; Connecticut Department of Health Services
612 Hunter, Paul; American Medical Student Association/Foundation
625 Goldstein, Bernard; University of Medicine and Dentistry of New Jersey, Robert Wood Johnson Medical School
628 Low, Lisa Kane; American College of Nurse-Midwives
633 Rosenfield, Allan; Columbia University
635 White, Francine; National Association of Community Health Centers
678 Arnold, Milton; American Academy of Pediatrics
690 Carr, Katherine; American College of Nurse-Midwives
694 Hagens, William; Washington State House of Representatives
717 Denno, Donna; University of Michigan
755 Blumenthal, Daniel; American Public Health Association, Medical Care Section
780 Sobel, David; The Permanente Medical Group
796 Black, Robert; Monterey, California

9. Health Promotion and Disease Prevention in Community Settings

Our world—and our neighborhoods—are instrumental in determining our health status. Education, access to services, family life, and work all play a role in shaping individual health and lifestyles. The kinds of health messages that people receive close to home, in their own "world," also are among the most influential in determining their health behaviors. Many witnesses, therefore, argued that interventions in schools, the workplace, and the community at large can be powerful tools in implementing the Year 2000 Health Objectives.

Many testifiers accepted this premise and focused some, if not all, of their proposed objectives on interventions within the school, the workplace, and other community settings. They addressed common health problems faced by people in these settings, as well as programs that have been implemented to deal with them.

In schools, for instance, the major immediate concerns are substance abuse, AIDS, and teen pregnancy, but testimony was also directed at the health-enhancing possibilities for education programs on nutrition, physical fitness, mental health, and general lifestyle awareness and skills to enhance behavioral change. On the worksite, the primary concerns are screening for chronic diseases and programs to deal with smoking, nutrition, and stress. In the community, testifiers paid special attention to programs aimed at substance abuse and the prevention of chronic diseases, and on ways to make them culturally relevant to the community they serve.

In addition to the needs and proposals specific to these three settings, a number of implementation issues cross the three areas, including the content of health education programs, financing issues, and the coordination of services. These are addressed at the end of the chapter.

HEALTH PROMOTION AND EDUCATION IN SCHOOLS

Many witnesses see both a great potential and a great need for school-based health promotion endeavors. Thirty-four of them focus their remarks on health education in schools, and another 135 mention the need for school-based health education interventions either in the context of a specific issue or in terms of special interventions for children and adolescents.

The American School Health Association (ASHA) presents a detailed analysis of the needs and opportunities for school health programs. Problems encountered in school-aged children include unhealthy lifestyles, chronic and episodic illnesses, emotional and behavioral problems, visual and hearing deficits, eating disorders, nutrition problems, teenage pregnancy, sexually transmitted diseases, and dental problems.

In the face of these problems, "the school, as a social structure, provides an educational setting in which the total health of the child during the impressionable years is a priority concern." No other setting approximates the magnitude of the school in terms of the number of children that can be reached. Thus, many witnesses see the school as a focal point for health planning in the community. (#196)

Given this orientation, the ASHA proposes specific objectives regarding

• periodic screening for hearing, vision and dental disorders; scoliosis; high blood pressure; and fitness levels;

• care and health promotion programs for students with chronic illnesses or problems;

• professional preparation and availability of school nurses;

• provision of primary health care clinics in schools;

• school breakfast and lunch programs;

• health education curriculum, class time, and the professional preparation of teachers;

• physical education programs and testing that emphasize cardiovascular fitness and lifetime sports;

• mental health programs that include the development of prosocial behaviors, stress management skills, and control of stress and violence;

• provision of worksite health promotion programs for faculty and staff and a healthful school environment. (#196)

Implementation of School-based Health Promotion

Testifiers feel that to meet many objectives, education must begin in the schools. However, school health programs need to be significantly improved if they are to serve this purpose. More comprehensive curricula are required, along with more hours spent on health education, better teacher training, and better availability of health professionals or health services to students. The involvement and support of parents are also viewed as critical to the success of many school-related activities.

Texas Commissioner of Education William Kirby writes:

> The public schools of America bear much of the burden to educate children about the physical, emotional, social and economic dangers of such health issues as drug abuse, school-age pregnancy, AIDS and smoking. We accept this responsibility, yet we know that the task is too great for education systems to bear alone. We are grateful to the federal government for its support in such programs as the Drug-Free Schools and Communities Act, to the Surgeon General for his comprehensive report on AIDS, and for federal funding to assist in the education of disadvantaged and handicapped children. We appreciate the philosophical and economic support and look forward to continued cooperation and coordination of education and health efforts among federal, state, and local governmental entities. We share a common goal—ensuring bright futures and long, healthy lives for our children. *(#305)*

Many testifiers suggest ways to improve the health education system so that it deals more successfully with adolescent health problems, including such far-ranging suggestions as environmental health issues; training in how to be an active and responsible medical consumer *(#105)*; issues of television exposure, "latchkey children," and homelessness *(#198)*; suicide prevention programs *(#500; #731)*; and art therapy and dance to deal with stress and to foster creativity *(#477; #595)*.

Underlying these specific programs is concern about the capability of elementary and secondary school faculty to teach health issues. Chet Bradley of the Wisconsin Department of Public Instruction writes:

I am convinced that unless a significant change in the professional preparation of elementary teachers in the area of health becomes a reality, the institutionalization of quality health instruction at the elementary level will never occur. I propose to you that the most meaningful and effective long-term approach toward successful school-based prevention and health promotion efforts for our young people is through an investment in outstanding teachers.

His testimony includes a proposal to train elementary school teachers to earn a three-year master's degree in elementary health education. *(#593)*

The American School Health Association supports Bradley's view and states that

> most health education is conducted by poorly trained, non-specialists who devote much less than the minimum of 50 hours necessary for success, and who see health education at the best as secondary to their primary functions. These teachers also are working without the benefits of the other components of a comprehensive school health program. Thus, school health education is generally a failure. *(#055)*

Some witnesses called for more use of tested and effective behavioral teaching models. According to the National Education Association:

> Attitudes and behavior are not changed by simple presentation of the facts—or by scare tactics. Regardless of race, creed, or socioeconomic status, young people believe in their own invulnerability—that "it" simply isn't going to happen to them. An effective preventive health curriculum must rationally counter this belief in invulnerability and build a youth culture that embraces healthful behavioral choices. *(#059)*

Similarly, Kenneth Kaminsky of the Wayne County Intermediate School District in Michigan writes that "the most successful programs today employ the social competency or 'life skills' model." This model emphasizes skill development in communication, assertiveness, resistance skills, peer selection, problem solving and decision making, critical thinking, making low-risk choices, self-improvement, and stress reduction skills. *(#426)* According to David Groves of Comerica Incorporated, "Social competency development programs emphasizing cognitive and social problem solving skills, perspective taking, and coping skills should be provided to all children as a part of their educational opportunities." *(#075)*

Williams argues that a comprehensive, preventive health curriculum in schools necessitates collaboration not only among "educators, parents, school boards, administrators, and communities," but also among teacher preparation institutions and the medical community. *(#059)* The effectiveness of a school health promotion and disease prevention program relies on the support of the entire community.

Community involvement is especially important when the more sensitive issues of AIDS education and school-based or school-linked reproductive health clinics for teenagers are addressed. Kirby emphasizes the need for local discretion in all health programming.

> We believe that where school-based clinics exist, they must be coordinated with existing health services and should be established and maintained to meet the specific needs and philosophy of the local community. It is imperative that school-based clinics be under the direct supervision of the campus administrator and that considerable flexibility be allowed at the local community level. Programs not supported by and congruent with local standards are not likely to be successful. *(#305)*

One problem with focusing on school-based programs, however, is that not all adolescents stay in school long enough to benefit from them.

> A large percentage of school age children are disenfranchised from the nation's schools. They are in jail, on the street, working, or on the run. Thus, the health objectives regarding school aged children are not realistic and lack sophistication. They have only focused on those children currently attending school or available to what is called "school site health education." *(#055)*

Specific Problems and Interventions

Much of the testimony on school health issues arose in the context of interventions in specific areas. Programs aimed at improving nutrition, physical fitness, and mental health, and also at preventing AIDS, teenage pregnancy, smoking, and other substance abuse were mentioned most frequently.

Nutrition. Testifiers proposed various nutrition objectives, many of which are designed to ensure both classroom education and cafeteria participation. Several witnesses also underlined the need for a nationwide monitoring system of school-age children's nutrition status; without this, setting objectives will be difficult. Many of those testifying about nutrition education referred to the Nutrition Education and Training (NET) Program, which came into being by an act of Congress in 1977. Its purpose is "to teach children the value of a nutritionally balanced diet through positive daily lunchroom experience and appropriate classroom reinforcement, to develop curricula and materials, and to train teachers and school food service personnel to implement nutrition education programs." *(#161)* Witnesses testified that this program should be supported and, in some cases, expanded.

Some testifiers, such as Carol Philipps representing the Midwest Region NET Program Coordinators, advocate "integrating nutrition concepts into other curricular areas as appropriate, for example biology, elementary language arts, mathematics, home economics, and social studies." *(#590)* Others place great emphasis on maintaining school lunch and breakfast programs and summer food programs in public and private schools. To actually maintain a nutritionally balanced diet, they argue, many children need school meals.

Physical Fitness. The discussion of physical fitness focuses on engaging children in vigorous health-fitness activity and on preparing children for healthy physical activity behaviors later in life. For instance, the American Alliance for Health, Physical Education, Recreation and Dance (AAHPERD) believes that thoroughly and appropriately integrating physical activity into one's life is possible only with a sound educational program as a starting point. *(#596)*

One of the current problems with physical education programs, according to Brian Sharkey of the University of Northern Colorado and others, is that physical fitness tests given to school children often dictate, at least in part, the content of the curriculum. Hence, it is important to select fitness tests that will lead to the desired behaviors. As an example, he cites the health-related fitness test developed by AAHPERD as being preferable to the athletic skills-related test of the President's Council on Physical Fitness and Sports (PCPFS). Unfortunately, he says, "well-meaning school teachers see the glitter and polish of the PCPFS award system" and forsake

AAHPERD's fitness test. This, Sharkey feels, prevents the establishment of a unified health-fitness related program in U.S. schools. *(#363)*

Others discuss the need to integrate physical education with other health-related programs. Guy Parcel of the University of Texas Health Science Center at Houston, for example, discusses a program called *Go For Health* that was designed to reduce cardiovascular risk factors in elementary school children. This program makes an organizational-level change in the school lunch and physical education programs to "create an environment supporting healthful diet and physical activity practices," which is then supplemented with classroom instruction and theory "consistent with the school environment."[1] *(#295)*

Charles Kuntzleman of Fitness Finders makes the argument that increasing the amount and time of current physical education programs as they now exist may not solve the problem of the poor physical condition of today's children. According to Kuntzleman, 75 percent of the time in a typical physical education class is spent on record keeping, roll call, listening to instructions, waiting to take a turn, and general management; only 25 percent of the child's time is devoted to motor activity. *(#121)*

Mental Health. Many witnesses stressed the necessity of providing mental as well as physical health education to children. Such programs can address a wide variety of issues ranging from stress management to the prevention of adolescent suicide.

The American School Health Association accents the pivotal role a school can play in fostering the mental health of a child and building skills for later life. The ASHA believes that stress management is an important part of a school health education curriculum. *(#196)*

Gaffney speaks of suicide and the potential of a teacher for identifying a suicidal child. She argues that "teachers are the children's first line of defense because they see behaviors before even parents do on occasion." *(#731)*

The school is also an important setting for dealing with problematic personality characteristics. Bruce Dohrenwend of Columbia University School of Public Health says that because problematic dispositions can be "laid down early in life," the school is a good place to provide "training and orientation toward mastery and control." *(#729)*

Family Planning and Reproductive Health. Many testifiers endorse the provision of family planning programs within the general school health curricula. They also agree that reproductive health or sex education should begin early in the school years. Testifiers acknowledge the sensitivity of these issues and recognize parental concerns, but most feel that ignorance of pregnancy and AIDS outweighs the concerns about sex education.

High teenage pregnancy rates indicate a failure of educational and service provision efforts, according to Deborah Bastien of Galveston, Texas. She underlines the disparity of adolescent pregnancy and abortion rates in the United States and in other industrialized countries, and concludes that the higher rates of both pregnancy and abortion here are due not to greater sexual activity but to lesser availability of contraceptive services and sex education. Despite this, "U.S. public policy still focuses on preventing sexual activity among teens." *(#236)* Sylvia Hacker of the University of Michigan supports this position: "Recognizing that adolescents are risk takers, espousing abstinence as the *only* choice will not work." Instead, she says, sex education could help adolescents realize that choices are possible in expressing one's sexuality, and intercourse is only one of them. *(#406)*

Jackie Rose of the Clackamas County Department of Human Services in Oregon suggests social motivations for teenage pregnancy: "We see teens for whom making a baby is one thing they can succeed in." To change these attitudes, she argues:

> We need comprehensive, coordinated teen-parent programs and teen pregnancy prevention programs to help them realize other options. We need to devise strategies to keep teens in school, for example, teaching teens and their families techniques for success and making available health services that minimize barriers to those services; that is make services available where the teens are—school-based health clinics. We need a goal to decrease the rate of repeat pregnancies during the teenage years. *(#343)*

When and how family planning education should begin, argues Susan Addiss of the Quinnipiack Valley Health District in Connecticut, are important questions. Even though "there is controversy about the content and timing of such education in communities around the country," Addiss urges "most strongly that an objective be developed with respect to some desired percentage of the nation's school systems having comprehensive family life education curricula in place by the year 2000." *(#460)*

The National Parents and Teachers Association also supports school-based sex education and says that because few parents actually discuss sex education, "schools and other public agencies and organizations must undertake this education." *(#578)* Similarly, Cathy Trostmann, a community school nurse in Texas, feels that sexuality education should begin in the first year of school and be presented at a level and in a manner that relates to the level of the child's development. She argues, however, that provisions be made for parents "to give their own instructions in the home with guidance provided by the school system," if they so desire. *(#302)*

The American School Health Association calls for school-based intervention programs to reduce not only teen pregnancy, but teen alcohol and substance abuse as well. According to ASHA, these programs must encompass more than just classroom education. The best way to decrease adolescent pregnancy and the incidence of sexually transmitted diseases among adolescents is to provide multiple channels: health and educational professionals, parents, and peers. The utilization of school-based clinics, school-linked clinics, and school- and community-based education programs is an example of an intervention that complements instruction and has been shown to be effective in reducing adolescent pregnancy. *(#232)*

Clinical services are a critical part of successful intervention programs for teenage reproductive health. As ASHA notes, in preliminary evaluation a few programs have shown dramatic efficacy in combatting teenage pregnancy.[2] It also cites studies that show widespread support for school-based clinics; the number of clinics across the United States has risen from 1 in 1970 to 120 in 1988.[3] *(#232)*

AIDS Education. Although the ideal content of AIDS education programs is controversial, most witnesses who address this issue call for aggressive school education. Wayne Teague of the Alabama Department of Education writes that when he was asked whether parents or the school system should decide the content of an AIDS education program, "I took the position that we do not give people an option for their children to commit suicide." *(#675)* However, although AIDS education is now mandatory

in Alabama state schools, across the nation—according to Ralph DiClemente of the University of California, San Francisco—few school systems currently provide AIDS education as part of a formal curriculum, and even fewer have evaluated program effectiveness. *(#273)*

DiClemente believes that AIDS prevention programs should "encourage health-promoting behaviors and eliminate or reduce high-risk sexual and drug behaviors. Adolescents cannot be coerced into changing behavior patterns." *(#273)*

AIDS education, however, is hampered by the lack of information on the epidemiology of behavior among at-risk groups. Lew Gilchrist of the University of Washington says that baseline information is lacking on the actual use of condoms among specific populations, including adolescents. To offer effective education, these programs must be grounded in an understanding of actual behaviors and attitudes in at-risk populations. *(#691)*

Smoking, Alcohol, and Substance Abuse. Some testifiers argue for early, school-based prevention activities for smoking, alcohol, and substance abuse. For example, according to the National Association of State Boards of Education:

> There should be a specific focus on alcohol and drugs beginning in the fourth grade and continuing until graduation. Providing accurate information is essential for a substance abuse prevention program. This includes knowledge about physiology, high-risk populations, high-risk situations, the actual prevalence of drug and alcohol use, family influence, peer pressure, stress, the role of the media, and cultural norms. *(#573)*

Kaminsky argues that students now view schools as the leading source of antidrug information. For this reason, schools must provide a program that can give adolescents information and influence healthy lifestyle behaviors. He outlines a program for substance abuse and lists as its components a grade-specific curriculum, in-service teacher training, counseling services for children, parent education programs, peer leadership and liaison work with community service providers, parent groups, and the media. *(#426)* Many of Kaminsky's components are reiterated by other testifiers, especially peer leadership and community-wide efforts.

HEALTH PROMOTION IN THE WORKPLACE

As the American Occupational Medical Association (AOMA) points out, virtually all the 1990 Objectives can be addressed effectively and efficiently in the workplace. Health problems having to do with "reproduction, child-rearing, immunization, mental health, substance abuse, hazard exposure, risk-taking, and self-destructive habits" are all appropriate and pertinent material for workplace health education and health promotion programs. *(#071)* Many other witnesses agree.

Business Roundtable spokesperson Paul Entmacher offers a sample list of health promotion programs to be found in businesses today which "amply demonstrates the extent that business health promotion activities are part of the nation's total effort." These include

- smoking cessation, general tobacco use abstention;
- coronary heart disease prevention, including nutrition education;
- stroke prevention and hypertension control;
- seat belt usage and auto crash injury prevention;
- diabetes screening and education;
- early identification and treatment of alcohol abuse;
- cocaine, heroin, and marijuana education and counseling;
- occupational safety standards and matching education;
- occupational toxicity education and control;
- weight control;
- physical fitness and exercise;
- cancer detection (cervical smears, mammography); and
- AIDS public education and worker counseling. *(#465)*

A survey of 48 companies by the Washington Business Group on Health identified the five priorities (and some reasons for them) among workplace health issues in the 1990s:

1. Detection of, and intervention against, *chronic diseases,* including cancer and heart disease (32 responses): because chronic diseases account for the bulk of health care expenditures and for considerable absenteeism and productivity losses. Although solutions require addressing multiple risks, chronic diseases are amenable to large-scale detection and prevention programs.

2. Reduction of *alcohol and drug abuse* (21 responses): because alcohol and drug abuse are a major source of health costs, absenteeism, and lost productivity; because abuse increases legal and security costs; and because abuse reduces the morale of coworkers.

3. Improvement of *mental health* (19 responses): because mental health costs continue to grow. Stress-related illnesses are becoming more prevalent and contribute to overall health costs; employee assistance programs at the worksite can be effective.

4. Control of *HIV infections and AIDS* (15 responses).

5. Prevention and control of *tobacco* use (14 responses): because no other single factor accounts for as much cost and loss of productivity.

Smaller numbers of respondents identified physical fitness (11 responses), maternal and infant health (8), occupational safety and health (8), maintaining health and quality of life in older people (8), nutrition (6), and other topics. *(#355)*

Many of those who addressed the question of worksite-based programs spoke of generic issues such as the need for comprehensive policies, the role of health professionals, and the special difficulties faced by small businesses. Others addressed specific activities, policies, and programs to deal primarily with smoking, nutrition, stress reduction, substance abuse, and physical fitness and exercise.

Implementation of Workplace-based Programs

Marilyn Rothert of Michigan State University targets three factors for developing a successful worksite health promotion program: (1) involvement of employees and management in the identification and development of all phases of the program; (2) expectation that successful programs will be sustained; and (3) working across populations and risk areas, and using multiple strategies. *(#394)*

Margo Gorchow of the Health Development Network at Botsford General Hospital in Michigan describes the problems encountered in a worksite risk reduction program at a General Motors plant.

To put up a poster announcing a smoking cessation program will not necessarily fill your classroom with eager, expectant students willing to give up smoking and pay money to do it. Offering free introductory sessions so groups can learn what the program is about does not necessarily make people want to give up a habit of eating potato chips, chocolate chip cookies, *et cetera.* Aggressive outreach and engagement strategies need to be developed and implemented, to reach out to the individuals, to raise their level of health awareness, and engage them in a program to support their own interests, rather than what we think is a good idea for their health, to make a lifestyle change. *(#386)*

Gorchow maintains that her program's success comes from keeping

a high profile of visibility, with our professional staff (R.N.s and R.D.s) periodically on the factory floor talking to employees and signing them up for risk reduction classes. This approach is working to engage the employees into a program as well as to provide follow up to assess their progress or relapse. There are on-site wellness coordinators at the plant as well. This proves to be an expensive, labor intensive approach. Still, in the first year of this study we were able to attract approximately 10 percent of the work force into behavior change programs. *(#386)*

A number of testifiers called for a comprehensive set of policies, interventions, and activities for work-site wellness. According to Rothert and others, these programs share three components: (1) employee education, (2) a knowledgeable and available health professional, and (3) incentives for sustained participation. *(#153; #394)*

For example, the Adolph Coors Company provides fairly complete wellness services to its employees, retirees, and their dependents. These include preventive dental coverage, smoking cessation programs, exercise programs, stress prevention programs, screening for high blood pressure, causes and solutions for low back pain, good nutrition, weight management, healthy pregnancy/prenatal awareness and education programs, and mammography screening for the company and the community. A cost benefit analysis of Coors' programs shows that for each dollar invested, the company can expect a return of $1.24 to $8.33. Max Morton, manager of the Coors Wellness Center, claims a high level of participation and success for the various programs. Morton underlines the need to reach production staff as well as management staff: "Our studies suggest a difference in where production and nonproduction workers get their health information. Production workers reported that the majority of their information comes from television, radios, and newspapers, in contrast to nonproduction workers information sources, which were their M.D.'s and our Wellness Center." *(#153)*

A similarly comprehensive health promotion program is being undertaken at Michigan State University. Rothert explains that its purpose is to "establish an institutional process to sustain health promotion as a broad-based commitment and component of the mission of Michigan State University and to develop a model of this process that can be deployed to other organizations." She adds, "Health habits can be contagious, and we are attempting to create a broad-based environment supportive of individual health promoting decisions." *(#394)*

Many testifiers who have or are developing work-site health promotion programs concluded that a knowledgeable health professional at the worksite is a necessity for success. For example, Pat Joseph, representing the American Association of Occupational Health Nurses, argues that workplace health education is most successful through occupational health nurses. "Approximately 75 percent of all occupational health nurses are the sole health care provider in the workplace," she says, and for this reason, they are "among the 'movers and shakers' in the activity to eliminate preventable disease and to promote optimum health in the workplace." *(#385)*

However, although a program under the direction of a health professional might be the ideal, it may be too expensive for most small businesses to staff and draft comprehensive workplace wellness programs. To overcome this difficulty, there are now a host of local business groups on health, community organizations, and coalitions that can aid small businesses. Companies, such as insurance providers, make programs available, and resources can be found that help provide at least some wellness information or services, according to witnesses.

Jack West, President of the Puro Corporation of America, illustrates what can be done. With 47 employees of his own, he argues that small businesses "can pick the low-hanging fruit" of employee health promotion programs. These are cheap interventions such as employee self-assessment questionnaires (at $12 per person), lunchtime cancer self-screening seminars, complimentary flu shots, a company newsletter on health and fitness, a company subscription to a local fitness club, and providing his company's product—bottled water—to pregnant employees or spouses. *(#734)*

The New York Business Group on Health, a not-for-profit coalition of nearly 300 organizations of which the Puro Corporation is a member, tries to help businesses obtain health information appropriate to the workplace. Its director, Leon Warshaw, says, "We have published a two-volume directory of available resources for health education/promotion and every issue of our bimonthly newsletter is replete with articles describing innovative and successful programs and capsule reviews of publications and educational materials suitable for use in the workplace." *(#448)*

Warshaw also talks about providing help and direction in the adaptability of projects.

One should remember that the work force is not a uniform population. Specific cohorts can be identified on the basis of age, sex, educational and ethnic backgrounds, health status, and disease predilections so that they can be targeted for specific programs. The economies of scale, ease of access, and the enhancing effects of peer pressure serve to increase the effectiveness of these programs. *(#448)*

Specific Problems and Interventions

As with school-based health promotion programs, many of those who testified on workplace wellness singled out specific health needs and programs that should be addressed effectively by employers. The most commonly mentioned programs involved screening for chronic diseases, smoking, stress reduction, and nutrition.

Screening for Chronic Diseases. Worksite screening for heart disease and cancer can be invaluable in identifying individuals at risk of developing either of these chronic diseases. Heart disease and cancer remain the two top killers in the United States despite the fact that, to a great extent, both can be prevented. As speaker Thomas Washam of the Aluminum Company of America (Alcoa) points out, worksite screening can save lives. For example, at Alcoa there are blood pressure monitoring programs and chronic health condition monitoring programs. These programs have found individuals who were in need of medical or surgical intervention, as well as individuals for whom better compliance with recommended medication was imperative. *(#307)*

The AOMA suggests as an objective that "90 percent of the Fortune 500 companies and 75 percent

of all employers with more than 100 employees should provide for on-site blood pressure screening and follow-up." Voluntary organizations, health care providers, and other organizations will have to assist employers that do not have their own assessment resources, AOMA adds. *(#071)*

Leslie VanDermeer, an occupational health nurse, says that "screening of total cholesterol levels should be made available to all employees who work in a company that has an on-site medical unit or nursing department." She argues that since the fingerstick method of measuring total serum cholesterol is "low cost, accurate and easily accessible," it would be "a scientifically sound and attainable goal for the year 2000 to have 100 percent of the worksites that contain employee health services offer this service." *(#217)*

Angelo Fosco, General President of the Laborers' International Union of North America, calls for making preventive services available through company-provided health plans. He suggests that these plans give particular emphasis to occupational diseases and work-related disorders, and that they be made available to retired workers as well. *(#586)*

Worksite screening for chronic conditions also can be useful in encouraging individual responsibility and coordinating other components of a worksite wellness program. Screening for cholesterol, high blood pressure, and breast cancer, for example, can help individuals to monitor their own health conditions. It also enhances the connection with other wellness programs for nutritional awareness, smoking cessation, physical fitness, and stress management. The Adolph Coors Company, in addition to blood pressure screening, cholesterol screening, and a cardiac rehabilitation program, provides a significant mammography screening program. The company has encouraged employees and their spouses to "spread the word" to the community that many breast cancer deaths can be avoided if detected early. Coors offers mammograms for $15 to all staff and dependents, and is now coordinating screening for the nearby community. *(#153)*

Smoking. Nonsmoking programs are the most frequently cited worksite interventions. Many large businesses in the United States are actively and effectively reducing smoking in the workplace. According to Alice Murtaugh of New York City, 36 percent of U.S. companies with 50 or more employees have smoking control activities.[4] *(#159)*

Charles Arnold, representing the Health Insurance

Association of America (HIAA), exhibited a step-by-step implementation plan as an example of what can be done for employers who want to reduce smoking among their employees. The manual entitled *Non-smoking in the Workplace: A Guide for Insurance Companies* is put out by HIAA and the American Council of Life Insurers, who have "resolved to make the provision of worksite smoking cessation programs a top priority for the employees of our industry." *(#440)*

Some in the business community are not content to limit their activities to the private sector, and address participation by the government, both as a regulator/lawmaker and as an employer. "More laws to ban smoking in the workplace must be enacted," says Murtaugh. *(#159)* However, Robert Rosner of the Smoking Policy Institute of Seattle adds, "Before the government can advise any other organization on the issue of smoking policy and cessation programs, it must get its own house in order." Although the government has made progress, Rosner says it still lacks consistent and comprehensive policies for its own employees and worksites. *(#349)*

Nutrition. Because of the link between nutrition and chronic disease, a number of testifiers described nutrition goals that would be appropriate for the workplace. Providing information about sodium, cholesterol, fats, and sugar in foods, and including cafeteria and other food providers in worksite nutrition programs were viewed as good policy. However, according to Marilyn Guthrie of the Virginia Mason Clinic in Seattle, "although there exists both professional and public awareness of nutrition's role in health, more concrete data on the cost versus benefit of initiating changes in eating patterns are needed to provide the impetus for more structured programs." *(#077)*

Loring Wood of NYNEX suggests combining nutrition and physical fitness objectives into a single objective to bolster the effect of education in the workplace. Specifically, he says that overweight, hypercholesterolemia, and exercise are closely related to each other and to cardiovascular risk. Thus, workplace initiatives that foster good nutritional guidelines in the cafeteria and at the same time actively encourage employees to exercise regularly either off site or in subsidized programs are likely to increase productivity, lower absenteeism, and help retain satisfied employees. Wood proposes that "by 2000, 25 percent of companies and institutions with more than

500 employees should actively encourage their employees to exercise regularly through subsidized programs or on their own time, and their cafeteria managers to be aware of and actively promote U.S. Department of Agriculture and Department of Health and Human Services dietary guidelines." *(#736)*

Stress Management. Stress management is also a common element in specific interventions suggested for the workplace. Because of its toll on productivity and the absenteeism stress produces, stress management has become a compelling health issue for the business community. James Henderson of Pacific Bell reiterates this: "Our fastest growing health care cost item is the price of stress and depression in Southern California." *(#761)* Harriette Zal of the Southern California Association of Occupational Health Nurses remarks, "It is predicted that 'stress' will be the occupational health disease of the 1990s." *(#230)*

As described in testimony, employer-sponsored programs for stress management can range from lunchtime classes to long-term education and relaxation classes. James Quick from the University of Texas at Arlington, representing the American Psychological Association, outlines how individual and organizational stress can be dealt with without causing "distress." He cites four basic components of a stress management program:

1. knowledge of what stress is, what causes it, and what constitutes the stress response;

2. knowledge of costs—"both individually and collectively"—of mismanaged stress;

3. familiarity with how to diagnose stress and its effects; and

4. knowledge of responsible individual and organizational prevention strategies that are beneficial in the management of stress. *(#176)*

Employee assistance programs (EAPs), which provide counseling services and resources for employees, are another work-based method of handling stress. The benefit of EAPs for employees is that it recognizes their total environment—in and out of work—as appropriate for interventions. As the AOMA says:

Such broad-based programs should provide the expertise to counsel on finances, parenting, interpersonal relations, marital discord, dislocation support, bereavement, AIDS, substance abuse, violent crime victimization, rape, etc. It is unlikely that many small businesses will have all counseling resources within their organization. Rather, the EAP counselor (whether contracted or employed, on- or off-site) should serve as an advisor and should guide employees to appropriate resources. *(#071)*

COMMUNITY-LEVEL INTERVENTIONS

More than 100 testifiers argue that behavior-related health problems—for individuals or entire populations—can be addressed most effectively through at least some degree of community-level intervention. Linda Randolph of the New York State Department of Health says that the increasing appreciation of "the role that communities play in supporting the individual" makes it necessary not only to empower individuals in the health arena, but to empower "communities as aggregates of individuals" as well. *(#177)*

As an organization with the resources necessary to provide support for community health plans, the New York State Department of Health has devised a five-step process that allows it to help communities "determine for themselves the means they will employ to realize optimal health" and to establish prevention interventions: (1) identify health problems, (2) determine the relative public health threat, (3) devise strategies to solve the problems, (4) implement strategies, and (5) evaluate the effectiveness of the strategies. *(#177)*

Other testifiers who outline community intervention strategies reiterate these five steps, perhaps using different terminology. Many argue that a key element of both devising and implementing prevention interventions is the realization that customs, mores, and socioeconomic status affect the health of individuals and communities. Effective programs, they say, must take these components into account.

Frank Bright of the Ohio Department of Health observes that "populations whose needs are being addressed should be brought into the planning process." Forcing an intervention upon a community from without or establishing an isolated intervention within an unsupportive community will not bring the same change in health status to that community as community-owned goals will. Bright says that community ownership of health objectives offers the potential of bringing necessary services into existing structures and making them acceptable to the population. *(#470)*

Most of those who testified about community interventions spoke about specific programs, but some addressed the opportunities that community-level programs offer to racial and ethnic minorities. Still others stressed the need to link community-level programs with wider efforts in society.

Specific Problems and Interventions

Witnesses mentioned a number of specific areas where community-level interventions are especially valuable. These areas include adolescent suicide and substance abuse, other adolescent issues, alcoholism, and the prevention of cardiovascular disease.

Problems of Adolescents. Robert Tonsberg, Director of the Wind River Health Promotion Program, reports that a community coalition to reduce adolescent suicide was developed when a series of suicides took place in the Wind River Indian Reservation in Washington State. In looking at the histories of the victims, it was found that there was a high incidence of substance abuse and depression among them. The Wind River Health Promotion Program approached this by developing stress-coping skills among young people and education programs for children and youth. The planners also decided to use the "Tupperware approach"—instead of having participants coming to them, they brought the services to the community. The program relies on community-based networking and on collaboration and coordination with community groups; schools; churches; and local, state, and federal organizations. It focuses on multiple targets for change and multiple strategies for intervention and evaluation. *(#711)*

In Seattle, a citywide program to provide education and services to urban children was developed with the aid of a survey distributed to adolescents in the city. Robert Aldrich of the University of Washington says that one of the most startling discoveries of this survey was "some very major differences between what kids thought and what the adults thought the kids thought." To deal with this, says Aldrich, "we put in place a kids' board, 30 teenagers who report to the mayor and who, with the officials of the city and the private sectors began to deal with each of the issues that have been brought up by the kids, and some we thought of ourselves." Aldrich also points out that this Kids' Place program is not a medical intervention program. Instead, it is "more socially driven so that the primary things that are being dealt with are things like housing, and facilitating a day-care system." Aldrich urges others who might be interested in organizing similar programs to conduct a citywide survey and then plan strategies around the results. *(#689)*

Alcohol-related Problems. Al Wright of the Los Angeles County Department of Health Services describes a county-level alcohol intervention program that supports "the prevention of, intervention in, and recovery from alcohol-related problems that occur at the individual, family, and community levels as a result of the relationship between alcohol, drinkers, and the environment." Among the strategies for primary, secondary, and tertiary interventions, Wright includes an "environmental approach to community-level prevention of alcohol problems," that is a counterattack on the social components of drinking. He lists price, product, place, and promotion as four areas in which there are industrial and societal pressures to drink. Los Angeles County's intervention program has developed four countermeasures: taxes, alternative beverages, planning/zoning, and norms/policies. Wright's testimony illustrates that through coordinated activities, social habits can be changed. *(#229)*

Cardiovascular Problems. Adrian Ostfeld of Yale University describes a statewide hypertension control program that was implemented with good results in Connecticut. After the organizers carried out a statewide survey of both health consumers and health providers in 1978, they decided to focus their efforts on controlling high blood pressure and reducing lifestyle-related risk factors, especially in younger men whose problems were more severe. They sought and received the cooperation of physicians, other health professionals, and provider agencies such as neighborhood health centers, public and private nursing agencies, the Red Cross, and family planning agencies. After four years, noticeable changes occurred in two areas. First, physicians and other health professionals became more active in screening for hypertension and helping their clients control it. Second, many residents of Connecticut reduced their behavioral risk factors for heart disease, including smoking and the consumption of salt and fat. *(#459)*

For Raymond Bahr of St. Agnes Hospital in Baltimore, Maryland, active participation of the community hospital is essential in a community program to prevent heart attacks. To enhance the link between early cardiac care and the community, Bahr says, "it is going to become important for each community hospital to have a coronary care system that moves into the community with educational programs focusing on chest pain and providing an early cardiac care center in the hospital." Bahr emphasizes the hospital's responsibility in this program.

> Coronary care is a community problem because a significant number of sudden deaths and myocardial infarctions take place in this environment. Before entering the hospital coronary care system, the public must interact with the emergency care delivery system as well as with the hospital emergency room. The ultimate fate of the community depends on the quality and effort available in these areas. *(#511)*

Bahr's plan also includes strategies for informing the community at large. He argues that people must be instructed in cardiopulmonary resuscitation and must recognize the early warning signs of a heart attack. "But what is more important," he argues, "is developing the concept of having an 'executive person' in each family to deal with the chest pain patient who is experiencing procrastination and denial of the heart attack." Bahr also targets high school education as an appropriate vehicle for teaching that late entry into care causes sudden cardiac deaths. *(#511)*

Racial and Ethnic Minorities

Because of the importance of culturally related health knowledge and attitudes, as described in Chapter 6, community-level intervention is thought to be an especially effective way to implement health promotion and disease prevention programs.

The Hispanic Agenda in Colorado, described by Rita Barreras of the Colorado Department of Social Services, is one such program that aims to develop community health objectives and programs for the Hispanic community. Its premise is that the responsibility "to insure that there is a coordinated, integrated and systematic approach to positive change" lies with the Hispanic community itself. *(#243)*

The steering committee for the Hispanic Agenda acted as impetus for the community-wide goal-setting process. It first identified eight component areas: education, higher education, labor and employment, economic development, housing and neighborhood, health and human services, political participation and leadership, and media. Next, experts were invited to submit papers and to draft goals for these eight component areas. Finally, criteria were developed to help planners identify and assess issues and strategies. *(#243)*

Margaret Hargreaves and her colleagues at Meharry Medical College's Cancer Control Research

Unit describe several cancer prevention strategies being undertaken by Meharry, Morehouse, and Drew universities for the Black community. Their awareness program

> aims to improve cancer knowledge of Blacks in the three consortium cities by developing a program to ensure the diffusion of cancer information throughout the community. The strategy will employ community organization, mass media, and personal contacts. The program will be provided through churches, worksites, and the community-at-large. (#615)

Hargreaves stresses the need to develop strategies that are culturally specific to the Black community.

> Blacks have been reported to exhibit a particular pattern in availing themselves of health care, delaying in utilization of the traditional health care system, and relying upon family, friends, and even spiritualists and healers during critical stresses in their lives. Such delays are compounded by medical care expenses that they are unprepared to meet. With their unique value systems and problems of access, it is apparent that different health promotion strategies should be used to reach Blacks. (#615)

Mario Orlandi of the American Health Foundation emphasizes the importance of designing substance abuse community intervention programs that are "culturally relevant and that address specific sociocultural barriers to effective cross-cultural program dissemination." He also notes, however, the need for more data and research studies in these communities. In an evaluation of two community intervention approaches and their applicability to minority cultures, Orlandi found difficulties and gaps in assessing the substance abuse intervention needs of Blacks, Mexican-Americans, Asian Americans, and Native Americans. For all four of these groups, he cites a lack of basic research or intervention development research projects. For Blacks, compared to other groups, although there have been a number of research studies on substance abuse, Orlandi argues that "despite this accumulated body of research, the relevant understanding of Black substance abuse is lacking," and especially absent are "the appropriate information and insight necessary to design effective preventive interventions for this population. The lack of systematic, longitudinal, multivariate studies, and

the failure to employ ethnographic and other culturally-sensitive data collection procedures also has impeded progress." Orlandi concludes that the problem is not that preventive innovations are not available for planners trying to develop programs for minority populations, but rather that "programs are not available that fulfill both criteria: demonstrated efficacy and cultural relevance for particular minority or ethnic groups." (#167)

Linking Community-level Programs with Larger Efforts

A number of testifiers argue the necessity of linking community intervention programs with wider state, regional, and national health goals. The importance of networks, linkages, broad-based support, and above all, mass communication should not be ignored.

Woodrow Myers of the Indiana State Board of Health says that state health departments have a role to play in helping communities link themselves "to statewide solutions that affect other communities' problems and ultimately to national solutions, whether private or public, to address those needs." Myers describes several injury prevention programs that Indiana has undertaken, which involve both government and community components. Two examples are the Hoosiers for Safety Belts program and the Indiana Poison Control Center. The first is a statewide nonprofit coalition of private citizens, professional groups, service clubs, corporations, public agencies, and trade associations. The second program is a regional center dedicated to the prevention and treatment of poisoning. The center maintains a 24-hour, toll-free poison information line to inform citizens about household products, chemicals, pharmaceuticals, and live plants that may be poisonous. In both these interventions, the communities and the state share common goals to increase the use of safety belts and to provide statewide poison control services. (#405)

In some cases, the resources for health promotion and disease prevention programs are already available, but poorly coordinated. For example, writing about adolescent health problems, Claire Brindis and Phillip Lee of the Institute for Health Policy Studies at the University of California, San Francisco note that "categorical programs that have followed traditional patterns and focused on a single aspect of an issue—family planning, drug abuse, counseling—have had limited success." Only a small portion of the adolescent population has responded to this categorical, medical-model approach. "Communities need to work toward comprehensive and coordinated services," according to Brindis and Lee. This means making health education, social services, and job-related services available in the same place, with combined funding from public and private sources, and conducting rigorous evaluation to document success or failure and to move away from policies and programs that are not effective. "This comprehensive approach increases the efficiency of currently available community resources; facilitates the formation of linkages among a variety of concerned groups, such as parents, religious organizations, service clubs, clinics and social service agencies; and spreads funding responsibilities among several concerned parties." *(#027)*

Karil Klingbeil of the University of Washington recognizes that community-level education, counseling, and services are very important for reducing violence but calls for national-level activity, as well. Klingbeil recommends six secondary prevention steps that would be national in scope:

1. implementation of a national family violence prevention week;

2. "major media campaigns utilizing billboards, newspapers, radios, buses and other public vehicles, that can be used by public and private agencies";

3. development and implementation of legislation on all forms of abuse;

4. mandated "training and education on all aspects of family violence in all professional schools and cross-training in substance abuse and alcohol";

5. "innovative approaches to interviewing and interrogating child as well as adult victims";

6. "establishment of cross-agency committees or boards whose sole purpose it is to alleviate system barriers for victims as well as the offender groups." *(#697)*

The array of lifestyle choices offered to individuals in today's society and the conflicting information available in the media about what constitutes healthy behavior lead some testifiers to target communication channels in their intervention programs.

The National Council on Alcoholism, for instance, discusses the need to look at alcohol problems as social, as well as individual, problems. Thus, there should be process objectives for each objective on "public and community education based on the principles of sound educational theory and mass media communication." According to the council, "The alcohol and beverage industry spends two billion dollars a year on alcohol marketing that encourages and glamorizes drinking and associates alcohol use with maturity, success, sexuality, and high-risk activities." To counter this, it recommends that broadcasters "grant equivalent air time for health and safety messages about alcohol." *(#467)*

Ruth Roemer of the UCLA School of Public Health states that the most effective legislative measures to reduce smoking are "(1) banning all advertising and promotion of tobacco products, and (2) raising the taxes on and prices of tobacco products very substantially."

> Government has an obligation to protect the health of the people, and a ban on advertising would promote the social norm of a nonsmoking society. It would counter the negative consequences of advertising, which are especially pernicious in influencing young people to smoke. *(#184)*

The American Medical Association calls for responsibility in the media. The AMA believes that the media can be of "inestimable value" in attaining objectives, but that to do a responsible job, the medical community and the federal agencies must provide them with factual data. The AMA notes that the media have made a "cooperative effort at banning or otherwise censoring counterproductive advertising and promotional practices that are harmful to the public's health." *(#095)*

CROSSCUTTING IMPLEMENTATION ISSUES

Michael Eriksen, representing the Society for Public Health Education, writes:

> As part of the effort to assure quality of health promotion interventions, it is important to remember that not all interventions should concentrate solely on the individual. In fact, often the most effective health promotion interventions are those directed at the changes in the behaviors of providers, environments, and systems. Organizational change is inherent in the definition of health promotion and should be considered an integral component. *(#309)*

A number of implementation issues are common to interventions proposed for schools, workplaces, and communities. Suggestions were made about the content of health promotion and education programs, their financing, and the coordination of available services.

Content of Health Promotion and Education Programs

Recognizing the importance of health promotion activities in nonmedical settings, many witnesses had suggestions about defining the scope and content of such programs. Sunny Chiu of the Michigan Department of Public Health, for instance, calls for (1) clearly defined policies, priorities, and strategies for health promotion; (2) scientific data and the opportunities to apply them through program planning and implementation; (3) the tools and resources for practitioners and the community; and (4) the information, educational processes, and a combination of motivational and supporting forces for behavioral change—both individual and collective—aimed at reducing preventable morbidity and mortality. *(#395)*

The National Education Association suggests that health education focus on "life-enhancing" behaviors. According to Williams, "Our nation's schools must put into place health education programs that engage students, ensure that they understand the scientific and medical facts, and motivate them to choose appropriate behavior." Education must motivate young people to adopt healthful, life-saving behavior. *(#059)*

According to the American School Health Association:

> The health education curriculum needs to be comprehensive and not content-specific or narrowly targeted. It should work to motivate health maintenance and promote wellness and not merely to prevent physical illness. In order to do this, it must possess the following characteristics: its activities should develop effective decision-making skills; it must be well-planned, sequential, and based upon the student's health needs and interests as they relate to national and local community health priorities; it must focus on health attitudes and feelings, as well as behaviors and practices; it must integrate all dimensions of human health and not focus only on the physical; it needs specific goals and objectives in addition to effective formative and summative evaluation procedures; it requires effective management and sufficient resources. *(#055)*

Igoe writes that "despite increasing pressure to participate in the management of their own health, consumers of all ages are often unable or unwilling to do so." Research shows, she says, that those people who strive for mastery over their own health needs and who are prepared to deal assertively with health professionals usually obtain the best health care. To overcome consumer passivity and conversational barriers between the health professional and the consumer, Igoe stresses self-responsibility and autonomy. Consumers must learn to approach health care as a "problem-solving endeavor that requires an active coping effort, rather than as a situation calling for passivity and submission." She suggests objectives to integrate "consumer activism" education into all school curricula, including medical schools; to make it a responsibility of state health implementation programs to provide public service materials for consumer activism; and to do more research and survey work on outcomes of consumer activism. *(#105)*

Charles Lange of Loyola University says that one of the greatest obstacles to improving health is the lack of understanding by the general public of science, its methods, and its accomplishments. Unless the general public becomes more conversant with science, Lange feels, the achievement of the health objectives will be impossible. *(#707)*

Financing Health Promotion and Health Education

Health promotion and health education programs often fall outside of the common fee-for-service medical system and, therefore, are especially difficult to finance. Witnesses addressed this issue in the context of schools, worksites, insurance companies, and the media.

William Kirby, the Texas Commissioner of Education, says that "health services and health education are critical components of the public school program." However,

> no education funds are specifically earmarked in the state budget for health services. Competition is steep for the funds that are provided in the form of general state aid to school districts, which must use those limited funds to meet the costly mandates of salaries, instructional provisions, and special programs as well as requirements for health services. With the exception of drug abuse education, no additional funding has been allotted to local school districts to help them meet these responsibilities. Those in the legislative and health arenas must understand that education cannot continue to be expected to provide services and health-related instruction

without some financial support. *(#305)*

Gorchow feels that financial support for health promotion must be sought from the private as well as the public sector. The insurance model in the United States has always been based on providing illness coverage rather than wellness coverage. With worksite-based intervention and education about prevention and management of chronic problems, it is possible to reduce the burden of illness on the individual as well as on the reimbursement systems. *(#386)*

Individuals should be encouraged to take responsibility for adopting and maintaining healthy lifestyles, says Jeannette Merijanian of the University of Montevallo. To do this, they need motivation to change their lifestyles, information on what and how to change, and support. Thus, "national resources and knowledge" should be linked together "with local organizations to promote, educate, and support citizens who want to improve their own health status." This will require insurance reimbursements for lifestyle changes and funding for health education programs, she says. Insurance reimbursements could be made either on self-reporting data or on quantifiable health changes, such as lower blood cholesterol and cessation or absence of smoking. *(#644)*

Kenneth Warner of the University of Michigan addresses the question of financing advertising efforts.

Television has aired one shocking documentary after another on drugs, while magazines have repeatedly featured the grim and stark imagery of crack and smack on their covers. Their *front* covers, that is; the back covers feature attractive, glossy ads for cigarettes and alcoholic beverages. The effect of this media hype is that teenagers believe that illegal drugs are the principal source of premature death in our society, while in fact cigarettes kill as many Americans in a single day as cocaine does in a year. We need a professionally designed paid broadcast media advertising campaign against tobacco use and alcohol misuse.

According to Warner, the hundreds of millions of dollars required for such an effort could not be raised voluntarily. One solution is to increase the excise taxes on cigarettes and alcohol to pay for the campaign. As little as one cent per pack of cigarettes would raise $300 million, he says, and the tax itself would reduce the demand for tobacco, especially among younger people.[5] *(#429)*

REFERENCES

1. Parcel GS, Simons-Morton BG, O'Hara NM, et al.: School promotion of healthful diet and exercise behavior: An integration of organizational change and social learning theory interventions. J Sch Health 57(4):150–156, 1987

2. Lovick SR, Wesson WF: School Based Clinics: Update. Washington, D.C.: Center for Population Options, 1986

3. Lovick SR: School-based clinics: Meeting teens' health care needs. J Sch Health 58(9):379–381, 1988

4. U.S. Department of Health and Human Services: National Survey of Worksite Health Promotion Activities: A Summary. Office of Disease Prevention and Health Promotion, 1987

5. Warner KE: Selling health: A media campaign against tobacco. J Pub Health Policy 7(4):434–439, 1986

TESTIFIERS CITED IN CHAPTER 9

027 Brindis, Claire and Lee, Phillip; University of California, San Francisco
055 Eberst, Richard; Adelphi University (Long Island)
059 Williams, James; National Education Association, Health Information Network
071 Givens, Austin; American Occupational Medical Association

075 Groves, David; Comerica Incorporated (Detroit)
077 Guthrie, Marilyn; Virginia Mason Clinic (Seattle)
095 Hendee, William; American Medical Association
105 Igoe, Judith; University of Colorado Health Sciences Center
121 Kuntzleman, Charles; Fitness Finders (Spring Arbor, Michigan)
153 Morton, Max; Adolph Coors Company
159 Murtaugh, Alice; New York
161 Neill, Carol; Alum Rock Union Elementary School District (California)
167 Orlandi, Mario; American Health Foundation
176 Quick, James; University of Texas at Arlington
177 Randolph, Linda; New York State Department of Health
184 Roemer, Ruth; University of California, Los Angeles
196 Seffrin, John, Allensworth, Diane, Eberst, Richard, et al.; American School Health Association
198 Sheps, Cecil; American Public Health Association
217 VanDermeer, Leslie; Hunter College (New York)
229 Wright, Al; County of Los Angeles Department of Health Services
230 Zal, Harriette; Southern California Association of Occupational Health Nurses
232 Allensworth, Diane; American School Health Association
236 Bastien, Deborah; Galveston, Texas
243 Barreras, Rita; Colorado Department of Social Services
273 DiClemente, Ralph; University of California, San Francisco
295 Parcel, Guy; University of Texas Health Science Center at Houston
302 Trostmann, Cathy; Houston, Texas
305 Kirby, William; Texas Commission on Education
307 Washam, W. Thomas; Aluminum Company of America
309 Eriksen, Michael; University of Texas Health Science Center at Houston
343 Rose, Jackie; Clackamas County Department of Human Services (Oregon)
349 Rosner, Robert; Smoking Policy Institute (Seattle)
355 Jacobson, Miriam; Washington Business Group on Health
363 Sharkey, Brian; University of Northern Colorado
385 Joseph, Pat; United States Air Force, Lowry Air Force Base, Denver
386 Gorchow, Margo; Botsford General Hospital (Farmington Hills, Michigan)
394 Rothert, Marilyn; Michigan State University
395 Chiu, Sunny; Michigan Department of Public Health
405 Myers, Jr., Woodrow; Indiana State Board of Health
406 Hacker, Sylvia; University of Michigan
426 Kaminsky, Kenneth; Wayne County Intermediate School District (Michigan)
429 Warner, Kenneth; University of Michigan
440 Arnold, Charles; Metropolitan Life Insurance Company
448 Warshaw, Leon; New York Business Group on Health
459 Ostfeld, Adrian; Yale University
460 Addiss, Susan; Quinnipiack Valley Health District (Connecticut)
465 Entmacher, Paul; Metropolitan Life Insurance Company
467 Aguirre-Molina, Marilyn and Lubinski, Christine; National Council on Alcoholism
470 Bright, Frank; Ohio Department of Health
477 Speert, Ellen; American Art Therapy Association
500 Medrano, Martha; University of Texas Health Science Center at San Antonio
511 Bahr, Raymond; St. Agnes Hospital (Baltimore)
573 Wilhoit, Gene; National Association of State Boards of Education
578 McGuire, Judi and Crowder, Aletha; The National PTA
586 Fosco, Angelo; Laborers' International Union of North America
590 Philipps, Carol; Wisconsin Department of Public Instruction

593 Bradley, Chet; Wisconsin Department of Public Instruction
595 Leventhal, Marcia; New York University and BrooksSchmitz, Nancy; Columbia University
596 Perry, Jean; American Alliance for Health, Physical Education, Recreation and Dance
615 Hargreaves, Margaret, et al.; Meharry Medical College
644 Merijanian, Jeanette; University of Montevallo (Montevallo, Alabama)
675 Teague, Wayne; Alabama Department of Education
689 Aldrich, Robert; University of Washington
691 Gilchrist, Lew; University of Washington
697 Klingbeil, Karil; University of Washington
707 Lange, Charles; Loyola University (Chicago)
711 Tonsberg, Robert; Indian Health Service/Wind River Indian Reservation (Fort Washakie, Wyoming)
729 Dohrenwend, Bruce; Columbia University
731 Gaffney, Donna; Columbia University
734 West, Jack; Puro Corporation of America (Maspeth, New York)
736 Wood, Loring; NYNEX Corporation
761 Henderson, James; Pacific Bell

10. Tobacco

By 1985, the midpoint in the 1990 Objectives process, it appeared that 12 of the 13 smoking objectives for which data were available would be met. Clearly, during the 1980s, the United States made progress in reducing smoking among all groups of Americans— except teenage girls.[1] Yet according to those testifying on the Year 2000 Health Objectives, much needs to be done: 19 individuals concentrated primarily on the issue of smoking, and 31 others included smoking as a major part of their testimony. Many others mentioned it in their discussion of chronic diseases and other issues.

Most witnesses agreed that cigarette smoking is the single most important preventable cause of death in our society and that efforts to reduce tobacco consumption will result in improved health. Each year, about 390,000 Americans die of tobacco-caused cancer, coronary heart disease, chronic obstructive lung disease, and other diseases.[2] Disease outcomes associated with the use of cigarettes include lung, laryngeal, esophageal, bladder, and pancreatic cancer; chronic obstructive lung disease; atherosclerosis, coronary heart disease, cerebrovascular disease, and myocardial infarction. (#002) However, according to Woodrow Myers, Commissioner of the Indiana State Board of Health, smoking habits are difficult to change because they involve not only personal habits and addictions, but also political will. (#405)

Many testifiers concentrated their remarks on the need to direct future objectives toward helping those groups who still have relatively high smoking rates, whose rates of smoking are increasing, or at whom tobacco advertising is directed. In addition to teenage girls, testifiers identified prime target populations as adolescents in general (see also Chapter 4); pregnant women; ethnic minorities, including Blacks, Hispanics, and Native Americans (see Chapter 6 for a more thorough discussion of racial and ethnic minorities); and the economically disadvantaged. Education, political action, and both local and federal legislation were identified most often as the avenues for reaching these audiences.

The potential for reaching large numbers of smokers through the workplace also received considerable attention from testifiers, as did the increased use of smokeless tobacco, which was not even addressed in the 1990 Objectives.

ADOLESCENT SMOKING

Gabrielle Acampora of the Greater New York Association of Occupational Health Nurses explains, and others agree, that adolescents, especially Black adolescents and those in lower socioeconomic groups, are more likely than others to initiate smoking and resist cessation. (#002) Kenneth Kaminsky of the Wayne County Intermediate School District in Michigan reports that nearly one-fifth of high school seniors are daily smokers and more convert from occasional to regular smokers in the years after high school.[3] He also notes that research and surveys indicate that smoking has increased especially among teenage girls. (#426) Surveys also tell us, according to Kenneth Warner of the University of Michigan, that teenagers believe illegal drugs to be the principal cause of premature death in our society, whereas in fact, cigarettes kill as many Americans in a single day as cocaine does in a year. (#429) The American Academy of Pediatrics says that more than 30 percent of high school seniors do not believe that a great health risk is associated with smoking.[4] (#115)

The early- to mid-teen years are important because smoking behavior tends to be formed (or avoided) during this period and retained over the life course. (#419) According to Diane Allensworth, the American School Health Association (ASHA) suggests that the 1990 objective about adolescent smoking be retained, namely, that "the proportion of children and youth aged 12 to 18 who smoke (or use tobacco products) should be reduced to below 6 percent." (#005) To help accomplish this by the year 2000, the ASHA proposes process objectives for kindergarten through twelfth grade for health education, teacher training, and "interventions that combine and coordinate multiple forces of the community with those of the school." (#005) It further suggests that schools ban all smoking by students and teachers. Acampora says that "by 2000, 85 percent of adolescents aged 15–18 should be able to state that they perceive great risk associated with frequent, regular cigarette smoking." (#002) Particularly important, because it is very difficult to unlearn addictive behavior, is the development of good smoking education programs early in life that involve not only families but also schools. As Harriette Zal of the Southern California

Association of Occupational Health Nurses mentions, the challenge is in developing programs that address "assertion skills, increasing self-control and self-esteem, and learning to cope with stress without drugs." *(#230)*

Kaminsky further recommends that "by the year 2000, students who enter elementary school in 1988 be smoke-free" and that "advertising for tobacco be banned." *(#426)* Furthermore, to help control the availability of tobacco to minors, Acampora suggests that "by 2000, 50 states have legislation restricting sale or distribution of tobacco products to minors." *(#002)*

The problem of smoking among working youth also was perceived as requiring attention. Acampora proposes that "by 2000 at least 40 percent of workers aged 15–18 years should be offered smoking education and smoking cessation programs." Those who drop out of school and then work in small enterprises without health programs might be reached by peer group teens trained as health educators, by occupational health nurses in outreach vans traveling to worksites, or by community agencies. *(#002)*

SMOKING AND PREGNANCY

Cigarette smoking is the most common drug addiction during pregnancy. It is associated with fetal growth retardation, premature delivery, and low birth weight. Those who testified on this issue were concerned with the limited amount of available data on the number of women who smoke during pregnancy. Data that do exist apparently show an increase in the last decade in the number of women smokers in the unmarried, under-24 age group. Data exist for married women, but collecting data on unmarried, especially young, women is also important because this subset may have more difficulty in quitting. Moreover, say Robert Welch and Robert Sokol of the Hutzel Hospital in Detroit and Wayne State University, "while public education appears to be reaching the married, over 24-year-old age group, we do not seem to be communicating the No Smoking message as well to the under-25-year olds." *(#421)*

Richard Windsor of the University of Alabama at Birmingham adds that "universal use of available smoking cessation methods by nurses, physicians, and patient educators in obstetrical settings, all of which need little adaptation or revision for different practice settings, has the potential to produce an additional 100,000 pregnant women quitting in the United States each year. This represents 10 percent of the total of

approximately 1,000,000 pregnant smokers."[5] *(#267)*

Welch and Sokol, who also spoke on behalf of the American College of Obstetricians and Gynecologists, propose as an objective that "by the year 2000, the prevalence of cigarette smoking in pregnant women be one half that of the U. S. population or approximately 12 percent, 50 percent below the projected 1990 level, with needed focus on educating the under 24-year-old age group about the hazards of smoking in pregnancy." *(#421)* Terry duPont of the American Association for Respiratory Care suggests that "the proportion of women who smoke during pregnancy should be no greater than 25 percent of women who smoke overall." *(#054)* Windsor suggests a revision to the 1990 objective on teaching smoking cessation to pregnant women, namely, that "by 1995, at least 80 percent of all pregnant women will be taught smoking cessation skills to quit or significantly reduce their intake." *(#267)*

WORKSITE SMOKING

Worksite smoking and the effect of passive smoking on workers who do not smoke were of particular interest to many testifiers. Alice Murtaugh of New York City emphasizes the concern of many others that nonsmokers, by common law, have the right to a safe and healthy workplace. *(#159)* Some testifiers felt that the 1990 Objectives paid too little attention to worksite health promotion. Murtaugh sees the problem as one that goes well beyond a simple question of whether or not workers should be allowed to smoke.

> In allowing people to smoke in the workplace, we are encouraging a basically healthy segment of the population to destroy their health. As we have recently observed, they are not only ruining their own health, but also the health of their families and coworkers. Since most adults spend a fourth of their time at work, smoke in the workplace is a serious problem for many individuals. A worker with a smoking habit will not only affect the health of his coworker, but may be responsible for the habit continuing into a new generation. *(#159)*

Loring Wood of the NYNEX Corporation says that "a strong workplace smoking policy delivers a clear message, and when this is combined with smoking hazard awareness publicity to employees, and the offering of smoking cessation programs on or off premises, this achieves reduction in numbers and intensity of smokers." *(#736)* Robert Rosner of the Smoking Policy Institute in Washington state says that Pacific Northwest Bell's stringent no smoking policy improved employee morale, improved the work environment, and most important, led to increased smoking cessation. He reports that "smoking policies have a positive impact on both the participation and success levels of company-sponsored smoking cessation programs. This has a great potential for impact on the smoking and health objectives for the nation." *(#349)*

Many specific worksite outcome objectives were suggested. Some call for a basic but far-reaching objective such as "a smoke-free workplace for every individual," a goal thought by some testifiers to be possible in view of recent reports on smokers' opinions, health findings, local legislation, and the growing pattern of smoke-free policies in a wide range of companies. *(#159)* Others suggest very specific objectives, for example, that worksite health promotion programs which include smoking cessation be present in 75 percent of the Fortune 500 companies and for 75 percent of government workers by the year 2000. *(#712)* Wood further recommends that the 1990 objective pertaining to employer/employee sponsored or supported smoking cessation programs at the worksite be changed to include that "35 percent of all businesses with more than 500 employees have smoking policies in place that ban smoking at all work stations, including private offices, whether or not they provide alternative smoking areas on site. In addition, 70 percent of employees of such businesses should have been offered smoking cessation programs by their employers by the year 2000." Wood adds that a national survey of worksite health promotion, which includes smoking in the workplace and data on access to smoking cessation programs, is necessary. *(#736)* Murtaugh confirms that many companies have recently implemented policies without studying their effects on smoking habits. *(#159)*

Some testifiers feel that health care facilities have a special responsibility to set examples as nonsmoking worksites. According to the National Hospitals Tobacco Policy Survey, conducted by the American Lung Association of Lancaster County and the Pennsylvania Academy of Family Physicians, 93.6 percent of responding hospitals agreed that they have a responsibility to discourage tobacco smoking within their physical confines. Yet only 5.3 percent were considered "smoke free," according to Terry duPont. She recommends that by the year 2000, 75 percent of

all health care facilities be smoke free and 100 percent have smoking policies in place. *(#054)* More emphasis also should be placed on training physicians to counsel patients against smoking, according to Robert Van Citters of the University of Washington. *(#779)*

SMOKELESS TOBACCO

Smokeless tobacco was not addressed in the 1990 Objectives. Moon Chen of Ohio State University says that this omission is not surprising because the resurgence in the use of smokeless tobacco is a recent phenomenon.[6] *(#039)* Conan Davis of the Alabama Department of Public Health explains, and others agree, that "scientific evidence is strong that the use of smokeless tobacco can cause cancer in humans. The association between smokeless tobacco use and cancer is strongest for cancers of the oral cavity."[7] *(#249)* Myers says that smokeless tobacco use also is associated with stained teeth, bad breath, tooth abrasion, leukoplakia, gingival recession, and bone loss. *(#405)* Data show that smokeless tobacco has made serious inroads among young people—primarily among males and particularly in the South. *(#419)* Myers mentions that among certain groups, children as young as kindergarten age are trying and using smokeless tobacco and that most youth who use it become regular users by the time they are 12 years old. *(#405)* Bernard Turnock of the Illinois Department of Public Health mentions a 1987 survey in Illinois schools which revealed that of the eleventh grade males in rural areas, 28 percent used smokeless tobacco and 28 percent smoked cigarettes. *(#215)*

Education in this area is important, according to Myers. *(#405)* Davis explains that attempts to reverse this increase must counter peer pressure, the influence of the media and advertising, endorsements by athletes and celebrities, the ease of obtaining and using smokeless tobacco, and the widespread misconception that it is safer than cigarette and other smoking. *(#249)*

Several outcome objectives were proposed. Linda Randolph of the New York State Department of Health suggests reducing the proportion of males who use smokeless tobacco in rural areas from 24 to 10 percent. *(#177)* Turnock adds that "by 2000, the proportion of youth aged 21 and under who use smokeless tobacco will be reduced to no more than 4 percent." *(#215)* Chen further mentions several objectives relating to reducing the prevalence of those who have ever smoked from 15.5 percent[8] to 8 percent. *(#039)*

Chen proposes that "by 2000, all U.S. legal jurisdictions should establish 18 as the minimum age to purchase tobacco products, including snuff and chewing tobacco, and ban distribution of free tobacco products in public places." He also suggests objectives dealing with the teaching of hazards due to smokeless tobacco in elementary schools, making health professionals and the public more aware of the hazards, and devoting more funds to education and research activities in this area. *(#039)*

IMPLEMENTATION ISSUES

To foster the success of the smoking outcome objectives for the year 2000, many suggestions for implementation, some in the form of process objectives, were offered by testifiers. Many testifiers recommended that new and more effective methods of educating the general public and specific target groups (including adolescents, especially girls; pregnant women; ethnic minorities; and the poor) be developed, sometimes in combination with political action or legislation.

Warner suggests that a professionally designed, paid broadcast media advertising campaign be developed against the use of tobacco and alcohol products, with increased excise taxes on cigarettes being used to pay for it. *(#429)* Ruth Roemer of the University of California, Los Angeles also sees the need to limit advertising and increase taxes.

> Government has an obligation to protect the health of the people, and a ban on advertising would promote the social norm of a nonsmoking society. Moreover, commercial speech enjoys less protection than other speech, and the First Amendment does not protect the right to promote death. Since tobacco is addictive, every influence promoting it should be eliminated. Taxes and prices of tobacco products need to be raised substantially and at regular intervals, and tobacco products should be excluded from the cost of living index, if a significant decline in smoking is to be achieved. *(#184)*

Business executive Jack West of Puro Corporation of America calls for rescinding farm subsidies for tobacco. "Do not use my tax dollars against me, against my employees' health. When my employees are sick, I do not make any money." *(#734)* Young says that "every state should have a coalition of organizations to combat proliferation of tobacco promotions." *(#712)* Action by health insurers to offer differential rates for nonsmokers also has the potential of decreasing smoking rates according to John Banzhaf of Action on Smoking and Health. *(#516)*

However, Rosner believes that "before the government can advise any other organization on the issue of smoking policy and cessation programs, it must get its own house in order." A report by his Smoking Policy Institute examining the response of various federal agencies to regulations on smoking in government facilities documented that "the government has made progress, but still lacks consistent and comprehensive policies." *(#349)*

In terms of research, testifiers said that more data are needed and should continue to be gathered on the health hazards of passive smoking to nonsmoking individuals, the evaluation of worksite smoking, the reduction of smoking among minorities *(#615)*, and cost containment. Because Blacks have been a special target for cigarette advertising, several testifiers point to the need for focused research into ways to attract Blacks into programs aimed at reducing smoking rates. *(#537; #615)* Wood believes that the impetus for collecting better information on the existence and effectiveness of worksite policies and cessation programs will come from three sources:

> First, the proliferation of municipal or state laws requiring increasingly stringent worksite smoking policies. Second, the pressure of media exposure and a word of mouth from top management about other businesses through trade associations, coalitions, etc. And third, the increasing voice of the nonsmokers within the company. *(#736)*

REFERENCES

1. U.S. Department of Health and Human Services: The 1990 Health Objectives for the Nation: A Midcourse Review. Washington, D.C.: U.S. Government Printing Office, 1986

2. U.S. Department of Health and Human Services: Reducing the Health Consequences of Smoking: 25 Years of Progress, A Report of the Surgeon General (DHHS Publication No. [CDC] 89-8411), 1989

3. Bachman JG, Johnston LD, O'Malley PM: Monitoring the Future: Questionnaire Responses from the Nation's High School Seniors, 1986. Ann Arbor: Institute for Social Research, University of Michigan, 1988

4. Ibid.

5. Windsor R: An estimate of the behavioral, obstetric and economic impact of smoking cessation methods for the annual U.S. cohort of pregnant women. Presented at the 75th Anniversary Meeting of the School of Hygiene and Public Health, Society of Alumni. The Johns Hopkins University, Baltimore, June 7, 1989

6. Connolly GN, Winn DM, Hecht SS, et al.: The re-emergence of smokeless tobacco. N Engl J Med 314(16):1020–1027, 1986

7. U.S. Department of Health and Human Services: The Health Consequences of Using Smokeless Tobacco: A Report of the Advisory Committee to the Surgeon General (DHHS Publication No. [NIH] 86-2874), 1986

8. Centers for Disease Control: Smokeless tobacco use in the United States: Behavioral Risk Factor Surveillance System, 1986. Morbid Mortal Wkly Rep 36(22):337-340, 1987

TESTIFIERS CITED IN CHAPTER 10

002 Acampora, Gabrielle; Greater New York Association of Occupational Health Nurses
005 Allensworth, Diane; American School Health Association
039 Chen, Jr., Moon; Ohio State University
054 duPont, Terry; American Association for Respiratory Care
115 King, Carole; American Academy of Pediatrics
159 Murtaugh, Alice; New York
177 Randolph, Linda; New York State Department of Health
184 Roemer, Ruth; University of California, Los Angeles
215 Turnock, Bernard; Illinois Department of Public Health
230 Zal, Harriette; Southern California Association of Occupational Health Nurses
249 Davis, A. Conan; Alabama Department of Public Health
267 Windsor, Richard; University of Alabama at Birmingham
349 Rosner, Robert; Smoking Policy Institute (Seattle)
405 Myers, Jr., Woodrow; Indiana State Board of Health
419 O'Malley, Patrick and Johnston, Lloyd; University of Michigan
421 Welch, Robert and Sokol, Robert; Wayne State University/Hutzel Hospital (Detroit)
426 Kaminsky, Kenneth; Wayne County Intermediate School District (Michigan)
429 Warner, Kenneth; University of Michigan
516 Banzhaf, III, John; Action on Smoking and Health (Washington, D.C.)
537 Greenberg, Michael; Rutgers University
615 Hargreaves, Margaret, et al.; Meharry Medical College
712 Young, "Snip" Walter; Colorado Department of Health
734 West, Jack; Puro Corporation of America (Maspeth, New York)
736 Wood, Loring; NYNEX Corporation
779 Van Citters, Robert; University of Washington

11. Alcohol and Drug Abuse

Experts who testified about the Year 2000 Health Objectives identified the use and misuse of alcohol and drugs as a major national problem. Substance abuse affects overall health status, contributing to intentional and unintentional injuries, heart disease, cancer, cirrhosis, AIDS, fetal and infant death, and many other health problems. Its direct and indirect mortality, morbidity, and impact on health care costs are tremendous, according to testifiers. Furthermore, the broad array of licit and illicit drugs now available carries a range of social costs that extend well beyond those suffered by the users themselves.

A total of 32 individuals focused their testimony on issues relating to the use and misuse of alcohol and other drugs, another 24 made major statements on these issues, and many others addressed them as part of their testimony on other subjects. Testifiers agreed, in general, that the nation has made progress on the 1990 Objectives but that, as William Wallace of the New Hampshire Division of Public Health Services says, "we have only scratched the surface." (#430) The National Association of State Boards of Education (NASBE) adds that upon reviewing the current status of the national health objectives for 1990 it is apparent "that our country still has far to go in some significant areas related to the misuse of alcohol and drugs." (#573)

Many testifiers advocate continuing and strengthening the objectives on alcohol and other drug use, including setting additional targeted reductions. In the words of Bob Dickson of the Texas Commission on Alcohol and Drug Abuse, "We must emphasize chemical dependency's significance as a major nationwide health concern." He also stresses the need to focus much energy on preventing the disease. That means not only finding "genetic markers" to warn susceptible individuals, but also changing attitudes in a society that still glorifies drinking. (#312)

Along with other witnesses, Al Wright of the Los Angeles County Department of Health Services calls for strong health protection measures to fight alcohol and drug abuse. (#229) Marilyn Aguirre-Molina and Christine Lubinski, speaking for the National Council on Alcoholism (NCA), say that an assertive public policy, systematic and coordinated educational approaches, and other interventions are required. Because alcohol control measures can be used to limit consumption, the control of alcohol availability is a public health issue.[1] The NCA strongly urges "the inclusion of economic incentives and other policy initiatives in the form of process objectives to facilitate the achievement of a number of outcome objectives. This can best be accomplished through the cooperation of the public, voluntary, and private sectors to advance the formulation of such policies and to advocate for their enactment." Issues that the NCA believes should be addressed include increased prices through tax policy and health and safety warning labels. (#467)

Anne Windle of the Department of Addiction, Victim, and Mental Health Services of the Montgomery County Government in Maryland, acknowledges that substance abuse is an emotional issue. Many of the potential solutions are highly political and have serious implications for this society. She adds that a national dialogue is needed to openly consider all options. "We must address the enormous financial incentives at every level of the drug trade. And we must acknowledge the societal realities that exclude some segments of our society from participating in means of earning a legal and acceptable living," she says. (#616)

Donald Gragg of the Southern California Permanente Medical Group suggests that "much of the progress made on the 1990 Objectives seems to be a result of a slight shift in societal attitudes particularly with regard to the acceptability of drinking and driving (and the use of illicit drugs). It is imperative that a major thrust be made to continue and accelerate this shift in societal values during the next decade, with special focus on adolescents and young adults." (#282)

Many testifiers focused their comments on several particular areas of concern surrounding alcohol and drug abuse. By far, the two most commonly discussed areas were problems associated with alcohol and the issue of substance abuse among adolescents. Many other witnesses addressed the special substance abuse problems in minority populations. These three areas are discussed in detail below.

Although not addressed in great detail, other topics were discussed that testifiers felt needed attention in the Year 2000 Health Objectives: substance abuse during pregnancy, especially the risk of fetal alcohol syndrome; cocaine, "crack," and heroin; and AIDS among intravenous drug users. Robert Welch and Robert Sokol of Wayne State University and the Hutzel Hospital in Detroit explain that even though nationwide efforts appear to have increased awareness of the adverse effect of alcohol consumption during pregnancy, "a segment of intractable, heavy drinkers who are unable to modify their behavior" still exists. With respect to cocaine, Welch and Sokol report that there is little mention of this drug in the 1990 Objectives and emphasize that since their publication, cocaine has "become more readily available and easier to take in the form of 'crack'." (#421) Finally, heroin is identified as important, not only because of the deleterious effects of addiction, but also because of perinatal AIDS.

Patrick O'Malley and Lloyd Johnston of the University of Michigan recommend, and others agree, that because of AIDS, reducing the prevalence of intravenous drug use should be a very important objective. (#419) The issue of AIDS is covered further in Chapter 19.

ALCOHOL PROBLEMS

Many witnesses testified about the problems caused by alcohol. Dave Anderson of the American Automobile Association, for instance, reports that about half of all highway fatalities—26,000 of the 52,000 deaths per year—are alcohol related.[2] (#008) Harold Jordan of Meharry Medical College adds that 18 million adults currently experience problems as a result of alcohol, and of these, 11 million suffer from the disease of alcoholism. The direct and indirect costs of alcoholism amounted to $117 billion in 1983, according to Jordan. (#254)

To deal with the problem, Wallace calls for more attention to the causative agent itself and would eventually like to see an alcohol-free society. Short of that, he recommends warnings on alcoholic beverage containers similar to those on tobacco products; a ban on radio and television advertising of alcoholic beverages; an increase in taxes on alcoholic beverages to be used for alcohol-related programs; and a "major and massive" educational effort aimed at health professionals, the schools, and the public. (#430)

The NCA recommends the enactment of comprehensive legislation that requires education and training for servers of alcoholic beverages, third-party liability laws, and zoning ordinances specifying the location and density of alcohol outlets, with considera-tion of their proximity to public and private transportation. (#467)

Linda Grant of the Washington State Association of Alcoholism and Addictions Programs says that "the information we have today is not the same as the information that was available when the objectives for 1990 were drawn up." For example, there is much evidence on the heavy genetic role of alcoholism. Thus, she says, drug abuse and alcoholism may require different approaches. (#692)

In addition, the NCA believes that the term "abuse" should not be used in discussions of alcoholism. The term is vague, and no clear-cut line exists between use and abuse; it should be replaced, when warranted, with the word "problem." Along with others, the NCA agrees that the title of any chapter or section on alcoholism should convey a broad approach to the problem, that is, the objectives must focus on issues resulting from, as well as factors related to, its use. (#467)

ADOLESCENT SUBSTANCE ABUSE

According to Wayne Teague of the Alabama Department of Education, "the most serious threat to the health and well-being of our children is drug abuse." (#675) Elaine Hill and Casey Clark of the University of Colorado Health Sciences Center add that "a recent national survey, the National High School Seniors Survey conducted in 1986, demonstrated that 92 percent of high school seniors had used alcohol, 15 percent had tried cocaine, 10 percent had used some hallucinogen, 1 percent heroin, 17 percent inhalants, and 50.2 percent reported using marijuana."[3] It appears that alcohol use continues to predominate over illicit drugs, and that cocaine and crack have replaced heroin. Statistics also clearly indicate, they say, that children are now using drugs at younger ages.[4] (#577) According to the American School Health Association (ASHA), adolescents involved in substance abuse are at high risk for many health problems, such as lack of physical endurance and respiratory problems. Furthermore, quoting Brenda Wagner, ASHA writes:

One of the greatest concerns of professionals working with adolescents involved in substance abuse is the delay of accomplishing the adolescent tasks necessary to reach emotional maturity. It is difficult to adequately accomplish these tasks if one's perception of self, time, and sequence is distorted or if one's interest and ability in evaluative thinking is impaired.[5] (#005)

Michael Jarrett of the South Carolina Department of Health and Environmental Control points out a problem with the 1990 objectives that address adolescent substance abuse, which must be corrected for the year 2000. "The problems and preventions needed for these age groups are quite different, and the 1990 objectives do not address rather significant problem areas. For example, the targeted ages in the plan are often too late to begin efforts to measure and reduce the problem." (#108)

Claire Brindis and Phillip Lee of the University of California, San Francisco foresee problems in reaching this group with interventions because "no one approach will respond to the various segments of the adolescent population and the different needs of new immigrants, refugees, the middle class, and the poor." To combat the problem, they suggest that "a diversity of programs under the umbrella of a common goal may be an effective way of responding to the needs of different individuals and groups in the community. For example, drug education programs directed at high school students may be more effective if programs also are available for parents and pre-high school students." (#027) Yet strategies for reaching youth must not rely solely on formal educational programs, according to Gragg. To be effective, they must also use everyday television, music, and other media. (#282)

To deal with the problem of substance abuse in adolescents, the ASHA calls for prevention interventions that "combine and coordinate multiple forces of the community with those of the school." (#005) Teague says that parents, school officials, and community leaders all must commit to the task. (#675) Health care professionals, including physicians, nurses, pharmacists, and dentists, need to be educated about the prevalence and availability of alcohol and illegal drugs to school age children, as well, add Hill and Clark. They also suggest that other states follow Colorado and legislate drug education in kindergarten through high school classes. (#577)

The NASBE calls for an even more comprehensive strategy in efforts to reach young people.

Health risk behaviors overlap and, equally important, are associated with low academic achievement, school failure, and dropout. For this reason, society cannot afford to address health problems piecemeal through discrete programs aimed at reducing substance abuse, teenage pregnancy, AIDS, and other issues. Rather, they must see these problems as part of a more general, at-risk syndrome that requires a comprehensive approach, including school and community.

To this end, the NASBE advocates the active involvement of parents, peers, law enforcement agencies, social service agencies, health care givers, the churches, business, industry, and the media in any programs aimed at adolescents. In addition, the NASBE says that education programs must be designed to alter knowledge, attitudes, and most important, behavior. "Mere public awareness of the risks associated with drinking is not sufficient. Knowledge must be transferred "into changed attitudes and changed behavior." (#573)

"Risk-taking adolescents do not believe that it is harmful, or that the risks outweigh the thrills in the areas of driving, drinking, drugs, and sex," says Herbert Rader of the Salvation Army in New York. Thus, it is also important that youth activities be organized to enhance self-esteem, promote new skills acquisition, and promote life skills that encourage healthy behaviors, as do the youth programs of the Salvation Army. (#432)

The NCA calls for legislation mandating equal time for health and safety messages to counterbalance alcohol ads on radio and television. (#467) Gragg suggests that by the year 2000, 75 percent of the references to alcohol or drugs in television, drama, film, and popular music reflect negative connotations about the use of these substances. (#282) Prevention strategy for the nation must send the message that "it's all right not to drink" and that the abuse of alcohol is unacceptable behavior, according to Jacqueline Morrison of Wayne State University. (#723)

SUBSTANCE ABUSE BY MINORITY GROUPS

Given the differences between ethnic and racial minorities and the rest of the population in the rates of alcohol morbidity and mortality, the NCA suggests the "development of sub-objectives with specific targets for minority populations." (#467) Mario Orlandi of the American Health Foundation in New York adds that "ethnic variability presents a dilemma to health planners who are responsible for developing substance abuse prevention initiatives." Programs, he continues, must have not only demonstrated efficacy but also cultural relevance for particular minority or ethnic groups and subgroups. *(#167)*

Blacks

Morrison, who also represented the National Black Alcoholism Council, calls alcoholism "the number one public health problem in the Black community, as it is related to cancer, vehicle accidents, domestic violence, homicide, school dropout, hypertension, fetal alcohol syndrome," and many other problems. Morrison calls for more culturally sensitive individual and community-level alcoholism awareness and education programs. She also calls for more attention to programs for children of alcoholics. In addition, Morrison calls for more data on Blacks and alcohol-related driving accidents and for public information and educational programs targeted to the Black community. *(#723)*

Hispanics

According to Sylvia Andrew of Our Lady of the Lake University in San Antonio, Texas, alcohol and drug abuse are problems among Mexican-American youth as well. In terms of prevention, attention should be given to the overaccessibility of alcohol in barrios. *(#495)*

Ricardo Jasso of Nosotros Human Services Development in San Antonio calls attention to the problem of inhalant abuse among Mexican-Americans. To deal with the problem, Nosotros is developing a comprehensive continuum of programs, including counseling for individuals, groups, and families, as well as psychiatric assessments; alternative activities; chemical abuse education, general educational programs, and job skill training; job placement programs; social services and referrals; and residential treatment programs for teenagers. *(#494)*

Native Americans

JoAnn Kauffman of the Seattle Indian Health Board reports that many deaths among Native Americans 45 years old or younger are alcohol related.[6] A large part of the Native American adolescent suicide problem, discussed in greater detail in Chapters 6 and 16, is alcohol related.

Currently there are not adequate resources to treat Indian alcoholism or substance abuse. There are even fewer resources available to

meet the treatment needs of children of alcoholics. The multi-generational cycle of family dysfunction perpetuates alcoholism, violence, sexual abuse and self-destructive behaviors. To break the cycle requires breaking through family and community denial, and striving for cultural revitalization and adequately trained treatment providers. *(#696)*

The Indigent, Homeless, and Disadvantaged

The terrible toll exacted by substance abuse, as seen in the breakdown of personal health and the breakup of families and neighborhoods, is even more pronounced among the disadvantaged. Rader reports that a major expansion of drug detoxification and rehabilitation programs, including adequate residential facilities, is needed for the large number of intravenous (IV) drug abusers who would be willing to come off the street. "Some recent surveys suggest that many IV drug abusers on the streets of New York would voluntarily enter residential drug treatment programs if they were available," says Rader. *(#432)*

Programs are successful, Rader explains, because

something has been kindled within a person. Attainment of this change of outlook, which results in a dramatic change in behavior, seems to create a contagious hope within others. The answer to a great deal of drug abuse is not education alone or provision of clean needles or addressing chemical dependency only, but providing emergency shelter, secure safe houses, psychosocial support and counselling, health care, education and training for living, camps away from the streets, community centers where opportunity for personal achievement, self-esteem, and respect for others are developed, employment counselling, etc. *(#432)*

IMPLEMENTATION

A variety of strategies were proposed for achieving the year 2000 alcohol and drug objectives. Dickson calls for a strong and focused attack on substance abuse.

It is time for the chemical dependency field, and the general public, to turn from the "drug-of-the-month" hysteria of the media, place our country's manpower and resources into the fray, and begin a major offensive against substance abuse. Everything that we have gained could well be lost if we once more are forced to endure the perception that chemical dependency is a weakness, a sign of moral deficiency, rather than a treatable neuro-chemical disease. Our progress depends on the final answering of this question that, indeed, it is a disease. *(#312)*

The NCA views "a policy to substantially increase the tax rates among alcoholic beverages" as an important element in a successful implementation strategy.

Tax rates among beverage classes should be equalized by alcohol content. Such a move would, in and of itself, raise four billion dollars and serve to undermine public perceptions that beer and wine are more "moderate" alcoholic beverages. *(#467)*

The worksite has great potential for combatting alcohol and drug problems, according to Dickson: "Random drug screening, to create a drug free workplace, coupled with an EAP (employee assistance program) is the most effective method so far for dealing with chemical dependency." *(#312)*

Many testifiers were concerned with uniformity in data collection. The NCA strongly recommends, and others agree, that the Year 2000 Health Objectives also include a process objective for implementing and monitoring an improved and coordinated information system within and between federal, state, or local governments and the private sector, and for both health and human services information. This would be based on the concept of uniform minimum data sets and would include greater precision and standardization in the definition of terms that describe drinking and levels of problem use. *(#467)*

Accurate surveillance of alcohol problems among minority groups also requires the implementation of a uniform demographic information collecting system, the NCA adds. It recommends that in addition to collecting data on age and gender, a uniform racial and ethnic identifier be included on all pertinent records. *(#467)*

Although prevention and treatment of both alcohol and drug problems, as well as data collection and surveillance, will be critical to the achievement of the year 2000 alcohol and drug objectives, society must "understand that factors of public policy, urban economics, family life, and education are among the risk factors for both these problems," states James Sall of the Detroit Department of Health. Putting it into an even broader framework, he adds that "while disease-specific objectives and monitoring of health status will continue to be legitimate, we are acting on the assumption that, at least among the urban underclass, the following health areas share a common group of underlying risk factors: sexually transmitted diseases, maternal and infant health, teenage pregnancy, internal injuries, stress-related mental illness, and alcohol and drug abuse." *(#389)*

REFERENCES

1. Bruun K, Edwards G, Lumio M, et al.: Alcohol control policies in public health perspective. Finnish Foundation for Alcohol Studies, vol. 25. WHO and Addiction Research Foundation, 1975

2. U.S. Department of Transportation, National Highway Traffic Safety Administration: Fatal Accident Reporting System 1988. A Review of Information on Fatal Traffic Crashes in the United States in 1988 (DOT Publication No. HS 807 507), 1989

3. Bachman JG, Johnston LD, O'Malley PM: Monitoring the Future: Questionnaire Responses from the Nation's High School Seniors, 1986. Ann Arbor: Institute for Social Research, University of Michigan, 1988

4. Ibid.

5. Wagner BJ: Intervening with the adolescent involved in substance abuse. J Sch Health 54(7):244–246, 1984

6. U.S. Department of Health and Human Services: Report of the Secretary's Task Force on Black and Minority Health. Washington, D.C.: U.S. Government Printing Office, 1987

TESTIFIERS CITED IN CHAPTER 11

005 Allensworth, Diane; American School Health Association
008 Anderson, Dave; American Automobile Association
027 Brindis, Claire and Lee, Phillip; University of California, San Francisco
108 Jarrett, Michael; South Carolina Department of Health and Environmental Control
167 Orlandi, Mario; American Health Foundation
229 Wright, Al; County of Los Angeles Department of Health Services
254 Jordan, Harold; Meharry Medical College
282 Gragg, Donald; Southern California Permanente Medical Group
312 Dickson, Bob; Texas Commission on Alcohol and Drug Abuse
389 Sall, James; Detroit Department of Health
419 O'Malley, Patrick and Johnston, Lloyd; University of Michigan
421 Welch, Robert and Sokol, Robert; Wayne State University/Hutzel Hospital (Detroit)
430 Wallace, Jr., William; New Hampshire Division of Public Health Services
432 Rader, Herbert; The Salvation Army in the United States
467 Aguirre-Molina, Marilyn and Lubinski, Christine; National Council on Alcoholism
494 Jasso, Ricardo; Nosotros Human Services Development (San Antonio)
495 Andrew, Sylvia; Our Lady of the Lake University of San Antonio
573 Wilhoit, Gene; National Association of State Boards of Education
577 Hill, Elaine and Clark, Casey; University of Colorado Health Sciences Center
616 Windle, Anne; American Public Health Association, Public Health Education Section
675 Teague, Wayne; Alabama Department of Education
692 Grant, Linda; Washington State Association of Alcoholism and Addictions Programs
696 Kauffman, JoAnn; Seattle Indian Health Board
723 Morrison, Jacqueline; Wayne State University

12. Nutrition

Nutrition plays a key role in the cause and prevention of many health conditions. As a result, topics covered by the 69 witnesses who concentrated on this area were many and varied. A significant amount of attention was given to the role nutrition plays in two physiological risk factors, hypertension and high serum cholesterol, which contribute to chronic diseases such as cancer, cardiovascular disease, diabetes, and others. Also of major interest were several nutrition-centered areas that are both risk factors for other diseases and health problems in and of themselves—obesity, anorexia and bulimia, and anemia.

Taking a somewhat different approach to the problems of nutrition, a number of testifiers focused on the basic problem of hunger, rather than on the need for a balanced diet. Special mention was made of hunger as it applies to the homeless and to migrant workers. Still others discussed the need for an overall balanced diet and the dietary needs of specific population groups such as pregnant women, infants and children, and hospitalized patients. The relationship of good nutrition to birth outcome, mental health, work performance, and the ability to recover from illness also was noted. (#057) Witnesses generally supported continuation and strengthening of the 1990 Objectives concerning nutrition, and pointed to the *Surgeon General's Report on Nutrition and Health*[1] and the National Research Council's *Diet and Health*[2] as examples of consensus-building documents that had contributed to progress toward the 1990 nutrition objectives.

The links between diet and health suggest clear opportunities for reducing disease. Also, as witnesses commented, history shows that given the opportunity, information, and time, Americans will change their eating habits. (#063; #462) However, they also emphasized that consumers must have the necessary tools. The Society for Nutrition Education comments:

> Dietary change is not easy, so that even though a food may be better for one's health, it may not be competitive in other factors of choice such as taste, history, ease of preparation, etc. Other strategies are needed to bring the public to actually choose foods that are most nutritious. (#462)

According to dietitian Marilyn Guthrie of the Virginia Mason Clinic in Seattle, if improvements in the nutritional and health status of Americans are to occur, "we need to do a better job at going beyond making people aware of relationships between food and health toward giving them the tools and skills to make changes in eating behavior." (#077) Testifiers also discussed strategies for surveillance and intervention to change diets.

HUNGER

The feelings of many testifiers about the problem of hunger in our country are best summed up by Eleanor Young of the University of Texas Health Science Center, San Antonio.

> Identification of health objectives for the nation relating to nutrition cannot possibly exclude the serious concern of increased hunger in the United States. In the 1960s and 1970s, identification of extensive hunger shocked the American people. In response, development of programs virtually eliminated this problem. Now, during the 1980s, hunger in the U.S. has returned. A fact that has now been well documented by some 20 studies conducted between 1982 and 1986 in major cities, including Boston, Dallas, and Chicago. (#496)

The Society for Nutrition Education notes that although the numbers may wax and wane, there always are hungry people in America. (#462) A 1987 report cited by Young estimated that 9 percent of the population is hungry, including 12 million children and 8 million adults.[3] (#496) Several witnesses cited local increases in the number of hungry people, as indicated by a growth in the number of emergency food sites, waiting lists for food services, and the number of people served. (#057; #462) In some states, residency and citizenship requirements block otherwise eligible migrant farm workers and unnaturalized immigrants from receiving food benefits. Similar requirements for a permanent domain within the state bar the homeless from participating in public assistance programs. (#462)

Several objectives were proposed to reduce or eliminate hunger. Dorothy Conway, representing the California Conference of Local Health Department Nutritionists, for instance, proposes that by the year 2000 no one in the United States will go without food for more than 48 hours. *(#043)*

Jean Egan, representing the Michigan Dietetic Association, addresses the importance of locating surplus food and getting it to needy populations. She says that national objectives relating to access to food should be strengthened substantially in the Year 2000 Health Objectives. Witnesses underscored the importance of maintaining government and private sector food programs, emphasizing the need for strong outreach and easy access. *(#043; #057)*

The Society for Nutrition Education calls for congregate facilities, such as school lunch rooms, to be used for feeding homeless people. *(#462)* School breakfast and lunch programs also can help to reduce hunger and are discussed in the section on special populations.

SPECIFIC NUTRITIONAL RISK FACTORS

Many nutrition goals are related to risk factors associated with specific diseases or disorders such as heart disease, stroke, cancer, diabetes, osteoporosis, and others. Two of these risk factors—high blood pressure (hypertension) and high serum cholesterol—are central nutrition goals, but they are the focus of Chapter 24 and therefore are discussed briefly here. Obesity, anorexia and bulimia, and anemia are directly related to food consumption; they are problems in themselves, as well as causes of other conditions. Food-borne diseases, foods that might cause dental cavities, and calcium intake as a factor in osteoporosis prevention also are nutritional issues; they are discussed in Chapters 18, 26, and 27, respectively.

Hypertension

Individuals with high blood pressure are at increased risk for cardiovascular disease. Much of the testimony on nutrition and hypertension focused on the role of sodium, and there was disagreement among the testifiers. The 1990 Objectives call for reductions in the average daily sodium intake to 3–6 grams and seek increases in the percentage of food that is labeled for sodium content. The American Heart Association (AHA) and other witnesses want to continue to target sodium intake, perhaps with quantitative changes; the AHA suggests that an adult's daily intake of sodium not exceed 3 grams. *(#636)* However, other witnesses, including the Salt Institute, say that recent research argues for eliminating sodium reduction goals for the general population. Only about one-third of the population is salt-sensitive, and for another third of the population, salt reduction may be harmful, it says. *(#053; #082)* Chapter 24 continues this discussion in greater length.

Cholesterol

An elevated blood cholesterol level is one major risk factor for cardiovascular disease. The testimony on nutrition as a way of reducing serum cholesterol levels focused on food labeling; public education; and reduction in the fat, saturated fat, and cholesterol content of manufactured food. Several witnesses favor adding cholesterol content to the objective dealing with food labeling; the 1990 objectives on food labeling included only sodium and caloric values. Other testimony calls for the food industry's cooperation in reducing the fat and cholesterol content of foods. One proposal, for example, says that by the year 2000, the saturated fat content (specifically coconut and palm oils) in processed and convenience foods should be reduced 50 percent from present levels. *(#178)*

Several witnesses suggested incorporating the AHA's dietary guidelines for reducing these risk factors into the Year 2000 Health Objectives. These guidelines call for an average daily consumption of cholesterol of 300 milligrams or less per day; the percentage of calories from fat should be less than 30 percent; the percentage of calories from saturated and polyunsaturated fat should each be less than 10 percent. *(#627; #636)*

A primary consideration in changing the public's consumption of fats and other substances must be education, according to Jennifer Anderson of Colorado State University.

> I would like us to think that as we translate the nutrition information, we also must think of practical messages, telling people how you eat to reduce the risk of chronic disease. I would like us to try and encourage people to think about how they decrease fat; how they can increase fiber; and how they, therefore, apply the dietary guidelines developed from the U.S. Department of Health and Human Services and the U.S.D.A. *(#739)*

Obesity

Obesity is an important risk factor for hypertension as well as for diabetes, cancer, and cardiovascular disease. Young describes it as the single most prevalent nutrition problem in the United States. According to the latest National Health and Nutrition Examination Survey (NHANES) study cited in her testimony, 34 million adults in the United States are overweight, which is defined as at least 20 percent above their desirable weight, and 13 million of them are severely overweight, or 40 percent over their desired weight.[4] (#496)

The 1990 Objectives include targets for reducing the proportion of the population that is overweight, and witnesses favored continued efforts in this area. One specific objective recommended for the year 2000 calls for reducing the prevalence of obesity in men by 20 percent and in women by 25 percent. Strategies to achieve these reductions include education, research into causes and interventions, and physicians' "prescribing" weight reduction. (#496) Another objective proposed is that pilot weight loss programs in which weight loss is rewarded be established for federal and state health workers. (#052)

George Bray of the University of Southern California reported that three European and two U.S. studies have now shown that fat distribution is a greater risk factor than total body fat, and that sufficient data exist to add maldistribution of fat to the objectives. Bray proposes that by the year 2000, the prevalence of individuals with waist-hip measurements above the tenth percentile for age, as defined by recent epidemiologic data from North America, should be reduced by 10 percent for both males and females, regardless of initial body mass index. (#238)

A number of witnesses note that pediatric obesity is a growing problem that should be included in the Year 2000 Health Objectives. (#228; #462) According to Nancy Wooldridge, representing the Alabama Dietetic Association, many overweight children remain overweight as adults. (#228) Physical activity is decreasing among youth while dietary intake remains high, according to testimony. Dodds proposed an objective for the year 2000 calling for the prevalence of obesity among children age 6–11 and girls age 12–17 to be reduced by 10 percent. (#462)

Anorexia and Bulimia

Some witnesses recommended that targets relating to eating disorders such as anorexia and bulimia be included in the Year 2000 Health Objectives. A survey of 300 middle- and upper-class shoppers in Boston found that 10 percent of them had a bulimic history.[5] (#216) Another study at a large, Eastern university found that only 1 percent of the women had bulimia. Part of the difficulty in determining the prevalence of this disorder, according to the authors of this latter study, is the definition of bulimia.

> Whether there is an epidemic of bulimia on the college campus or not depends on the definition of bulimia. If bulimia is defined as self-reported overeating in combination with occasional purging, then the answer is an emphatic "yes." If, however, the term bulimia is restricted to the diagnosis of a clinically significant disorder, the answer is "no." Its prevalence rate did not exceed 1.3 percent in a sample of university women, those presumed to be at highest risk.[6]

The incidence of anorexia is steadily increasing, with nearly 1 percent of women now affected, according to the Utah Nutrition Council. A proposed goal for the year 2000 is to prevent and reduce the incidence of eating disorders. The strategies recommended to achieve this include media campaigns, outpatient clinics, and a hotline to prevent relapse. (#216)

Anemia

Conway notes that the use of iron-fortified infant formulas is declining and suggests that this could result in an increase in infant and child iron deficiency anemia. Education and iron supplementation are required to prevent the condition. Conway proposes that the year 2000 objectives on anemia target all age groups. (#043) Sharon Hoerr of Michigan State University echoes Conway's point by calling for the identification of "additional population subgroups at risk for impaired iron status." Specifically she states that "the prevalence of impaired iron status as defined by low iron stores in children aged one to two years, in males aged 11 to 14, and in females aged 15 to 44 years, should be reduced to at least 50 percent of those levels estimated for these groups in NHANES II." (#100)

SPECIAL TARGET GROUPS

In addition to identifying objectives for several nutrition-related conditions, testimony produced recommendations for targeting populations with special nutritional needs. Pregnant women, infants and children, and hospitalized patients received special attention in the testimony. Others suggested that this list be expanded to include the elderly and some subgroups within the minority population.

Pregnant Women

For pregnant women, nutrition counseling was seen as a critical part of prenatal care. The Michigan Dietetic Association recommended that objectives relating to access to comprehensive prenatal care specifically mention nutritional services. (#057) The federal Special Supplemental Food Program for Women, Infants, and Children (WIC) was hailed as an important way to improve the nutritional status of pregnant women. (#057; #063) According to the Grocery Manufacturers of America:

The WIC program is a vivid example of how health objectives can be achieved through cooperation with government, the food industry, the banking industry, local communities, and health professionals. This program has now developed into a food assistance program remarkable both in its degree of personal nutrition services, as well as its ability to produce measurable improvements in the nutritional status of its clients, and has had an economic impact that is continuing to be viable. (#063)

However, several witnesses pointed to the lack of adequate resources as a real obstacle to the potential impact of WIC. The March of Dimes Birth Defects Foundation states, "There is no state in the country that services all of its WIC-eligible women and children. In 42 states, fewer than 50 percent of those eligible are served." (#203) The Society for Nutrition Education adds that "high volume WIC programs are seldom able to consistently provide individual attention." (#462)

Several states are attempting to supplement the WIC program. A study by the Michigan Food and Nutrition Advisory Commission looked at admissions between 1978 and 1982 to a Flint hospital in which children, age two or less, failed to thrive. Shirley Powell, who represents the group, reports that even though these children were in the WIC caseload, their results were poor.

Growth failure had nearly doubled [1978–1982] and the increases closely paralleled rising unemployment and deepening recession. The doctor continues to see serious problems, and she is involved in piloting an intervention in which close counseling on infant care and feeding is provided, in addition to WIC's food supplementation. (#390)

The Massachusetts Department of Public Health also has tried to go beyond WIC, according to its Commissioner Deborah Prothrow-Stith, but it is still not enough.

We are one of the states that significantly supplements our WIC funding, and we do that not only in the monetary reward, but also in looking at foods and agriculture. We have made an alliance with our Department of Food and Agriculture, and women are eligible to receive fruits and fresh vegetables. But even with those initiatives, we have an infant mortality rate that concerns us. (#735)

Among the suggested objectives aimed at improving nutrition for pregnant women is one from the Utah Nutrition Council supportive of "goals and objectives that would improve the quality and quantity of sound nutrition education programs," including those targeting pregnant teen girls delivering low-birth-weight infants, who "increasingly need nutritional help and guidance." (#216)

Infants and Children

Many witnesses emphasized the nutritional benefits of breast-feeding for infants; Chapter 22 provides more detail. Testifiers in this area called for maintaining or increasing the 1990 targets for the percentage of mothers that breast-feed.

Many testifiers emphasized the importance of school meal programs for preschoolers and school-age children. According to Carol Neill of the California School Food Services Association, school children who are hungry or malnourished suffer a range of effects from permanent neurologic defects to behavior problems, inability to concentrate, and other learning problems. (#161)

The National School Breakfast Program serves about 4 million children, 89 percent of them at no charge or at a reduced price.[7] In addition, approximately 24 million children receive a school lunch each school day, many of them free or at a reduced price.[8] Food assistance programs are directly related to improvements in dietary habits and nutritional status of children, according to testimony. (#161) Witnesses supported maintaining and extending these programs. Specifically, according to Jacqueline Frederick of the New Jersey Department of Education:

> The National School Lunch Program should have guidelines for feeding special populations. In essence, the school lunch program must consider the nutrition requirements of the pregnant teen, the problems of refugee children with marginal nutritional status, and children with various physical and mental handicaps. Nutritious, well-balanced meals should not only be available to each student, but should be tailored to meet their specific nutritional needs. (#618)

Witnesses also feel that dietary guidelines are needed for preschoolers and school-age children. They say that adult guidelines sometimes are used to determine appropriate levels for children, but this is not the best approach. (#161; #590) For example, Egan points out that "the progress of the USDA/ DHHS Dietary Guidelines promotion in school lunches has been greatly hampered by the lack of availability of the revised school lunch recipes that have been adapted to comply with the Dietary Guidelines." (#057)

In an attempt to get dietary guidelines designed for children, Neill requests that Congress require a study on "how to apply the USDA/DHHS Dietary Guidelines to children, including, in particular, sodium, fat, and sugar recommendations." The group asks that all food companies that supply the school lunch programs review their specifications to maximize compliance with the guidelines. (#161)

The Nutrition Education and Training Program (NET), designed to teach children the value of a nutritionally balanced diet through positive daily lunchroom experiences and appropriate classroom reinforcement, also drew support. Carol Philipps of the Midwest Region NET Program Coordinators praises NET not only for contributing to the improvement in nutrition topic areas of the objectives, but also for helping in the related areas of dental caries, periodontal disease, obesity and overweight, eating

disorders, and intervention against certain chronic diseases. (#590) In addition to its role in training teachers and school food service personnel, Ann Buller of the Texas Department of Human Services sees the NET network as having the potential to "conduct school food service research, develop workshops and training materials, and provide technical training," in order to offer "an educational framework that would ultimately improve children's nutritional status." (#606)

Hospitalized Patients

A number of testifiers suggested that malnutrition is a serious problem among hospital patients, even those in general hospitals. Estimates vary according to the criteria used, but they agreed that about half of all patients suffer from malnutrition, and longer-stay patients are more likely to be malnourished than shorter-stay patients.[9] Also, according to Joel Kopple of the Harbor-UCLA Medical Center, poor nutritional status is associated with increased morbidity and mortality. (#681) Testifiers suggested as objectives that the prevalence of hospital malnutrition be reduced by 25 to 50 percent. (#238, #496) To reduce hospital malnutrition, Kopple called for an increase in the number of hospital personnel who can assess the nutritional status of patients and for training medical students and other health care providers to be more sensitive to nutritional disorders. (#681)

EDUCATION AND OTHER PREVENTIVE STRATEGIES

Educating both the public and health professionals about the role of nutrition in disease prevention is an important part of the effort to achieve nutrition objectives. However, witnesses also emphasized the need to go beyond merely informing consumers about good nutrition; they also must have the ability and the will to change their dietary habits. (#007; #077)

Nutrition education can come from a variety of sources: schools, health providers, mass media, community organizations, professional and trade associations, and health professionals. Powell suggests that by the year 2000, every state should have a broad-based, interdisciplinary commission to provide advice, advocacy, and networking on health-related food and nutrition issues for consumers. (#390)

Making nutrition counseling a part of school meal programs, the WIC program, or elderly meal programs is very effective, according to the Society for Nutrition

Education, which reported findings that when WIC clients were counseled about nutrition, the birth weight of their babies increased by 15 to 60 grams.[10] (#462) Several witnesses called for the inclusion of nutrition education in the school health curriculum; this is discussed more fully in Chapter 9.

Education also must be targeted toward health professionals. Young pointed out that a 1985 National Academy of Sciences report found nutrition education in medical schools inadequate.[11] She says that not even one-third of medical schools have a required full course in nutrition and suggested, along with other witnesses, that the objectives be expanded to include nutrition education for health professionals. (#496) According to the Grocery Manufacturers' Association, the 1990 objective that virtually all contacts with health professionals include a nutritional component is unrealistic. Instead, efforts should begin with the education of health professionals and then address their contacts with high-risk patients or those with a disorder in which nutrition plays a role. (#063)

Once consumers are aware of good nutritional habits, food labels can help them make dietary changes. The importance of clear labeling of fat (saturated and unsaturated), calories, cholesterol, and sodium content was mentioned repeatedly. Health claims permitted on labels should be worded so they do not confuse consumers, and efforts should be made to eliminate health fraud. Kathy Duffy of Harborview Medical Center in Seattle noted that with a large fraction of the population unable to read English, nutrition information should be presented with pictures, signs, colors, or logos. (#052) Restaurant menus and fast-food outlets could also provide information on nutritional content. (#462)

Other testifiers said that nutrition education and counseling should be part of general fitness programs; these should include the availability of healthy foods, especially in the workplace where exercise programs are sometimes offered and where cafeteria or vending machine food is available. (#100; #736)

IMPLEMENTATION

The goal-setting process must take into account some fundamental issues critical to progress in preventing nutrition-related problems. According to witnesses, these include funding, data needs, adequate staffing with nutritional specialists, and involvement of a variety of players.

Many witnesses spoke of an urgent need for a national system to monitor progress toward the nutrition objectives. According to Conway, a data system should be integrated at the federal, state, and local levels including, perhaps, a tie-in between local systems and NHANES. (#043) Such a system should have a core set of commonly identified data items, says the Society for Nutrition Education. (#462) Hoerr notes, as an example, the current use of different definitions of obesity and ways to measure it. (#100)

In addition to surveillance objectives, several types of research were proposed. Examples include studies of the cost and benefits of dietary changes (#077); research into food-borne disease and individual susceptibility (#733); exploration of food processing techniques that do not require harmful additives (#228); and general nutrition research, especially by the federal government. (#733)

Testimony involved discussion of the roles of many different types of organizations in improving nutritional status. These include the federal government through the National Institutes of Health, the Food and Drug Administration, and the Department of Agriculture; the Institute of Medicine's Food and Nutrition Board; state and local health departments; professional associations of dietitians and other health providers; community and social service groups; schools; employers; and the food industry. Representatives of many of these groups testified about their involvement in preventing nutrition-related health problems. Dietitians, for example, emphasized the role they can play in education and counseling. The National Dairy Council, in particular, emphasized its public education efforts. (#571)

The American Dietetic Association noted that 33 state health agencies have established dietary recommendations but that barriers to implementation, such as inadequate funding, personnel, and administrative structure, interfere with progress in meeting objectives. (#007) Others made clear that meeting nutritional objectives will require putting in place the resources upon which effective strategies can be built.

REFERENCES

1. U.S. Department of Health and Human Services: Surgeon General's Report on Nutrition and Health (DHHS Publication No. [PHS] 88-50210), 1988

2. National Research Council, Committee on Diet and Health: Diet and Health. Washington, D.C.: National Academy Press, 1989

3. Brown, JL: Hunger in the U.S. Sci Am 256(2):37–41, 1987

4. Najjar MF: Anthropometric reference data and prevalence of overweight, United States, 1976–1980. Vital and Health Statistics Series 11, No. 238 (DHHS Publication No. [PHS] 87-1688), 1987

5. Pope HG, Hudson JI, Yurgelun-Todd D: Anorexia nervosa and bulimia among 300 suburban women shoppers. Am J Psychiatry 141(2):292–294, 1984

6. Schotte DE, Stunkard AJ: Bulimia vs. bulimic behaviors on a college campus. J Am Med Assoc 258(9):1213–1215, 1987

7. Radzikowski J, Gale S: The national evaluation of school nutrition programs: Conclusions. Am J Clin Nutr 40(2)(suppl.):454–461, 1984

8. Radzikowski J, Gale S: Requirement for the national evaluation of school nutrition programs. Am J Clin Nutr 40(2)(suppl.):365–367, 1984

9. Roubenoff R, Roubenoff RA, Preto J, et al.: Malnutrition among hospitalized patients: A problem of physician awareness. Arch Intern Med 147(8):1462–1465, 1987

10. Rush D (Principal Investigator): Evaluation of the Special Supplemental Food Program for Women, Infants and Children (WIC), vol. 1: Summary. Research Triangle Institute, New York State Research Foundation for Mental Hygiene, 1987

11. Committee on Nutrition in Medical Education: Nutrition Education in U.S. Medical Schools. Washington, D.C.: National Academy Press, 1985

TESTIFIERS CITED IN CHAPTER 12

007 Lechowich, Karen, et al.; The American Dietetic Association
043 Conway, Dorothy; California Conference of Local Health Department Nutritionists
052 Duffy, Kathy; Harborview Medical Center and Wilkins, Jennifer; Pullman, Washington
053 McCarron, David et al.; The Oregon Health Sciences University
057 Egan, M. Jean; Michigan Dietetic Association
063 Fletcher, Carol; Grocery Manufacturers of America
077 Guthrie, Marilyn; Virginia Mason Clinic (Seattle)
082 Hanneman, Richard; Salt Institute
100 Hoerr, Sharon; Michigan State University
161 Neill, Carol; Alum Rock Union Elementary School District (California)
178 Reid, Elaine; Sacred Heart Medical Center (Spokane, Washington)
203 Smith, Richard; Henry Ford Hospital (Detroit)
216 Utah Nutrition Council
228 Wooldridge, Nancy; Alabama Dietetic Association
238 Bray, George; University of Southern California

390 Powell, Shirley; Southeastern Michigan Food Coalition
462 Dodds, Janice; Society for Nutrition Education
496 Young, Eleanor; University of Texas Health Science Center at San Antonio
571 Speckmann, Elwood; National Dairy Council
590 Philipps, Carol; Wisconsin Department of Public Instruction
606 Buller, Ann; Texas Department of Human Services
618 Frederick, Jacqueline; New Jersey Department of Education
627 Stokes, III, Joseph; Boston University
636 Ballin, Scott; American Heart Association
681 Kopple, Joel; University of California, Los Angeles
733 Morse, Roy; Institute of Food Technologists
735 Prothrow-Stith, Deborah; Massachusetts Department of Public Health
736 Wood, Loring; NYNEX Corporation
739 Anderson, Jennifer; Colorado State University

13. Physical Fitness and Exercise

Although some say the United States is caught up in a fitness craze, with Americans taking to jogging tracks, swimming pools, and aerobics classes, 38 witnesses made clear that many physical fitness and exercise goals are yet to be met. According to testimony, only a small fraction of adult Americans are exercising at optimal levels as specified in the 1990 Objectives and by the American College of Sports Medicine. About half are quite sedentary, despite the fact that sedentary adults have double the risk of cardiovascular disease.[1] (#021) Youth also are failing to meet exercise goals, and their fitness is declining. (#121)

Steven Blair of the Institute for Aerobics Research in Dallas notes that although much is known about the kind of exercise needed to achieve physical fitness, considerably less is known about the level of activity required to achieve positive health effects. (#021) Nevertheless, current knowledge prompted Blair and many other witnesses to propose new directions in the health objectives for the year 2000, including a greater emphasis on moderate levels of exercise. According to David Sobel of the Permanente Medical Group, the myth of "no pain, no gain" needs to be firmly debunked in the public mind.

> The image and standard of vigorous, sweat-soaked exercise has discouraged many sedentary individuals from even trying to become more active. The bulk of benefit may come from expending as little as 500 kilocalories a week in moderate physical activity. And such activity need not be an arduous bout of exercise, but can be pleasurable, enjoyable activities: walking, gardening, bowling, dancing, golf, and so on. (#780)

Others called for more attention to musculoskeletal fitness, the contribution of exercise to controlling certain diseases, and the potential adverse effects of exercise. (#021)

The fitness of our nation's youth—or, more precisely, the lack thereof—concerned a number of witnesses. According to American College of Sports Medicine:

> Over one-half of our children do not get enough exercise to develop healthy hearts and lungs, and

a significant number of our school age youth already have established risk factors for cardiovascular disease. A conservative estimate suggests that adolescent obesity is prevalent among 20 to 30 percent of our youth. In our opinion, the majority of this can be attributed to significant reductions in physical activity, both at school and at home, the adoption of sedentary lifestyles, and the promotion of poor nutritional habits. (#534)

Among the recommended improvements to be addressed through Year 2000 Health Objectives are more and better-quality physical education programs in school and agreed-upon standards for fitness tests. Witnesses spoke with almost one voice about the need to stress health-related fitness—rather than motor fitness or power or sports-related fitness—for children.

NEW EMPHASES NEEDED

Much testimony about physical fitness and exercise includes proposals that would significantly alter the approach of the 1990 Objectives which, many witnesses believe, focused quite narrowly on attaining relatively high levels of cardiovascular fitness.

A major shift called for by many witnesses is to deemphasize high-intensity exercise and focus instead on getting more people involved in moderate exercise. (#021; #187; #534) James Ross fears that the emphasis on high-intensity exercise "has turned off a lot of people" who cannot or will not exercise long or hard enough. The past emphasis on intense exercise, according to Ross, probably has resulted in a lot of injuries to people who felt compelled to stick to exercise programs *at all costs*. From a public health perspective, encouraging more people to exercise at various levels of intensity—and in various ways suited to their own needs, interests, and abilities—might be better. (#187)

Taking a slightly different approach, Blair suggests that the 1990 objectives aimed at producing relatively high levels of physical fitness be retained but that new objectives be formulated to promote gains in moderate activity. A reasonable target for the year 2000 could be to reduce the percentage of extremely sedentary people to 20–25 percent. (#021)

Witnesses also say that the emphasis on cardiovascular fitness in the 1990 Objectives shortchanged other aspects of physical fitness. Several suggest adding objectives relating to the musculoskeletal system. (#021; #248; #534) Blair notes that musculoskeletal fitness is especially important in older individuals to prevent disability and preserve functional capacity for routine occupational, recreational, and daily tasks. (#021)

Witnesses also note other effects of exercise that should be reflected in the Year 2000 Health Objectives. Ross refers to the impact of exercise on non-insulin-dependent diabetes, the control of depression and anxiety, weight control, and the cessation of addictive behaviors. (#187)

David Siscovick of the University of Washington sounds a note of caution by pointing out that none of the 1990 Objectives addressed the responsibility to minimize the adverse effects of exercise, which can range from sore muscles to sudden death. Studies suggest that 15 percent of sudden cardiac deaths occur during moderate or vigorous exercise,[2] and that this is not a random event: vigorous exercise can precipitate sudden cardiac death. Nevertheless, he adds, among men who engage in regular vigorous exercise, the transient risk during activity is outweighed by a decreased risk at other times, so that the overall risk to vigorous exercisers is still less than among sedentary men. (#200)

Siscovick proposes that the Year 2000 Health Objectives place greater emphasis on the importance of reducing risks through pre-exercise evaluation and counseling, controlling extremes of temperature around exercise periods, and reducing cigarette smoking and alcohol use. He cites Kenneth Powell and Ralph Paffenbarger: "The potential overall beneficial impact of physical activity on health will be poorly served if activity patterns are recommended indiscriminately for all groups without regard for the subgroup's specific benefits and risks."[3] (#200)

SPECIAL POPULATIONS

A number of populations were identified as having special physical fitness needs and problems that require attention in the Year 2000 Health Objectives. The American College of Sports Medicine (ACSM) comments that the fitness boom has affected primarily highly educated, affluent suburbanites; blue collar and minority populations have not been affected much by pressures to exercise and maintain a healthful diet. In

setting new objectives, ways must be found to influence these groups. (#534)

Several witnesses propose objectives specifically targeted to older adults. According to the ACSM, because of major physiological changes in the nerves and muscle fibers, muscle mass in older individuals is decreased by approximately 50 percent compared to younger adults. James Breen of George Washington University proposes that by the year 2000, 50 percent of adults 65 years and older participate three or more times per week for sessions of 30 minutes or more in activities designed to promote or maintain flexibility, ambulatory skills, arm and hand strength, or other skills of daily living, and in physical activity at least as vigorous as a sustained slow walk. (#550)

However, physical health after age 65 is related integrally to earlier lifestyle habits. Thus, the ACSM states, "our target for the year 2000 should be to stimulate all adults to maintain their strength by incorporating strength-type training activities into their daily lives. In addition, more research into the benefits of strength training on cardiovascular and skeletal muscle injuries needs to be performed." (#534)

The need to pay special attention to those with developmental disorders, especially children, and to individuals who are physically, mentally, or emotionally disabled also was discussed. (#248; #313)

REVISING GOALS FOR CHILDREN AND YOUTH

America's children are not physically fit, according to many witnesses, who place much of the blame on the poor condition of physical education programs. Many recommendations for Year 2000 Health Objectives reflect the need to shift the focus of physical education classes from the quantity of time spent in class (the focus of the 1990 Objectives) to the quality of the program.

The child of the 1980s is less fit and fatter than the child of the 1960s, according to Charles Kuntzleman of Fitness Finders. (#121) Today's child typically gets less than 15 minutes of vigorous exercise a day. Kuntzleman says that only 25 percent of a child's time in the physical education classroom involves motor activity, and only 1 to 3 minutes of that time is of sufficient intensity to train the heart and make the child fit, whereas a minimum of 20 minutes is necessary. In addition, students do not tend to develop skills that promote lifelong physical fitness. "It is time for schools to recognize that the traditional curriculums developed in the early part of this century do not have application today." (#121)

Kuntzleman and others made specific recommendations about improving the quality of physical education classes by the year 2000. (#021; #121; #171; #187; #534; #596) Many suggestions emphasize activities that build strength and muscular flexibility, and teach lifelong fitness values and skills. The American Alliance for Health, Physical Education, Recreation and Dance (AAHPERD) also says that physical education should be taught every day for 30 to 55 minutes, depending on the grade, and classes should be no larger than those of other academic programs. The AAHPERD says that by the year 2000, all physical education classes in seventh through twelfth grades, and 75 percent of classes for kindergarten through sixth grades, should be taught by a certified physical educator. (#596)

Blair emphasizes the importance of teaching health and fitness concepts and deemphasizing motor performance, or sports skills instruction. He notes that most vigorous exercise among children takes place outside the physical education class and indicates that increasing enrollment in physical education classes is not a priority. (#021) Others propose targets for increased participation but emphasize the importance of improving the quality of the courses. Kuntzleman, for instance, recognizes the "Feelin' Good" program, sponsored by the W.K. Kellogg Foundation, as a model for improving aerobic and muscle fitness levels, flexibility, cardiovascular knowledge, exercise participation, and other positive outcomes. He also criticizes the trend toward reducing physical education classes as money becomes tight. (#121)

Several witnesses note that a serious impediment to improving youth fitness is the lack of agreed-upon standards and programs. For example, according to Russell Pate of the University of South Carolina:

The greatest current deficiency in the field of youth fitness testing is the lack of widely accepted criterion-referenced standards for physical fitness in children and youth. The lack of such standards greatly retards our ability to interpret the results of physical fitness tests and limits our ability to communicate effectively to children, their parents, and the public the meaning of fitness test results.

By the year 2000, there should be widely accepted criterion-referenced standards for physical fitness tests in children and youth, testifiers say. (#171; #187) The AAHPERD proposes that by the year 2000, more than 75 percent of schools should test all their students for physical fitness and recognize student progress. Only about 50 percent of students in the first to fourth grades currently attend schools that provide such testing.[4] (#596)

Numerous witnesses commented on the importance of using tests that assess activities that will lead to improved health, rather than just greater strength or athletic prowess. Brian Sharkey points out that the President's Council on Physical Fitness and Sports favors a fitness test that is not health related. The AAHPERD, on the other hand, promotes a health-related test. The inconsistency is confusing and should be resolved in favor of the health-related test, Sharkey says. (#363) Pate supports Sharkey's conclusions and believes progress already is being made.

Through the mid-1970s, the traditional motor performance tests that emphasized measurement of speed, power, and agility were dominant. However, over the past 10 years, virtually all newly developed tests have emphasized health fitness, including cardiorespiratory endurance, body fatness, flexibility, and muscular strength/ endurance. This approach to physical fitness testing seems to indicate that the physical education profession's operational definition of physical fitness is becoming more health-oriented. (#171)

Several witnesses said that objectives for the year 2000 should include goals for children as young as age five or six; the 1990 Objectives include only children ten and older. (#171; #248; #313) "The growth and development literature suggest that behavior patterns are established several years prior to age ten," according to Jeanette Winfree of the American Physical Therapy Association. (#313) The importance of physical fitness for children with developmental disabilities also was mentioned. (#248)

IMPLEMENTATION

Testifiers identified a number of specific sites with the potential to reach large numbers of adults. Loring Wood of the NYNEX Corporation and others endorse the value of worksite fitness programs. (#021; #550; #736) However, Winfree urges more worksite programs that address flexibility and muscle strength and place special emphasis on the serious problem of back injuries. *(#313)* Witnesses representing the National Recreation and Park Association encourage increased public support for, and utilization of, recreation facilities in promoting health and wellness. Recreational and health professionals should work together to "jointly develop and pursue a plan and strategy to define practical goals, policies, and means to achieve improved health and recreation." *(#538; #620)*

The need to do a better job of training certain professions about exercise and physical education was mentioned by several testifiers. Kuntzleman believes that an underlying cause of the lack of fitness in our youth relates to the need to upgrade the quality of physical education teachers.

> Our graduates seem to be so tuned in to sport skills development that they have neglected the basic vocabulary of the sport of fitness and acquisition of basic motor skills. We need a vocabulary of fitness, just as we have a basic vocabulary for teaching kids how to read, write, do math, etc. *(#121)*

There also were calls for expanding the education of physicians about exercise physiology and the value of physical activity so that they can encourage their patients in health-related activities. *(#021; #541)* Physicians also should instruct patients in ways to minimize the risk of sudden cardiac death during vigorous exercise. *(#200)*

Several witnesses cite the need for additional data to set or monitor progress in goals. Blair says current surveys are doing "reasonably well" in tracking physical activity, at least for adults; however, a better tracking system is needed for physical fitness. *(#021)* Breen identifies several goals relating to the need for increased knowledge about the relationship between exercise and health outcomes. *(#550)* Siscovick says that by the year 2000, a methodology for identifying all exercise-related sudden cardiac deaths and monitoring age-, gender-, and race-specific incidence rates should be established. *(#200)* Breen says that by the year 2000, the incidence of injuries from the most popular adult exercises should be known. *(#550)*

The ACSM calls for more research into the benefits of strength training in relation to cardiovascular and skeletal muscle injuries, noting that the greater elasticity of blood vessels in the young enables them to better compensate for cardiac overloads; it is not known whether strength training leads to greater elasticity in later years. *(#534)* Marilyn Gossman and Jane Walter, representing the American Physical Therapy Association, also say that more research on exercise and the musculoskeletal system is necessary. They call for additional risk-benefit data on fitness programs by the year 2000, with special emphasis on their effect on the musculoskeletal system. *(#248)*

In addition to its specific proposals for improving physical education courses, the American Alliance for Health, Physical Education, Recreation and Dance requests action by the federal government. The AAHPERD proposes substantial federal funding for research aimed at improving physical education courses, as well as establishment of an Office of Physical Education in the Department of Education. The organization also calls for providing women equal opportunities to compete in school and college athletics and sports programs as a way of encouraging lifelong fitness. *(#596)*

REFERENCES

1. Powell KE, Thompson PD, Caspersen CJ, et al.: Physical activity and the incidence of coronary heart disease. Annual Review of Public Health, vol. 8. Edited by L Breslow, JE Fielding, LB Lave. Palo Alto: Annual Reviews, 1987

2. Vuori I: The cardiovascular risks of physical activity. Acta Med Scand Suppl 711:205–214, 1984

3. Powell KE, Paffenbarger RS: Workshop on epidemiologic and public health aspects of physical activity and exercise: A summary. Pub Health Rep 100(2):118–126, 1985

4. Ross JG, Pate RR: Summary of findings from the National Children and Youth Fitness Study II. J Phys Educ Rec & Dance, 50-96, November–December 1987

TESTIFIERS CITED IN CHAPTER 13

021 Blair, Steven; Institute for Aerobics Research (Dallas)
121 Kuntzleman, Charles; Fitness Finders (Spring Arbor, Michigan)
171 Pate, Russell; University of South Carolina
187 Ross, James; Maryland
200 Siscovick, David; University of Washington
248 Gossman, Marilyn and Walter, Jane; American Physical Therapy Association
313 Winfree, Jeanette; Physical Therapy Services (Galveston, Texas)
363 Sharkey, Brian; University of Northern Colorado
534 Raven, Peter and Drinkwater, Barbara; American College of Sports Medicine
538 Curtis, Joseph; City of New Rochelle Department of Human Services (New York)
541 Sheehan, George; The Second Wind (Red Bank, New Jersey)
550 Breen, James; George Washington University (Washington, D.C.)
596 Perry, Jean; American Alliance for Health, Physical Education, Recreation and Dance
620 Tice, R. Dean; National Recreation and Park Association
736 Wood, Loring; NYNEX Corporation
780 Sobel, David; The Permanente Medical Group

14. Mental Health

Mental and emotional disabilities, according to the National Mental Health Association (NMHA), "consume an astounding portion of our nation's resources." The NMHA states that more than 19 percent of adults suffer from some mental or emotional disorder. The direct costs of mental health care were $24 billion in 1981, and the lost productivity costs were $29 billion.[1] Despite these high costs, many persons in need of care are not treated; still others with underlying mental or emotional problems are treated through the general health care system, at a cost of many billions of dollars, without ever being properly diagnosed. The NMHA reports that many "patients seeking medical help do so because of physical symptoms related primarily to stress reactions or emotional problems." On the positive side, however, the NMHA reports that "a substantial and rapidly expanding knowledge base exists to direct efforts in the prevention of mental-emotional disabilities." (#070) The combination of the high costs of mental illness and the potential benefits to be attained through prevention led 75 testifiers to address their remarks primarily to this subject and another 18 to make substantial comments.

According to Joan Reiss of the Sacramento-Placer Mental Health Association in California:

Ask a group of people to tell you what they think when they hear the words, "physical health." Responses often include: exercise, muscle tone, running, fitness, diet. Now ask the same individuals to free associate with the words "mental health." After a brief embarrassed silence the thoughts flow: crazy, depressed, headache, psycho, nuts, insane asylum. Physical health conjures up positive images and mental health brings on negative ones. Why? For most of the population, mental health does not mean health at all but refers to mental illness. A major goal of the National Mental Health Association by the year 2000 is to have the general public believe that mental health refers to a state of wellness as opposed to illness. (#179)

Others, however, object to the NMHA's focus on mental health and would prefer to see efforts concentrated on "severe mental illnesses" such as schizophrenia. Fewer people are afflicted with these disorders, but they suffer much more. Although these testifiers acknowledge that there are no proven prevention strategies for severe mental illness, they see great potential in biological, rather than psychosocial, research. (#088; #278)

According to the NMHA, the risk factors for mental and emotional disabilities "include genetic heritage, physical vulnerability, family circumstances, disruption of family stability and child nurturing, and critical events such as bereavement, marital disruption, or unemployment. Particularly at risk are those who experience multiple stressors." The identification of these risk factors is important because it can help target information and possible preventive interventions. (#070)

The NMHA reports, however, that the current application of this knowledge "in preventing mental-emotional disabilities is creditable, but far from sufficient." Many resources exist in state and local government, businesses, health and mental health agencies, and communities. These services, however, "tend to be scattered, without comprehensive planning and coordination, and are subject to funding cuts. Diversity of programming is fruitful, but coordination of efforts, with a clearer definition of prevention outcomes, improved taxonomy and standards of effectiveness, is needed to move the field forward." (#070)

The NMHA suggests four organizing principles to serve as a framework for considering prevention efforts:

1. Biological integrity: Because of the indivisibility of physical and mental health, "good health care addresses both medical and psychological concerns."

2. Psychosocial competence: "We can prevent some mental-emotional disabilities by ensuring that individuals have skills for relating to others and capabilities to handle crises."

3. Social support: "We can prevent some mental-emotional disabilities by helping people be involved with others who provide nurturance, support, and encouragement."

4. Societal policies and attitudes: "The practices and policies of organizations with which we are involved through[out] life—the hospital at birth, child

care centers, schools, work, health care and social service systems, and legal and government agencies—can either enhance or hinder mental health by affecting the development of competence or because they are closely involved in critical life events that result in greater risk for mental-emotional disabilities." *(#070)*

The witnesses also identified a number of groups in the population that are especially vulnerable to mental health problems, particularly children, adolescents, and older people. Prevention and early intervention are of critical importance in the mental health area, says Ernest Dahl of American River College. Because of this, intensive prevention efforts on behalf of children are needed; waiting to deal with the adult is too late. *(#047)* For adolescents, suicide *(#500)* and teenage pregnancy *(#070)* are seen as the critical mental health problems (see also Chapters 4, 11, 16, and 23). For older adults, physical illnesses associated with old age and the medication that people take for these illnesses increase the risk of mental-emotional disability. Older people also face such stressful life events as forced retirement, death of a spouse, death of relatives or friends, or moving or loss of home. *(#070)*

PARTICULAR PROBLEMS

Much of the testimony on mental health issues focused on three areas: stress, depression, and more severe mental illnesses such as schizophrenia. Stress and depression are more prevalent, and the witnesses saw a greater potential for primary and secondary prevention. Schizophrenia and similar disorders are less prevalent, but more devastating to the individuals affected and their families. The current potential for prevention of these disorders, however, is less promising, so many of the testifiers called for more research, better treatment modalities, and better services.

Stress

"Despite its failure to conform to the medical model of disease, stress illness is growing in impact and importance," says George Benjamin of the National Safety Council. "Because of fast changes in social, job, and personal environments, more and more people are reporting unbearable feelings of stress, of just feeling sick," he says. *(#019)* The Laborers' International Union of North America also calls for more attention to the mental health impacts of job loss and job change, to work-related and work-associated mental health problems, and to the organization of work and its influence on stress. *(#586)*

According to James Quick of the University of Texas at Arlington, representing the American Psychological Association:

Stress is neither a disease process nor necessarily bad. Used wisely, the stress response is a very useful asset in responding to legitimate emergencies and in achieving extraordinary peak performances, such as in athletic competitions. It is mismanaged stress that leads to a host of health disorders.

Thus, Quick calls for stress education of the public and of professionals, particularly for secondary school students, college and university students, employees in corporations, and members of professional associations. According to Quick, educational programs should cover (1) knowledge of stress and its causes, (2) knowledge of individual and collective costs of mismanaged stress, (3) how to diagnose stress and its effects, and (4) knowledge of "responsible individual and organizational prevention strategies that are beneficial in the management of stress." *(#176)*

Depression

Roseann Scott and others from the University of Colorado Health Sciences Center report that depression affects millions of people per year. They suggest a number of strategies for dealing with depression, including training school counselors and teachers to recognize its symptoms, comprehensive psychiatric evaluations of adolescents with drinking problems, counseling new mothers at risk for postpartum depression, and providing follow-up treatment for hospital patients with identified depressive symptoms. *(#015)*

Stephen Goldston of the University of California, Los Angeles says that bereavement is a major cause of depression. Community mental health centers could help by providing (1) specific preventive services for widows and widowers, parents who have lost a child, children who have lost a parent or sibling, and the family of a suicide victim; (2) death education programs for parents and teachers; and (3) training programs on death, dying, grief, and bereavement for care givers. *(#280)*

Schizophrenia and Other Serious Mental Illnesses

Writing about schizophrenia, Dale Johnson of the University of Houston reports:

Each year from 100,000 to 200,000 Americans, mostly adolescents or young adults, develop this dread disorder. For nearly all, the onset is marked by psychiatric hospitalization, and for the vast majority this is followed by a life of recurrent psychotic episodes, impaired social relations, joblessness, and abject poverty. The mentally ill are profoundly lonely, isolated, and vulnerable to stress. (#325)

Antipsychotic medications that were introduced in the 1950s, reports Johnson, have provided some relief from major symptoms and protection from stress, but have not altered the basic course of the disease. (#325) Floyd Bloom of the Scripps Clinic and Research Foundation, however, estimates that prompt treatment will reverse, significantly improve, or reduce relapse in one-quarter to one-third of schizophrenia cases.[2] The NMHA reports:

We do not yet know how to prevent schizophrenia or major depressive disorders. Encouraging advances are being made in epidemiological, biomedical, neurological, and behavioral science research. Eventual success in preventing these disorders will require support or research in all these approaches and active collaboration among researchers. (#070)

Johnson, representing the National Alliance for the Mentally Ill and the American Psychological Association, sees the hospital relapse rate for schizophrenia as too high and calls for action on this front. Lowering the relapse rate will entail less restrictive treatment and rehabilitation environments; continuity of care; adequate housing and protection against economic need; better education and training for caretakers, including family members; use of social learning methods to decrease unacceptable behavior and increase desirable behavior; and rehabilitation services, including supported employment, education, and skills training. (#325)

Many of the witnesses focused on the stigma associated with mental illness. Donald Richardson, representing the National Alliance for the Mentally Ill, says that "stigma contributes to insurance dis-crimination, housing discrimination, employment discrimination, and fosters client resistance to treatment. The public must be made aware of the fact that mental illness is a no-fault physical illness and not a character defect." (#278)

INTERVENTIONS

The NMHA identifies four program areas that have "immediate potential for reducing mental-emotional disabilities: wanted and healthy babies; prevention of adolescent pregnancy; school programs; and support, information, and training for those in situations of extreme stress." (#070)

Wanted and Healthy Babies

According to the NMHA:

Preventing mental-emotional disabilities can begin before birth by ensuring healthy, wanted, full-term babies. Society can increase the chances that a pregnancy is wanted by fostering the development of responsible decision making, providing reproductive and sex education at home and in schools, and making family planning services accessible. The media can play an important role by portraying responsible, rather than glamorous or casual, sexual attitudes and behavior. (#070)

According to Betty Tableman of the Michigan Department of Mental Health, facilitating attachment and parent-infant interaction would reduce low birth weight, cultural mental retardation, and damage from child abuse or neglect, as well as emotional and conduct disorders. Prenatal care settings and hospital maternity units should screen women for psychosocial risk. (#418)

The Mental Health Association in Texas calls for voluntary parenthood education programs to prevent mental, emotional, and health problems in the child's first years and unemployment or dependency in the longer term. Services should be available from pregnancy through preschool years, according to association representative Betty Jo Hay, and should provide "developmental screening and training and support services to help parents to enhance their children's intellectual, language, physical, and social development." One such program, the Perry Preschool Project in Michigan, reported that 19 years after the project, participating children had graduated from high school and gone on to jobs or further education at twice the rate of children without the program.[3] *(#091)*

Prevention of Adolescent Pregnancy

Adolescent pregnancies result in more than half a million births each year, 50 percent of them to unmarried teens;[4] these pregnancies constitute a significant risk factor for mental-emotional disturbances in both mother and child. *(#070)* Several witnesses saw the prevention of adolescent and teen pregnancies as a key factor in helping ensure the mental health of current and future generations.

The effect of teen pregnancy and parenting touch not only the mother and child, but also the father, their families, and society as a whole, says Jackie Rose of the Clackamas County Department of Human Services in Oregon. Among the problems resulting from births to young parents are low educational achievement, unemployment, single parenting, divorce, poverty, welfare dependency, pregnancy-related health risks, infant mortality, neglect, abuse, out-of-home placements, and juvenile court placements. *(#343)*

Some groups of adolescents may require special attention, according to Peggy Smith, representing the American College of Obstetricians and Gynecologists, whose data suggest that "biological and sociological factors may interact to generate a group of Hispanic teens especially vulnerable for early pregnancy." To effectively address the needs of these young girls, Smith calls for the use of bilingual staffs in state agencies dealing with them, as well as research into the effect of acculturation and its impact on health care practices, including contraceptive use and maternity needs. *(#308)*

Some programs already have proven success in reaching juniors and seniors, according to the American School Health Association. One program of education, counseling, and medical and contraceptive services offered at a clinic located near the school resulted in a 30 percent decline in the pregnancy rate for those in the school program after 28 months, but a 57.6 percent increase in pregnancies among those not in the program during the same period.[5] *(#006)*

To help prevent adolescent pregnancies, the NMHA calls for "cooperative efforts by parents, schools, and other social service agencies to prevent adolescent pregnancy, through programs to develop responsible decision making, provide health and sex education programs that emphasize the consequences of sexual activity, and ensure access to counseling about contraception and health services." *(#070)* Such programs are discussed at length in Chapter 23.

School Programs

"Programs in schools—preschool through high school—that incorporate validated mental health strategies and competence building as an integral part of the curriculum" can help prevent mental-emotional disorders, according to the NMHA. *(#070)*

Kevin Dwyer of the National Association of School Psychologists advocates prevention of mental health problems of children through a cascade of interdisciplinary, interagency, community-based preventive and treatment interventions. Such programs would "help children's social and interpersonal adjustment, increase their resistance to mental health problems, and improve their long-term ability to contribute meaningfully to society." Schools must help address the personal, emotional, and social development and concerns of students. Programs should include community awareness efforts; parent and care-giver education; preschool programs to teach social skills, problem solving, and communication; programs for school-aged children and youth that stress problem solving and building self-esteem; teen programs that focus on problem solving, conflict resolution, positive peer socialization, and the responsibilities of adulthood; and crisis intervention programs. *(#802)*

Other testifiers suggested more specific programs for the schools, namely art and dance therapy. According to Ellen Speert of Los Angeles, "Art therapy aids in the integration of a healthier sense of self. By increasing creativity, it enhances both effective problem solving and self-esteem." *(#477)* Marcia Leventhal of New York University and Nancy BrooksSchmitz of Columbia University report that dance can increase self-esteem and self-awareness, relieve tension, heal and strengthen the body, and provide a means of social communication. *(#595)*

Support, Information, and Training in Situations of Extreme Stress

According to the NMHA, "programs that help children and adults to anticipate and manage adverse life circumstances or critical life events—programs such as home visits to high-risk families with infants, training in coping skills and mutual support groups" also offer potential for reducing mental-emotional disabilities. *(#070)*

Reiss says that 15 million people in the United

States are currently involved in a half million self-help or mutual support groups.[6] (#179) Audrey Gartner of the National Self-Help Clearinghouse adds, "Over the past decade, self-help mutual support groups have become an important way of helping people cope with various life crises. Groups have organized to help individual members deal with a wide range of health-related and other problems." (#427) For instance, the NMHA reports that "mutual help groups, such as Widow to Widow programs, have been found effective in dealing with bereavement. Programs to increase the social involvement of older people in the community have shown positive effects on mental health and life satisfaction." (#070)

IMPLEMENTATION

A number of implementation issues were raised by testifiers, especially the integration of mental health and other health services, the overall organization and funding of prevention programs, and the need for better surveillance data and more research.

Henry Leuchter, President of the Mental Health Association of Franklin County in Ohio, and others say that mental health services should not be treated as separate from other health services. Adequate planning for all health services requires integration, consensus, and communication. (#130)

Goldston points out that "the number of state departments of mental health with a designated unit responsible for prevention, with adequate budget and administrative structure, should be increased"— there are currently five. "The number of employers and insurers supporting prevention efforts by including coverage for prevention activities in benefit plans and insurance packages should be increased," says Goldston. (#280)

The American Association of Child and Adolescent Psychiatry is particularly concerned with services for children. The number of children and adolescents at risk for psychiatric illness is overwhelming and growing, they say, whereas federal resources for services and training are shrinking. Prevention programs that do exist are highly fragmented; a systems approach is needed to combine outreach programs, needs assessment, treatment training, and technical assistance options. (#009)

The NMHA suggests an objective based on the belief that no adequate surveillance system exists for mental health issues.

By the year 2000, the federal government shall establish a periodic process for determining the extent and scope of mental health problems relative to general health. The 1984 Epidemiological Catchment Area (ECA) Study conducted by NIMH provided valuable information on the prevalence of mental disorders. Unfortunately such data are unusual; there is not adequate, accessible data on mental health needs, services, and so on. The value of the ECA study is heightened by the general difficulty in obtaining mental health data. Factors such as consistency in diagnostic terminology, confidentiality, and involvement of multiple agencies can affect the validity of mental health statistics. (#070)

Most witnesses agreed that more federal funds should go to research on mental illness. For example, Beverly Long of the World Federation for Mental Health says that "it makes no sense to allocate 5 percent of the health research dollars to mental health when one-fourth to one-half of the hospital beds in the U.S. are occupied by those diagnosed as 'mentally ill'." (#270)

Beverly Banyay, representing the Mental Health Association in Pennsylvania, points out that prevention interventions take time to develop and must be carefully evaluated. She calls for more well-designed, multidisciplinary research and demonstration projects on screening, diagnosis, and evaluation strategies for all age groups. Longitudinal research is especially necessary because the effects of prevention programs occur over lifetimes, not months. (#014)

REFERENCES

1. Commission on the Prevention of Mental-Emotional Disabilities: The Prevention of Mental-Emotional Disabilities. Alexandria, Va.: National Mental Health Association, April 1986

2. Warner R: Recovery from Schizophrenia. Boston: Routledge & Kegan Paul, 1985

3. Barnett WS: Benefit cost analysis of the Perry Preschool Program and its implications. Education Evaluation and Policy Analysis 7(4):333–42, 1985

4. Wallace HM, Ryan G Jr., Oglesby AC (Eds.): Maternal and Child Health Practices (3rd Edition). Oakland, Ca.: Third Party Publishing Company, 1988

5. Zabin LS, Hirsch MB, Smith EA, et al.: Evaluation of a pregnancy prevention program for urban teenagers. Fam Plann Perspect 18(3):119–126, 1986

6. Gartner A, Gartner A, Kobasa SO: Self help. Handbook of Behavioral Medicine for Women. Edited by EA Blechman, KD Brownell. New York: Pergamon Press, 1988

TESTIFIERS CITED IN CHAPTER 14

006 Allensworth, Diane; American School Health Association
009 Anthony, Virginia; American Association of Child and Adolescent Psychiatry
014 Banyay, Beverly; Community College of Beaver County (Pennsylvania)
015 Scott, Roseann; University of Colorado Health Sciences Center
019 Benjamin, George; National Safety Council
047 Dahl, Ernest; American River College (Sacramento)
070 Garrison, Preston; National Mental Health Association
088 Havel, Jim; The National Alliance for the Mentally Ill
091 Hay, Betty Jo; Mental Health Association in Texas
130 Leuchter, Henry; Mental Health Association of Franklin County (Ohio)
176 Quick, James; University of Texas at Arlington
179 Reiss, Joan; Mental Health Association, Sacramento-Placer
270 Long, Beverly; World Federation for Mental Health
278 Richardson, Donald; Los Angeles, California
280 Goldston, Stephen; University of California, Los Angeles
308 Smith, Peggy B.; Baylor College of Medicine
325 Johnson, Dale; University of Houston
343 Rose, Jackie; Clackamas County Department of Human Services (Oregon)
418 Tableman, Betty; Michigan Department of Mental Health
427 Gartner, Audrey; National Self-Help Clearinghouse
477 Speert, Ellen; American Art Therapy Association
500 Medrano, Martha; University of Texas Health Science Center at San Antonio
586 Fosco, Angelo; Laborers' International Union of North America
595 Leventhal, Marcia; New York University and BrooksSchmitz, Nancy; Columbia University
802 Dwyer, Kevin; National Association of School Psychologists

15. Unintentional Injuries

The harm, disability, and death resulting from injury can be reduced by coordinated community prevention and control measures and individual awareness of risk factors for injury, according to many testifiers. *(#368; #378)*

"Injuries are not accidents or random events. They are predictable and therefore preventable. Injury prevention can be effective, but there are many players, and little direction," states Patricia West of the Colorado Department of Health. *(#368)* Frederick Rivara, Director of the Harborview Injury Prevention and Research Center in Seattle, believes that "injury control is coming of age, and will have a significant impact on the morbidity and mortality due to trauma in the coming decade." *(#334)* Steven Macdonald of the University of Washington quotes the 1985 National Academy of Sciences report *Injury in America*, which states that "injury is the principal public health problem in America today."[1] Macdonald echoes this view and calls for a concerted local, state, and national approach: "Linking injury epidemiology and health policy is the key." *(#322)*

Over the past decade, adds Rivara, the increasing attention paid to controlling injury has allowed this attitude of preventability to take root. It is likely that aggressive goals in injury control can be set and reached by the year 2000. *(#334)* Forty-eight testifiers addressed unintentional injuries and suggested objectives to reduce injury from motor vehicle accidents, falls, fires, poisoning, drowning, and violence.

The Year 2000 Health Objectives distinguish between intentional and unintentional injuries. Speakers gave specific objectives for each category and outlined many prevention strategies. For a few testifiers, separation of the two categories in the Year 2000 Health Objectives is problematic. Not only is the intentionality of many injuries hard to assess, says Macdonald, but if trends and prevention measures are to be reliable, injury reporting must include all injuries, regardless of cause. *(#322)*

Because of the nature of much of the testimony and many of the suggested prevention strategies, this chapter presents injury prevention goals popularly grouped under "unintentional" injuries. Chapter 16 deals with injury prevention as it relates to violence, homicide, suicide, child abuse, and so on, which come under the heading of "intentional" injury in the Year 2000 Health Objectives outline. Disabling injuries, especially as they affect children and teens, are seen by many witnesses as deserving special attention, as are implementation problems related to manpower and organization and to surveillance and data collection.

MOTOR VEHICLE INJURIES

The American Automobile Association (AAA) reports that 44,241 people died nationwide in 1984, from motor vehicle crashes. Of these fatalities, about half were alcohol related.[2] *(#008)* Trauma from motor vehicle crashes is the fourth leading cause of death in the United States, the leading cause of death for ages 5 to 34, and the second leading cause of death for ages 1 to 4. The vehicular-crash-related death rate for a 15-year-old male is many times that of polio at its worst. *(#011)* In terms of potential years of life lost, motor vehicle fatalities rate above both cancer and heart disease.

To reduce the number of motor vehicle deaths, says Karen Tarrant of the Michigan Department of State Police, the problem must be seen as an important public health priority. *(#425)* Traffic injuries are more than just a "highway safety problem," echoes James Saalberg of the CUNA Mutual Insurance Group, and individuals must be encouraged to think of them as a health problem. *(#190)*

According to Tarrant, prevention and control of motor vehicle accidents involve five components: drinking and driving, proper restraint, speed, roadway design, and vehicle design. Of these five, drinking and driving, proper restraint, and compliance with speed limits reflect individual attitudes. Although law enforcement agencies can take measures to increase compliance with traffic rules, health promotion efforts in the community are necessary to bring about significant and long-lasting reductions in injury rates. Such programs should teach the importance of "buckling up," not driving after or while drinking, and obeying speed limits. *(#425)* Robert Haggerty of the William T. Grant Foundation reports that driver competence (or incompetence) is also a factor in some motor vehicle accidents, (e.g., older drivers with vision or hearing deficiencies) and should be addressed through both increased compliance and health promotion efforts. *(#784)*

Richard Austin, chairman of the Michigan State Safety Commission, adds that education on traffic safety has to include personal decisions about interacting with other vehicles as pedestrians, bicyclists, or drivers. *(#011)* Such education is especially important for children. As pedestrians and bicycle riders, many children do not have a proper understanding of how a car operates or how long it takes to stop. *(#058)* For five to nine year olds, pedestrian and bicycle injury is the most important cause of trauma that leads to death.[3] *(#334)*

Education, however, is not sufficient by itself to reduce fatalities from motor vehicle crashes. David Sleet of San Diego State University says that failure to use seat restraints may be the single most important preventable risk factor for motor vehicle trauma. This trend must be countered and reversed through policy and legislation, as well as through health promotion and incentives. "With 100 percent safety belt use in front seats, an additional 10,000 lives could have been saved and 120,000 injuries prevented in 1986," he says. *(#285)* Leo Gossett of the Texas Department of Public Safety also sees the proper use of occupant restraints as "the most identifiable and measurable factor" in the reduction of motor vehicle injuries and deaths. *(#296)*

State and local police should enforce seat belt use and be strict with alcohol-related offenses. According to Gary Trietsch of the Texas Department of Highways and Public Transportation, public awareness programs coordinated with a law enforcement program, including new safety belt and driving-while-intoxicated (DWI) laws, have contributed to a decline in traffic deaths to a 10-year low in Texas. *(#563)* Health professionals also should be involved in the effort to increase seat belt use and to strengthen legislation requiring such use at all times. *(#190)*

The successful implementation of laws in all 50 states and the District of Columbia requiring the use of child safety seats is a notable victory, achieved through the efforts of state and local traffic enforcement agencies, health professionals, organizations, and communities. Joseph Hill of the Detroit Department of Health, however, reports that the number of injuries to infants and small children is still unacceptably high due to lack of compliance and incorrect use of the seats. Continuing public awareness campaigns are still of vital importance. *(#404)*

One method of increasing compliance with child safety seat use, says Sleet, is to require that all newborns leave the hospital in child safety seats. *(#285)* Auto insurance companies also could offer free child safety seats to policy holders who have children. According to Saalberg, League General Insurance Company of Michigan offers such a program to its policy holders. Begun in 1979, this program is now available in five states and has distributed 17,000 seats. A four-year evaluation of this program showed increased restraint use and a substantial drop in injuries.[4] *(#190)*

Mandatory helmet laws for motorcyclists in all states were encouraged. *(#296)*

Enforcement of speed limits is another component of traffic safety, cited by Trietsch as one factor (along with safety belt and DWI laws) in the success of the Texas program. He underlines the role of police training and coordination between state and local levels in bringing about compliance. *(#563)*

To help provide safer conditions for all who use the roadways, an effective management system must be in place, according to the Highway User's Federation. A comprehensive management system would include road upkeep, pavement improvement, roadside obstacle removal, and pedestrian and bicycle access. *(#517)*

Finally, vehicle manufacturers themselves have a role to play. According to the Highway User's Federation, improved technology is making cars more crash resistant. Manufacturer changes include brake enhancement, side impact protection, use of on-board electronics, improved vehicle stability, and automatic restraints. Laboratory testing and field experimentation on better restraint systems are occurring, which include "improved belt designs, passive belts, air bag applications, and electronic accident avoidance technology." *(#517)*

OTHER CAUSES OF INJURY

Beyond automobile accidents, witnesses identified falls, fires, and drownings as key preventable causes of injury.

Falls

Children and elderly adults have the highest risk of death or injury due to falling, according to William King and colleagues of the Children's Hospital of Alabama. *(#266)* To reduce injury and mortality from falls, Michael Oliva of Aurora, Colorado urges funding for fall prevention programs for older people. Providers of health care should recognize, he says, that many falls are not unexpected events.

For example, you can identify those who have a high risk of falling when they get up at night to use the bathroom. They may have had prior falls, and their disabilities and medications may increase their risk of falling. Fall prevention in the elderly is closely related to their health problems and it should be included in their plan of care. *(#378)*

Fires

Residential fires took 3,900 lives in 1984. This makes fires the second leading cause of death in the home after falls.[5] From a public health perspective, a critical intervention to reduce residential fires is the installation of smoke detectors in all homes. Rivara says that smoke detectors should be installed in all households, but particularly in the households of the poor. "It is the poor who are at greatest risk of fire deaths," he says, "particularly poor children." *(#334)* West writes, "I would like to see legislation at the national level, but also state legislation that says that all new housing will have smoke detectors built in. But I think that any housing units that receive federal funding—and this is, specifically, low income housing—also should have smoke detectors in them." *(#368)*

Rivara points out that approximately one-half of residential fires are started by cigarettes.[6] Thus, development of a self-extinguishing cigarette would be an effective countermeasure. *(#334)* Sleet indicates that cigarette lighters in the hands of children cause between 120 and 200 childhood deaths annually, primarily to children under five years of age.[7] He stresses the need for federal standards to require that all cigarette and novelty lighters be child proof. *(#285)*

Poisoning

Poison control centers can reduce the number of emergency room visits made by poison victims. These centers should be set up regionally, says Lewis Schwarz of Morristown Memorial Hospital in New Jersey, and should be reachable through a standard toll-free number, publicized nationally. By keeping a data base on the many and frequently updated drugs and products on today's market, poison control centers can offer up-to-date information over the telephone. By monitoring calls nationally, they also

will be able to provide data for analysis of use and misuse patterns. *(#446)* The use of child-proof caps for medicines and household products has also proved to be a successful passive prevention technique, according to Haggerty. *(#784)*

Drowning

In 1983, over 5,000 persons died from drowning. More than half of the persons were under 25,[8] and 82.4 percent of those drowned were male.[9] To pursue the goal of no more than 1.5 drowning deaths per 100,000 people, Rivara encourages the use of multiple strategies and more studies; for example, "it is not known whether toddler and child swim classes are a positive or a negative risk factor for drowning." He also points out that "interventions for pool drownings may not be applicable to those occurring in natural bodies of water." *(#334)*

DISABLING INJURIES

Most injuries are nonfatal, according to Macdonald, but some severely disabling injuries are "perceived as worse than death." Of the eight 1990 objectives dealing with accident prevention and injury control, only one measures nonfatal injuries, and that is "based on unreliable data." Macdonald calls for the year 2000 objectives to measure the incidence of severe injuries, the prevalence of disability, and the rates of disability days. *(#322)* Samuel Stover of the University of Alabama at Birmingham refers to "this epidemic of injuries with permanent disabilities" and concludes that "we really don't pay much attention to them." *(#674)* In 1983, for instance, nearly 8,000 children age 15 or under died from injuries sustained in accidents,[10] and many more were permanently disabled, according to Martin Eichelberger of the Children's Hospital National Medical Center. *(#058)*

Injuries to the spinal cord, head, or brain are especially disabling. Approximately 8,000 new cases of spinal cord injury occur yearly, and these are concentrated in the late-teen, young-adult age group.[11] There is a lack of information on the effects of immediate treatment and rehabilitation on patients with spinal cord and head injuries, says Stover, and more applied research is critical to increase the rehabilitation rates of these patients. *(#674)*

Even mild or moderate head injury victims experience significant cognitive, emotional, and social disabilities, according to Thomas Boll of the University of Alabama Hospital. As yet, no systematic program exists in the United States for the diagnosis and treatment of noncatastrophic brain injury. The importance of primary prevention, however, is manifest, says Boll: many head injuries in childhood could be prevented if children always used restraint devices in vehicles, including school buses. *(#264)*

Several speakers were concerned with reaching children through injury prevention education. Jill Floberg of Olympia Physical Therapy Service writes:

> I often stand and wonder at how today's youth survive to adulthood with an apparent false sense of invincibility. High-tech toys with high-tech risks and the viewing of unreal responses to injury in various media, lead to an expectation that no matter what happens, someone can fix it.

An important intervention, Floberg says, is to assess the "recklessness" profile of 6 to 15 year olds. Collecting such information could help to design effective educational efforts in the schools on personal protection. *(#317)* Eichelberger sees a need for nationwide education efforts on the preventability of childhood injury. "Instill a conviction among Americans," he says, "that most childhood accidents can be prevented—and that this country has a responsibility to take the steps necessary to prevent them." *(#058)*

IMPLEMENTATION

Manpower and Organization

The sweep of environmental and control factors involved in injuries, and the necessary crosscutting strategies that must be undertaken to curb them, mandate a combination of local and statewide prevention efforts with individual and professional awareness efforts. Public health approaches, with an emphasis on social marketing and broad-based collaboration, are appropriate for implementing injury prevention, according to West. Collaboration between different groups reduces fragmentation of effort and increases use of the same message throughout a community. *(#368)*

Law enforcement officers, public health officials, and health professionals all have roles to play in enforcing or publicizing injury prevention measures and in educating the public on individual risk factors. Trietsch underscores the usefulness of interdisciplinary "teams" in the Texas effort to reduce traffic injury rates. For example, the Texas Department of Highways and Public Transportation provides funds directly to the Texas Department of Health for the promotion of safety belts, child safety seats, and DWI reductions. In return, the Department of Health "activates its extensive network of health professionals, clinics, and outreach programs to provide training, education, and materials where needed." *(#563)* According to Saalberg, health professionals also are invaluable in identifying, treating, and controlling those who suffer from alcoholism and problem drinking; expanding the availability of emergency medical services; and making further advances in trauma treatment. *(#190)*

West strongly urges the development of statewide programs for injury control, which could serve as umbrella organizations for the activities of different sectors of society. The minimum criteria for a statewide injury prevention and control program are

1. establishment of a statewide plan for injury prevention and control that encompasses (a) technical assistance to communities; (b) surveillance and data collection; (c) a broad-based coalition; and (d) a comprehensive focus that includes prehospital and acute care, as well as rehabilitation;

2. maintenance of statewide poison control services;

3. enforcement of existing legislation;

4. development of other legislative/regulatory approaches as needed; and

5. integration of injury prevention and control content into the education and training of a variety of populations, including health care providers and the media. *(#368)*

"Roughly 50 percent of injury deaths are immediate," says Macdonald. Of the remaining 50 percent, 30 percent occur within the first four hours after injury. This presents a compelling need to provide quality prehospital emergency services and trauma care as an important tertiary prevention strategy. *(#322)* Many testifiers supported Macdonald's argument, claiming that the quality and immediacy of intervention can determine mortality rates. *(#257)*

Surveillance and Data Collection

It is essential to ongoing injury control to have a statistical data base capable of producing comprehensive and reliable injury information. *(#019)* To establish and improve information collection for such data bases, speakers unanimously encouraged a more standard format of injury reporting and a regional collection system for this information. Currently, says the National Safety Council, "knowledge in this field is characterized by proliferating and redundant efforts in some areas and near absolute neglect in others." *(#019)*

One step in making reporting procedures more standard would be to have hospitals, emergency medical service units, trauma centers, and police reports record the same types of information with the same or similar coding schemes. *(#322)* Several witnesses called for the use of the ICD-9 External Cause of Injury codes, or E-codes, to identify risk factors from the physical environment. Without such coding, "head injuries from motor vehicle crashes cannot be distinguished from those due to falls," points out Rivara; with them, however, "the existing systems would serve as a feasible and extremely useful surveillance tool for injuries requiring medical care." *(#334)* Currently, only four states (Maryland, New

York, Pennsylvania, and Virginia) require hospitals to use E-codes. However, even the use of E-codes may not be enough, according to Macdonald, because they "do not allow for identification of risk factors that are behavioral (such as alcohol use or seatbelt non-use) or those from the social environment (such as occupational or recreational settings)." He advocates the incorporation of an "activity code" into the fifth digit of the ICD-10 version of the E-codes as a further refinement of the system. *(#322)* Schwarz's recommendation for regional poison information centers with a national 800 number is another example of how to collect the necessary data. *(#446)* Testifiers believe that having such information and control measures in place and available through a central organization, at either a state or a national level, could significantly increase the opportunities for large-scale prevention measures.

REFERENCES

1. National Research Council, Committee on Trauma Research: Injury in America: A Continuing Public Health Problem. Washington, D.C.: National Academy Press, 1985

2. U.S. Department of Transportation, National Highway Traffic Safety Administration: Fatal Accident Reporting System, 1988. A Review of Information on Fatal Traffic Crashes in the United States in 1988 (DOT Publication No. HS 807 507), 1989

3. Fingerhut LA, Kleinman JC, Malloy MH, et al.: Injury fatalities among young children. Public Health Rep 103(4):399–405, 1988

4. Saalberg JH: Second Evaluation of the League General Insurance Company Child Safety Seat Distribution Program. U.S. Department of Transportation, National Highway Traffic Safety Administration, 1985

5. National Safety Council: Accident Facts, 1985 Edition. Chicago, 1985

6. Baker SP, O'Neill B, Karpf RS: The Injury Fact Book. Lexington, Ma.: Lexington Books, 1984

7. Ibid.

8. U.S. Department of Health and Human Services: Disease Prevention/Health Promotion: The Facts. Palo Alto, Ca.: Bull Publishing Company, 1988

9. National Safety Council: op cit., reference 5

10. National Safety Council: Accident Facts, 1986 Edition. Chicago, 1986

11. Young JS, Burns PE, Bower AM, et al.: Spinal Cord Injury Statistics: Experience of the Regional Spinal Cord Injury Systems. Phoenix: Good Samaritan Medical Center, 1982

TESTIFIERS CITED IN CHAPTER 15

008 Anderson, Dave; American Automobile Association
011 Austin, Richard; Michigan Department of State Police
019 Benjamin, George; National Safety Council
058 Eichelberger, Martin; Children's Hospital National Medical Center (Washington, D.C.)
190 Saalberg, James; CUNA Mutual Insurance Group
257 Johnston, Carden; American Academy of Pediatrics
264 Boll, Thomas; University of Alabama at Birmingham
266 King, William; Kohaut, Edward C.; Johnston, F. Carden, et al.; The Children's Hospital of Alabama
285 Sleet, David; San Diego State University
296 Gossett, Leo; Texas Department of Public Safety
317 Floberg, Jill; Olympia Physical Therapy Service
322 Macdonald, Steven; University of Washington
334 Rivara, Frederick; Harborview Injury Prevention and Research Center (Seattle)
368 West, M. Patricia; Colorado Department of Health
378 Oliva, Michael; Aurora, Colorado
404 Hill, Joseph; Detroit Department of Health
425 Tarrant, Karen; Michigan Department of State Police
446 Schwarz, Lewis; Morristown Memorial Hospital (New Jersey)
517 Livingston, Charles; Highway Users Federation
563 Trietsch, Gary; Texas Department of Highways and Public Transportation
674 Stover, Samuel; University of Alabama at Birmingham
784 Haggerty, Robert; William T. Grant Foundation (New York)

16. Violent and Abusive Behavior

Violence and intentional injury are rampant in the United States. Homicide is the leading cause of death for Black males age 15 to 44;[1] suicide and homicide rank second and third, nationally, as causes of death among all adolescents;[2] of all the emergency room visits made by women seeking treatment for injury, 19 percent involve battering;[3] and more than 1.9 million children nationally are abused each year.[4] (#420; #697)

To put an end to endemic violence in communities across the United States, more than 40 testifiers who addressed violence and intentional injury asserted that public health must help focus attention on the problem, help screen victims and perpetrators, and participate in the difficult behavior modification strategies necessary to change interpersonal relations, especially within families. Primary prevention of family violence is an important element of any effort to reduce overall abusive behavior and is "often very elusive," states Karil Klingbeil of the University of Washington. Klingbeil recommends that we

> reassess our childrearing practices and our socialization patterns. We know politically that violence begets violence. We know about the generational aspects of behavior. It's time that we broke the cycle of violence. (#697)

Among those groups identified by witnesses as being vulnerable to violence were children, women, and the elderly, most often as victims; and males, most often as perpetrators. Minorities were identified as being at an especially high risk as both victims and perpetrators. Adolescents, especially as suicide victims, also received attention from testifiers.

"Although we tend to think of police and the criminal justice systems when we think of homicide and assault," writes Allen Bukoff of Wayne State University, "health professionals are the front lines of violence in our society." According to a study in Cleveland, of those individuals treated in emergency rooms for violence, only one-fourth made reports to the police.[5] (#715) Patience Drake of the Michigan Department of Management and Budget and Robert Dolsen, Chairperson of the Statewide Health Coordinating Council, echo the belief that "leaving the resolution of these difficult dilemmas to the criminal

justice system" will not prevent more violent behavior. To reduce intentional injury, the broader social context in which violence occurs must be explored. Childhood family relations, socioeconomic status, weapons availability, social acceptance of certain behaviors, and community structures can all adversely affect individuals and lead to an inappropriate conception of how to interact with others. (#420; #537) All sectors of society must establish and maintain value systems and social relations that do not support or lead to violence and intentional injury, according to testifiers.

Many witnesses called for implementation of the recommendations of the Surgeon General's Workshop on Violence and Public Health held in October 1985.[6] (#420) Recognizing the complex nature of the problem, the workshop's main recommendation was reduction of unemployment and poverty. Other recommendations emphasized a multidisciplinary approach to injury control, including changing views of appropriate behavior, especially conceptions of masculinity; reducing media violence and inappropriate views of sexuality; increasing community intolerance for violence; teaching conflict resolution skills; reducing alcohol and drug consumption; reducing the availability of firearms; providing stress reduction and support services for families and parents, as well as community intervention centers; identifying and treating abused children and adults who were abused as children; teaching parenting skills; and reducing the level of violence in schools. (#420) This chapter focuses on three types of violence: homicide and interpersonal violence, suicide, and family violence, and examines several implementation issues.

HOMICIDE AND INTERPERSONAL VIOLENCE

To prevent homicide, it is essential to look at the etiology of interpersonal violence. According to Bukoff, at least half of all homicides occur among family and persons acquainted with the victim.[7] (#715) Risk factors for homicide among "intimates" (husband/wife, boyfriend/girlfriend) include prior wife abuse and dating violence; therefore, education programs for high school students aimed at relationships without violence could be especially beneficial, says Jacquelyn Campbell of Wayne State University.

It also is important to note that the majority of murders, regardless of the sex or race of the victim, are committed by men. (#402) Several testifiers underline the lack of self-esteem, sense of social uselessness, or feelings of alienation that may influence aggressive or violent tendencies in individuals, especially young males. The homicide toll is especially great in minority communities, according to Carl Bell, Executive Director of the Community Mental Health Center (CMHC) in Chicago. (#018)

Bell describes homicide and interpersonal violence intervention strategies that have been implemented in a poor, Black Chicago community. The overall plan is to provide primary, secondary, and tertiary prevention programs to the community. Key elements are (1) to publicize and provide education on the causes of homicide and violence and how to cope with stress and violence, and (2) to get the medical community involved in recognizing and stopping cycles of violence.

Myths, ethnic tensions, and ignorance of homicide dynamics must be overcome, according to Bell. In CMHC's community, the task of clarifying the reality of homicide dynamics was undertaken through several steps: developing a series of radio talk shows on the facts and fables of homicide, distributing several thousand T-shirts with a slogan to "Stop Black-on-Black Murder," and persuading the staff of a local hospital emergency room to wear these T-shirts to awaken their coworkers to the possibilities of intervention. Other primary prevention resources have been used to redirect activities of young men, such as a karate class that Bell teaches which, he feels, "has done more to constructively influence the lives of young Black males away from violent tendencies" than has his work as a psychotherapist. (#018)

The importance of drug traffic-related violence was brought up by the Public Health Education Section of the American Public Health Association. Using the recent Washington, D.C., experience of 100 drug-related murders in just four months as an illustration of the magnitude of the problem, the group suggests a year 2000 objective "that addresses a reduction in violent drug-related deaths and injuries." (#616)

Primary prevention of homicide must strive to establish positive value systems in community members, testifiers say. Youth gangs, for instance, give social cohesiveness to young men, but accept murder and violence as appropriate ways to resolve conflict. These gangs, says Nancy Allen of the UCLA Neuropsychiatric Hospital, should be targeted for homicide reduction activities. (#240) The Los Angeles Gang

Violence Reduction Project, for example, employs gang member consultants who are respected members of youth gangs in their communities to intervene in potentially dangerous situations to prevent escalation.[8] (#240) Jeff Roth of the National Research Council suggests, however, that ideally interventions need to begin long before the ages of gang membership: with nutrition and parent training for expectant mothers during the prenatal period, and continuing through preschool with parental bonding; social learning about how to deal with frustrating situations nonaggressively; Head Start; etc. (#785)

In addition to the psychosocial strategies useful to communities, testifiers believe that handgun control legislation could significantly reduce homicide rates. "United States citizens are the most heavily armed in the world," says Allen. A great danger with private ownership, she warns, is that gun owners are often unfamiliar with their weapons and sometimes kill unintended victims, usually family members. (#240) Steven Macdonald of the University of Washington says that an enraged person with a gun is much more likely to kill someone than an enraged person who lacks ready access to a firearm. (#322) However, given the reality of current gun ownership, Bukoff calls the 1990 objective to reduce the number of privately owned handguns by 25 percent "naive" and Carl Bell calls it "idealistic." Instead Bell asks for a "major media effort to encourage handgun owners to unload their readily available deadly weapons," and Bukoff advocates outlawing plastic handguns in all 50 states. (#018; #715)

SUICIDE

Adolescent suicide rates have nearly tripled in three decades, says Martha Medrano of the University of Texas Health Science Center at San Antonio.[9] (#500) Among Native American communities, adolescent suicide already has become a local health priority.

According to Tom Barrett of the Center for Psychological Growth in Denver, American youth are finding it difficult to cope with the pressures of growing up in a rapidly changing society. (#702) Stress and substance abuse are widely prevalent and are two of the leading factors in adolescent suicide. Donna Gaffney of Columbia University emphasizes that it is not one particular stress that emerges as a significant correlate of suicidal behavior but rather "an entire constellation of life stresses that differ in severity from non-suicidal children." (#731) Adults must "create a less threatening and more supportive setting for youth, one with less social isolation, despair, and depression" in order to prevent suicide and other intentional injuries, says Michael Greenberg of Rutgers University. (#537)

Damien Martin of the Hetrick-Martin Institute in New York says that reducing communication barriers is especially vital in preventing suicide among adolescent homosexuals. Many of these adolescents have no cognitive, emotional, or social role models. Many are afraid to admit their homosexuality for fear of rejection. Educational interventions in the school, counseling for those who have attempted suicide, and research into the reasons for suicide, should all include "the possibility of social and psychological factors related to the stigmatization of homosexuality as contributing to teenage suicide." (#466)

Education against suicide must take place in the schools and in the community, argues Medrano. Stress-coping and communication skills need to be taught. Teacher strategies should include "breaking the taboo of keeping a suicide secret, especially for the students themselves." (#500) In the community, health professionals need to be informed of the signs of suicidal behavior, how to deal with them, and where to refer potential suicidal individuals. Because drug and alcohol abuse also are related to suicide among adolescents, intervention programs in these areas should include a component of suicide intervention, according to Barrett. (#702)

The media need to be made aware of what factors increase the "contagious" phenomenon of suicide and what factors decrease this effect. (#500) To do this, greater understanding of the role of the media in so-called copycat suicides is required, says Greenberg. For example, did the media coverage of recent widely publicized teen suicides increase the likelihood of similar incidents, or did it reduce them by conveying calming messages? (#537) Although Lou Large of Houston believes that television has the potential for "improving the physical, emotional, and intellectual health of this nation," she also says it can contribute to violent behavior, especially among young children. Large proposes objectives for the year 2000 to reduce violence in children's programming and during hours when children watch television, along with a campaign to educate parents and children about appropriate selective viewing for youngsters. (#304)

After a suicide has occurred, schools and communities must move quickly to prevent other suicides, according to Medrano. This involves "assisting students, staff, and parents to ventilate feelings of grief, guilt, rejection, and anger" produced by the suicide. (#500)

Meyer Moldeven of Del Mar, California, says that volunteer training is an important component of successful suicide interventions for all ages: "A community's suicide intervention and prevention resources—of which the suicide prevention center, crisis center, and 'hotline' are elements—depend to an enormous degree on local paraprofessionals and trained volunteers." In the workplace, employers already provide programs for stress management, as well as cardiopulmonary resuscitation and first-aid training. Thus, "why not a lay worker on the job site who is trained to function in an emergency suicide intervention?" asks Moldeven. The United States Army and Navy already have established formal suicide prevention programs, and the groundwork laid can be used to tailor programs for other employers. (#602)

FAMILY VIOLENCE

Millions of people a year are affected by family violence, and the majority are women and children. A history of abuse, early parenthood, low socioeconomic status, and poor coping skills for stress—all can produce aggression and violent conflict resolution within households. Children of battered mothers also are at high risk for stress-related physical problems, as well as behavioral and developmental problems, and show a propensity for family violence in adulthood, especially if male, according to Jacquelyn Campbell. (#402) David Besaw, representing the Wisconsin Tribal Health Directors, says that most domestic violence in Native American populations occurs under the influence of alcohol or other drug abuse. (#514) The single biggest correlate of interpersonal violence, say witnesses, is poverty. (#420; #715) According to Bukoff, reductions in poverty would improve our ability to prevent violence. (#715)

The community, especially health professionals, can intervene in domestic violence by recognizing perpetrators and victims. Emergency rooms could screen for victims of abuse, and alcohol and drug abuse programs could screen for violence, as well as provide stress-coping techniques. One such model emergency room program has been established at Rush-Presbyterian-St. Luke's Medical Center in Chicago. (#402) Community programs involving health professionals, in tandem with criminal justice efforts, could effectively change the nature of conflict resolution and childrearing in many communities. (#293)

Child Abuse

According to Blanche Russ of Parent-Child in San Antonio, child abuse destroys individuals and families, and the victims of child abuse often become abusers of their own children. Russ stresses the need to "break the cycle of repeated abuse and to stop or reduce the devastating effects of sexual, physical, and emotional abuse and neglect for victims, survivors, and perpetrators." To achieve this, she suggests several strategies: (1) provide parenting education for new parents to help them understand the stress involved in parenting and how to deal with it, and (2) involve health care providers in the screening and treatment of child abuse. (#748) A number of other witnesses call for parenting education, which is discussed in Chapter 14.

Comparisons of two large, national surveys conducted in 1975 and 1985 show a reduction in the rate of violence against children.[10] Among the possible reasons for this reduction, suggests Blair Justice of the University of Texas Health Science Center at Houston, are methodological differences in the two surveys, increased reluctance to report abuses, economic factors, and changes in family structure. However, Justice believes at least some of the credit must be given to treatment and prevention programs established during the decade. She recommends that the Year 2000 Health Objectives specify that hospitals and communities put in place programs that have been found to be effective for preventing child (and spouse) abuse. (#293)

Anne Helton of Bellaire, Texas, calls for protective services for children who have been abused. Battered children often are returned home to their abusers, she says, even when it has been determined that they have been abused. She agrees with Justice that "health care providers should be involved in every aspect of the problem of child abuse, assessment, education, research, intervention, and advocacy. I feel it is appropriate for health care providers to call for more proactive approaches to the problem of the abused child." (#094)

Spouse Abuse

Campbell is "dismayed" that there are no current objectives relating to battered women. (#402) Judith McFarlane of Texas Woman's University says from 2 to 4 million women are physically battered each year.[11] The problem is especially severe for pregnant women. "Although research documents that battered women report spontaneous abortions and stillbirths following episodes of battering, and battered women begin alcohol and drug use to cope with the violence, battering still is not included as a prenatal risk factor meritorious of surveillance and prevention." (#310)

Justice reports that police and community policies reduced the incidence of wife abuse between 1975 and 1985. In 1975, there were few shelters for battered women; in 1985, there were 700.[12]

A carefully-evaluated change in police policy also came about in many parts of the country. In 1975, the traditional police approach at the scene of domestic violence was to separate the warring parties and to leave. By 1985, laws and policies had changed so that police were mandated to deal with wife abuse the same as with any other assault, by arresting and jailing the alleged offender. A significant effect on recidivism has been demonstrated by such action. (#293)

Women need to have community resources and be aware of them; battered women need to perceive health care providers as resources. Community awareness and education can prevent violence. Routine assessment by health care providers is essential to prevent further abuse. (#310)

According to Campbell, the community must provide protective and social services because the risk of being killed is greatest when the woman attempts to leave the battering relationship. (#402)

Elder Abuse

"Far too many of our nation's senior citizens are victims of crime," states Allen. In the White population in Los Angeles, those 65 and over have the highest rate as victims of homicide.[13] Objectives to prevent and treat elder abuse and neglect, and to focus on the impact of this abuse on the quality of life of the elderly, are very important. (#240)

Melanie Hwalek of SPEC Associates in Detroit emphasizes the need for valid and reliable measurement instruments both to assess the risk of elder abuse in community populations and to substantiate elder abuse among suspect cases that arise in state reporting systems and human service agencies. She also advocates developing professional and public educational programs on detection, assessment, and treatment of elder abuse; community outreach programs; research on incidence and prevention; a national clearinghouse for coordinating research; training and program development; and services to elder abuse victims and to families caring for older people. *(#403)*

IMPLEMENTATION

One hindrance to the development of prevention programs, especially primary interventions, is inappropriate assessment of the level of injury and the cost to families and society. Klingbeil refers to confusion about definitions, terminologies, classifications, and psychologies: "If we can't count it it doesn't exist." *(#697)* In addition, "we don't even know what the cost of these injuries are," says Bukoff. "We don't have good methods yet of estimating the health costs, economic costs, in terms of days of work lost, etc." *(#715)*

Clinical protocols for the prediction, assessment, and diagnosis of various forms of family violence, and better definitions of family violence nationwide will permit better reporting and provide better statistical evaluation, according to Klingbeil. *(#697)* Hwalek offers an example of a definition of abuse for one population, the elderly, that consists of six distinguishable categories: physical abuse, physical neglect, psychological abuse, psychological neglect, material abuse (exploitation), and violation of personal rights. "Each component of this comprehensive definition of elder abuse can be related to important health implications," she says. *(#403)*

Several testifiers encouraged the establishment of a national center for the study and prevention of homicide. It would, among other things, coordinate and fund research projects on homicide; promote the use of standardized reporting methods and records; establish a state and national homicide registry; coordinate homicide information and education; assist communities in establishing homicide prevention services; coordinate and develop restitution and victim-assistance programs; and develop hypotheses and theories regarding perpetrators and victims. *(#240)* Other suggestions for more and better data collection and surveillance included a comprehensive data capability to monitor and evaluate the status and impact of substance abuse on criminal behavior because of the "links known to exist" between the two *(#093)*; more information about external causes and circumstances surrounding injuries, particularly internal injuries *(#715)*; the establishment of trauma registries in all states *(#108)*; and the use of E-codes (external cause of injury codes) in hospitals *(#322; #334)*.

REFERENCES

1. Centers for Disease Control: Homicide Surveillance, High-Risk Racial and Ethnic Minorities. Draft report. Atlanta: 1986

2. National Center for Health Statistics: Health United States, 1987 (DHHS Publication No. [PHS] 88-1232), 1988

3. Amler RW, Dull HB (Eds.): Closing the Gap: The Burden of Unnecessary Illness. New York: Oxford University Press, 1987

4. Flanagan TJ, Jamieson KM (Eds.): Sourcebook of Criminal Justice Statistics, 1987. U.S. Department of Justice. Bureau of Justice Statistics Publication No. NJC-111612, 1988

5. Barancik JI, Chatterjee BF, Greene YC, et al.: Northeastern Ohio trauma study: I. Magnitude of the problem. Am J Pub Health 73(7):746–751, 1983

6. U.S. Department of Health and Human Services: Surgeon General's Workshop on Violence and Public Health: A Report (DHHS Publication No. [HRS-D-MC]86-1), 1986

7. Federal Bureau of Investigation: Uniform Crime Reports for the U.S., 1987

8. Allen NH: Homicide Perspectives on Prevention. New York: Human Sciences Press, 1980

9. National Center for Health Statistics: op. cit., reference 2

10. Straus MA, Gelles RJ: Societal change and change in family violence from 1975 to 1985 as revealed by two national surveys. J Marriage Family 48(3):465–479, 1986

11. Hotaling G, Sugarman D: An analysis of risk markers in husband to wife violence: The current state of knowledge. Violence and Victims 1(2):101–124, 1986

12. Straus MA, Gelles RJ: op. cit., reference 10

13. University of California at Los Angeles, Centers for Disease Control: The Epidemiology of Homicide in the City of Los Angeles, 1970–1979. U.S. Department of Health and Human Services, August 1985

TESTIFIERS CITED IN CHAPTER 16

018 Bell, Carl; Community Mental Health Council (Chicago)
093 Heckmann, Glenn; Texas Board of Pardons and Paroles
094 Helton, Anne; Bellaire, Texas
108 Jarrett, Michael; South Carolina Department of Health and Environmental Control
240 Allen, Nancy; University of California, Los Angeles
293 Justice, Blair; University of Texas Health Science Center at Houston
304 Large, Lou; La Porte Independent School District (Texas)
310 McFarlane, Judith; Texas Woman's University
322 Macdonald, Steven; University of Washington
334 Rivara, Frederick; Harborview Injury Prevention and Research Center (Seattle)
402 Campbell, Jacquelyn; Wayne State University
403 Hwalek, Melanie; SPEC Associates (Detroit)
420 Drake, Patience; Michigan Department of Management and Budget, and Dolsen, Robert; Statewide Health Coordinating Council
466 Martin, A. Damien; Hetrick-Martin Institute (New York)
500 Medrano, Martha; University of Texas Health Science Center at San Antonio
514 Besaw, David; Wisconsin Tribal Health Directors
537 Greenberg, Michael; Rutgers University
602 Moldeven, Meyer; Del Mar, California
616 Windle, Anne; American Public Health Association, Public Health Education Section
697 Klingbeil, Karil; University of Washington
702 Barrett, Tom; Center for Psychological Growth (Denver)
715 Bukoff, Allen; Wayne State University
731 Gaffney, Donna; Columbia University
748 Russ, Blanche; Parent-Child, Inc. (San Antonio)
785 Roth, Jeff; National Research Council

17. Occupational Safety and Health

For some of the nearly 104 million men and women in our nation's work force, "living is hazardous to your health. Working is even more hazardous to your health." *(#337)* An estimated 10 million traumatic injuries occur on the job each year. In addition, about 400,000 workers become ill from exposure to hazardous substances in the workplace, and some 100,000 die prematurely from this exposure.[1]

Many of the 43 testifiers on occupational health issues call for improved or stepped-up cooperative efforts between public and private sectors to help achieve the nation's occupational safety and health objectives. Stronger regulatory measures and, equally important, stronger and more consistent implementation of existing regulations are high on many witnesses' agenda. The Occupational Safety and Health Administration (OSHA), the Food and Drug Administration, and the Environmental Protection Agency, along with numerous state agencies, are seen as the governmental groups with the greatest responsibility for improving occupational safety and health in the next decade. However, many testifiers recognize that these groups can be only as effective as their funding allows.

A Detroit Department of Health spokesperson identifies several trends that will have some impact on the year 2000 objectives, including continued cigarette smoking, which greatly magnifies the effects of toxic agents; excessive government regulatory programs that have led to an inhibition of new technologies for hazardous waste treatment; more women in the workplace, which has led to the emerging importance of possible mutagens and teratogens; and illegal dumping of toxic wastes, which has led to an increase in the probability of contact with toxic agents. *(#210)*

Among the worker protection issues discussed were toxic agent exposure, injury control, reproductive effects (for both women and men), and noise reduction.

Human immunodeficiency virus (HIV) infections and AIDS were identified as an important occupational health focus for the year 2000, especially for health care workers and law enforcement officers. A compelling case was made for directing some objectives to the special plight of farm workers, including migrant workers. Farmers tend to work alone and

"do not have a collective voice" to represent their complaints to equipment manufacturers or to government regulatory agencies. *(#540)* They are excluded from many laws and regulations such as some state workers' compensation laws. Other occupations singled out for special attention were construction workers, fire fighters, working children, and retired workers who could benefit from improved notification procedures regarding hazards inherent in their former jobs.

The need for more research into both the cause and the effects of occupationally related diseases, and the need for better data collection and analysis, were common themes throughout much of the testimony.

Testimony on occupational safety and health issues covers two separate but interrelated issues: the protection of workers from injuries and illness attributable to the workplace itself, and the workplace as a site for health promotion and disease prevention activities. This chapter deals primarily with the former; the latter issue is dealt with in more detail in Chapter 9.

The first section of this chapter examines the special needs of particular groups of workers: agricultural workers, health professionals, and so on. The second section highlights some particular problems to be addressed in workplace protection: toxic agents, injury control, etc. The third section describes briefly the testimony on the workplace as a site for health promotion and disease prevention activities. The final section deals with implementation issues, including surveillance and manpower needs.

GROUPS WITH PARTICULAR NEEDS

Several witnesses addressed specific occupations at high risk for particular problems, including agricultural workers, health care workers, construction workers, law enforcement officers, and fire fighters. Others were concerned about those who have retired from occupations that may have exposed them to risk and about children who are employed.

Agricultural Workers

David Pratt of the New York Center for Agricultural Medicine and Health, at Bassett Hospital in New

York, reports that agriculture has become the most dangerous occupation in the United States. Individuals who work in agriculture are injured or killed at a rate that is substantially higher than the mean for all U.S. workers. Pratt sees a problem of social equity here.

Why do these men and women not deserve the same safe working conditions on the job as other Americans? How can we allow those who produce the food we eat to finance it by squandering human capital? Why should they pay with their lives for the right to work? *(#540)*

A number of testifiers, such as Mary Ellis of the Iowa Department of Public Health, believe that the 1990 Objectives focused primarily on industrial hazards and injury control with little attention to farm-related injuries and hazards. *(#569)* In Colorado, rural areas have a higher occupational mortality rate than do urban areas, according to William Marine of the University of Colorado School of Medicine; from 1982 to 1984, for example, 20 percent of the work force employed in rural areas suffered 48 percent of the occupational injury deaths in the state.[2] *(#382)*

Chuck Stout, Director of the Colorado Migrant Program in the Colorado Department of Health, is particularly concerned about the conditions under which migrant workers labor. He cites a lack of access to potable water, toilets, and hand-washing facilities as serious and common problems in such settings. Although OSHA recently (under court order) set standards of basic hygiene conditions for agricultural workers, Stout charges that the agency has not developed mechanisms for inspection, enforcement, handling of complaints, or informing growers of their new responsibilities. "America's farm workers still suffer from diseases that may be controlled very easily by the application of the most basic sanitation measures that have been taken for granted for decades by the rest of this country's labor forces." *(#710)*

Paul Monahan of the Yakima Valley Farm Workers Clinic in Washington State recommends the identification and elimination of legislative and regulatory policies that discriminate against farm workers. Exclusionary features of many laws and regulations, he says, "have an adverse impact on the health of farm workers." For example, some 20 states provide no protection for farm workers under their workers' compensation laws, and another 15 states

protect only restricted categories of temporary workers. Unemployment benefits also are limited for workers on small farms, according to Monahan; in the off season, medical care for these workers is often inaccessible because of the cost. *(#330)*

Health Care Workers

The American Society of Hospital Pharmacists is concerned with the frequent use of cytotoxic and hazardous substances in health care settings, with a concomitant potential for toxicity to pharmacists, nurses, and other health care personnel. The society's Director of Clinical Affairs, Marie Smith, says that employees who come in contact with such materials should be made more aware and should adhere more strictly to procedures for the safe handling of these substances. *(#574)*

William Wilkinson of the University of Washington addresses the risk of HIV infection to health care workers: needlestick injuries and handling blood or blood products are the primary sources of HIV infection for health workers. Wilkinson calls for more research to determine the level of risk and for more education of workers about research findings. *(#319)* Similarly, the American Association of Occupational Health Nurses (AAOHN) points to hepatitis B as a major infectious occupational health hazard in the health care industry. They cite unpublished data from the Centers for Disease Control (CDC) indicating that each year 500−600 health care workers whose jobs involve exposure to blood are hospitalized with acute hepatitis B and that more than 200 deaths occur among health workers from this cause. Use of the universal barrier precautions recommended by the CDC should greatly diminish the risk of infection from blood-borne pathogens, including both hepatitis B and the HIV virus. In addition, the AAOHN indicates that significant numbers of at-risk health workers do not take advantage of the available vaccine against hepatitis B. *(#558)*

Other Hazardous Occupations

Several occupations, including construction, law enforcement, and fire fighting, require workers to undertake tasks on a daily basis that are both physically and emotionally hazardous.

The Laborers' International Union of North America (LIUNA) reports that construction workers suffer significantly more injuries, fatalities, and diseases than other workers. At the same time, according to LIUNA, federal government efforts to protect construction workers have been lagging. The union believes that specific objectives should be established to eliminate the differential in injury and illness rates between these workers and others. *(#586)* Some construction workers also have been exposed to very high levels of lead. For example, according to Harvey Collins of the California Department of Health Services, well over 3,000 individuals in that state are reported each year to have blood lead levels higher than 40 milligrams per deciliter. It is suggested that these workers be included in the standards for general workplace exposure to lead. *(#783)*

Fred Toler, Executive Director of the Texas Commission on Law Enforcement Officer Standards and Education, is concerned with the health of law enforcement workers. "People frequently view the felon as the greatest threat to the law enforcement officer's health and safety, when he or she actually is much more likely to die from heart disease, stroke, automobile accident, cancer, or suicide," he says. Law enforcement officers are widely perceived as heavier users of tobacco than many other professionals, and Toler calls for research to determine the accuracy of this perception and to identify approaches that would reduce such use. Law officers often are less physically fit than is good for their health, which makes them more susceptible to stress-related illnesses that may result in premature death or a reduced quality of life. Toler recommends training for this group in coping and stress reduction to help reduce the incidence of suicide, in handling hazardous substances, and in proper techniques for protecting themselves against AIDS and other contagious diseases. *(#297)*

Fire fighters, too, face high-stress situations daily and encounter work-related hazards such as heat stress, threat of physical injury, and exposure to toxic gases emitted from the combustion of synthetic materials in fires. *(#108)*

Retired Workers

Rebecca Richards of the North Woods Health Careers Consortium in Michigan notes that a number of the 1990 Objectives relate to identification, notification, and follow-up of workers at risk "while employed"; she suggests that this be extended to retirees as well. *(#183)* Because retired workers may have been exposed to materials capable of inducing diseases of long latency, LIUNA also urges that retirees be included in any programs of information and educa-

tion about occupational risks. Prevention-oriented health programs aimed at retirees, LIUNA notes, may mitigate the adverse health effects attributable to prior workplace exposures and help workers with work-related disease to avoid further disability and complications. *(#586)*

Working Children

The health and safety of children who work on family farms, in family businesses, or in other parts of the economy not covered by federal requirements for occupational safety and health are also of concern to LIUNA. Child labor under the age of 14 is legally prohibited in the United States and should be eliminated in those segments of the economy where it still exists. At a minimum, LIUNA suggests a goal to eradicate job-related injuries and illnesses in children under age 14, and states that there were hundreds of such claims under workers' compensation in a recent year. *(#586)*

WORKPLACE PROTECTION ISSUES

From among the many specific workplace protection issues, most witnesses focused on exposure to toxic agents. Some, however, did address injury control, reproductive effects, and noise. Occupationally related dermatitis was also noted as among the most commonly occurring illnesses in the workplace. *(#569)*

Toxic Agent Exposure

Robert Spear of the University of California, Berkeley submits that the greatest risks to health from exposure to chemical agents occur in the workplace, with rare exceptions involving accidental releases to the general environment. Therefore, toxic agent control in the workplace should be emphasized. "We must face the fact that, whatever the toxic hazard, the odds are very high that workers will or have experienced it first, and it is only sensible to have a strong preventive program focussed on the occupational environment." *(#275)*

George Gaines, representing the Detroit Department of Health, reports that toxic agents that produce acute or chronic illness are not new to the workplace, but the rapid growth of new technologies and new, potentially toxic, substances has led to a situation in which "what we do know continues to be far outweighed by what we do not know concerning all of the effects produced by toxic agents." He further notes that, although the specific effects of some individual materials are known, very little information is available about the synergistic effects of toxic agents on workers. It has become clear, for example, that smoking tends to magnify the effects of other toxic agents. Gaines recommends the increased use of multiphasic health testing to aid in identifying possible and multiple effects of toxic agents. *(#210)*

Employee right-to-know programs are vital in instructing employees about the procedures for handling a toxic substance and the actions to take in the event of accident with such a substance. *(#210)* Bernard Turnock of the Illinois Department of Public Health says that worker right-to-know legislation should be extended to include on-the-job instruction about occupational hazards. He feels that it is unreasonable to expect a prospective employee to research workplace hazards, and applicants believe that asking too many questions may result in being denied a job. *(#215)*

Lawrence Kenney, President of the Washington State Labor Council, AFL-CIO, reports that millions of workers are exposed to neurotoxic agents in the workplace and that many die or are disabled as a result of this exposure. *(#345)* Raymond Singer of the Mount Sinai School of Medicine notes that the effects of neurotoxicity are subtle and when symptoms caused by exposure to these agents appear, they may be attributed to "normal aging." Few U.S. workers are currently monitored for signs of neurotoxicity, although most of those who work with toxic chemicals are exposed to neurotoxic substances; if toxicity is detected early, permanent brain and nerve damage can be prevented, according to Singer. *(#638)* Kenney believes that worker education is the most effective means of reducing the rate of occupational disease and injury. *(#345)*

Turnock suggests a revision of a 1990 objective to reduce occupational lung diseases because "assessing [achievement of] the objectives in 1990 might create a false sense of security." The current objective calls for no new cases of asbestosis, byssinosis, silicosis, and coal worker's pneumoconiosis by 1990. Because of the long latency period between exposure and development of the disease, Turnock believes that many cases would not be detectable by 1990. He suggests that the deadline for assessing this objective should be 2010. *(#215)*

Injury Control

Jeanette Winfree, representing the American Physical Therapy Association, suggests that ergonomically designed jobs can prevent injuries. She reports, however, that employers are often reluctant to redesign tasks due to the cost, although "data are beginning to reveal ergonomically-designed jobs do prevent costly injuries and allow the worker a safe environment." *(#313)*

Michael Jarrett, Commissioner of the South Carolina Department of Health and Environmental Control, comments that as the work force ages, occupational injuries or days lost due to injury may increase. He suggests that specific objectives about occupational injuries to those over 50 may be appropriate. *(#108)*

Many industries report that the greatest number of work days lost are due to back complaints, according to Marilyn Gossman and Jane Walter of the American Physical Therapy Association. They suggest that fitness programs could serve as a preventive measure against these injuries. *(#248)* Kenneth Kizer of the California Department of Health Services reports that carpal tunnel syndrome "is second only to back injury as a cause of lost time from repetitive motion injuries" and suggests that model reporting systems and an intervention system be expanded to 50 percent of the counties in the country. *(#591)*

Reproductive Effects

Several witnesses addressed the occupational effects on reproductive health. According to the Centers for Disease Control, at least 50 chemicals widely used in industry have been shown to impair reproductive function in animals; these chemicals include heavy metals such as lead and cadmium, glycol ethers, organohalide pesticides, and organic solvents. Studies have shown increased rates of spontaneous abortion among laboratory and chemical workers and other workers exposed to lead, ethylene oxide, and anesthetic gases.[3]

Joan Bertin and others from the American Civil Liberties Union Foundation suggest that occupational exposures may account in part for the large proportion of infertility, miscarriages, infant mortality, and birth defects that are labeled as idiopathic or "cause unknown." They underscore the importance of looking at reproductive effects in men as well as women. "The practice of using selective data to ban one group of employees, always women, from an occupational hazard that is deleterious to the health of both sexes creates only the illusion of workplace safety." *(#617)*

Noise Reduction

The American Occupational Medical Association (AOMA) reports that many U.S. production workers have been exposed to high levels of noise and, as a result, have varying degrees of hearing impairment. In the future, noisy industries such as steel mills, machine shops, and foundries will make up a smaller proportion of jobs in the country; because of this fact, as well as improved technology, acoustic engineering, and better enforcement of laws, a lower rate of hearing loss from such causes is to be expected. *(#071)*

THE WORKPLACE AS A SITE FOR HEALTH PROMOTION AND DISEASE PREVENTION ACTIVITIES

When programs are properly designed, says Leon Warshaw of the New York Business Group on Health, the workplace is a uniquely advantageous site for health promotion; employers may undertake such programs to improve employees' well-being, morale, and work performance, as well as to minimize the company's costs for health services. *(#448)* Jill Floberg of Olympia Physical Therapy Service is less certain about the economic value of worksite prevention programs. "Although there are some data available, follow-up studies of in-house programs are as yet inconclusive in showing long-term decreases in health-related time loss and injury costs." *(#317)* Pat Joseph, a representative of the American Association of Occupational Health Nurses, says that the degree of voluntary participation in workplace health promotion programs is often higher than in similar community-based programs. According to Joseph, the increased participation is due to employee convenience, the presumption that programs are of good quality if they are sponsored by the employer, the employees' viewing the programs as a benefit, and the availability of social support for a desired change in behavior. *(#385)* Any objectives requiring more occupational safety and health services from businesses should also recognize that smaller businesses may need "ready access" to resources in order to provide

the services, according to Dorothea Johnson of AT&T. *(#450)* Workplace health promotion and disease prevention are discussed in greater detail in Chapter 9.

IMPLEMENTATION

The AOMA stresses the importance of a collaborative effort between government and the private sector toward reaching occupational health goals. This effort should include jointly designed and sponsored educational programs, plant health and safety committees, and jointly designed and operated employee assistance programs. *(#071)* Floberg, who represented the American Physical Therapy Association, would like to see the development of a labor-management relationship that removes health and safety issues from the politics of contract negotiation. *(#317)* Givens and Floberg agree that, in general, rewards are more effective than punitive measures. Thus, the AOMA wants to see rewards that encourage win-win attitudes between management and labor applied to the development and implementation of environmental hazard controls. *(#071)* Floberg specifically suggests that financial incentives through insurance or tax measures be used to reward companies and individuals for successful prevention and promotion programs. *(#317)*

Harvey Checkoway of the University of Washington suggests that the primary targets for occupational safety and health objectives be those diseases and injuries that have unambiguous occupational etiologies and are truly preventable. He urges concentration on selecting objectives that can be met realistically; developing methods for monitoring the occurrence of occupational diseases and injuries; and developing approaches for remediation of unacceptable risks. Among the conditions or diseases that should be monitored, he includes occupational asthma, lead poisoning, silicosis, carpal tunnel syndrome, noise-induced hearing loss, disabling injuries at the worksite, asbestosis, byssinosis, coal workers' pneumoconiosis, occupational hepatitis, solvent-induced encephalopathy, and peripheral neuropathy. *(#245)*

Surveillance

A number of people testified about the inadequacy of statistics on occupational health, which LIUNA refers to as "the failure to recognize the woeful inadequacy of occupational injury and illness statistics." The union cites a 1987 National Academy of Sciences report in support of its claim that the United States does not have a timely, accurate assessment of morbidity or mortality associated with job-related injuries, occupational diseases, and work-related disorders.[4] (#586)

Joseph suggests a standardized, ongoing occupational health hazard injury and illness coding system. (#385) Checkoway would establish regional centers for disease surveillance and research, because "workers' compensation claims, hospital discharge summaries and death certificates vary in quality and quantity of information" and "some of the important adverse health events occur in small workplaces where exposures often are not monitored and may be excessive." With good regional centers, nationwide monitoring is possible, and surveillance should then be supplemented by specifically designed industrial hygiene and safety remediation programs, he says. (#245) Marine suggests a computerized linkage of state workers' compensation data with state death certificate files to provide a more complete count of fatalities than either source alone. (#382) Ellis recommends the expansion of statistical, surveillance, and epidemiological studies related to farm injuries and diseases. She also advocates the use of hospital discharge data—including E-coding and information about a patient's occupation and industry—for occupational illness and injury surveillance. (#569) This type of information tracking requires that health workers take occupational histories and correctly interpret their findings. Kizer cautions, "There is no easy way to determine whether health care providers currently do this." (#591)

Manpower

Kenney urges increased emphasis in medical schools on the identification of occupational diseases. Many workers' compensation claims go unfiled each year, he says, because neither the doctor nor the patient can identify the cause of a particular condition. (#345) Steven Levine of the University of Michigan also calls for more training in occupational fields. He advocates developing an adequate supply of qualified personnel to carry out the purposes of the Occupational Safety and Health Act by maintaining and expanding the Educational Resource Centers program, which trains various occupational safety and health specialists. (#392) Bernard Goldstein of the University of Medicine and Dentistry of New Jersey calls for more trained public health professionals and better geographic distribution and outreach of existing graduate-training facilities in public health. (#625)

Wilkinson would like to see the number of occupational health professionals at industry sites increased and suggests that occupational health nurses assume the majority of these positions. (#319) The AAOHN agrees that occupational health nurses are well suited to be worksite health promotion professionals and recommends that every state health department hire at least one occupational health nurse as a consultant to local industries. (#558)

REFERENCES

1. U.S. Department of Health and Human Services: The 1990 Health Objectives for the Nation: A Midcourse Review. Washington, D.C.: U.S. Government Printing Office, November 1986

2. Colorado Department of Health, Health Statistics Section: Colorado Population-based Occupational Injury and Fatality Surveillance System Report, 1982–1984. Denver, n.d.

3. Centers for Disease Control: Leading work-related diseases and injuries—United States. Morbid Mortal Wkly Rep 34(35):537–540, 1985

4. Pollack ES, Keimig DG (Eds.): Counting Injuries and Illnesses in the Workplace: Proposals for a Better System. Washington D.C.: National Academy Press, 1987

TESTIFIERS CITED IN CHAPTER 17

071 Givens, Austin; American Occupational Medical Association
108 Jarrett, Michael; South Carolina Department of Health and Environmental Control
183 Richards, Rebecca; North Woods Health Careers Consortium (Wausau, Wisconsin)

210 Gaines, George; Detroit Department of Health
215 Turnock, Bernard; Illinois Department of Public Health
245 Checkoway, Harvey; University of Washington
248 Gossman, Marilyn and Walter, Jane; American Physical Therapy Association
275 Spear, Robert; University of California, Berkeley
297 Toler, Fred; Texas Commission on Law Enforcement Officer Standards and Education
313 Winfree, Jeanette; Physical Therapy Services (Galveston, Texas)
317 Floberg, Jill; Olympia Physical Therapy Service
319 Wilkinson, William; University of Washington
330 Monahan, Paul; Yakima Valley Farm Workers Clinic (Toppenish, Washington)
337 Sugarman, Jule; Washington State Department of Social and Health Services
345 Kenney, Lawrence; Washington State Labor Council, AFL-CIO
382 Marine, William; University of Colorado Health Sciences Center
385 Joseph, Pat; United States Air Force, Lowry Air Force Base, Denver
392 Levine, Steven; University of Michigan
448 Warshaw, Leon; New York Business Group on Health
450 Johnson, Dorothea; AT&T
540 Pratt, David; Mary Imogene Bassett Hospital (Cooperstown, New York)
558 Babbitz, Matilda; American Association of Occupational Health Nurses
569 Ellis, Mary; Iowa Department of Public Health
574 Smith, Marie; American Society of Hospital Pharmacists
586 Fosco, Angelo; Laborers' International Union of North America
591 Kizer, Kenneth; California Department of Health Services
617 Bertin, Joan and Taras, Ana; American Civil Liberties Union Foundation, and Stellman, Jeanne; Columbia University
625 Goldstein, Bernard; University of Medicine and Dentistry of New Jersey, Robert Wood Johnson Medical School
638 Singer, Raymond; Mount Sinai School of Medicine
710 Stout, Chuck; Colorado Department of Health
783 Collins, Harvey; California Department of Health Services

18. Environmental Public Health

For several years, Denver, Colorado, has led the Environmental Protection Agency's (EPA) list of cities with serious carbon monoxide air pollution problems. At the state level, Colorado has the fourth highest rate of death from chronic obstructive pulmonary disease.[1] Bradley Beckham of the Colorado Department of Health says that researchers can speculate that these two phenomena are related, but no model based on reliable data exists to definitively relate one to the other. (#469)

This situation is mirrored around the country with many environmental concerns. The most common observation of the 50 testifiers on environmental health goals for the year 2000 is that for a wide range of environmental problems, the data that might guide public health policy are sorely deficient. Most of the 1990 environmental health objectives are unquantifiable. According to the majority of testifiers, research and monitoring are needed to gauge how much of a particular substance the population at large, or a certain group, is exposed to and what health risk this exposure induces.

Testimony reported in this chapter illustrates the scientific and political problems involved in such issues as toxic agents, hazardous waste, water pollution, air pollution, lead poisoning, food purity, electric and magnetic fields, and noise pollution. Several testifiers call for interdisciplinary research, whereas others go further and identify the kinds of private and public action needed now.

One speaker, however, is very circumspect in committing more public health resources to environmental issues. Environmental health priorities should be guided by better surveillance data and weighed against priorities for known risks found in the occupational setting, argues Robert Spear of the University of California, Berkeley. Most toxic agent or radiation harm involves workers at specific sites. Thus, from a quantitative or population-based perspective, public health should devote more of its environmental efforts toward high-risk populations and to surveillance of the health outcomes of environmental conditions on populations such as these. Conversely, public health should not be expending as much of its limited funds, Spear urges, on "programs whose health benefits are difficult to justify on the basis of procedures like quantitative risk assessment, let alone on epidemi-

ological grounds." (#275)

Although most witnesses addressed either the immediate environment of the home and workplace or the proximate physical environment in terms of land, water, and air, Malcolm Watts of the University of California, San Francisco pointed out that to help ensure health for all people in the year 2000 and beyond, attention also must be paid to longer-term issues related to protecting our global environment. If these problems are neglected in the next 10 years, Watts says, they will be even more pressing—and possibly overwhelming—by the year 2000. (#781)

TOXIC AGENTS

Much of the testimony on environmental health issues involved toxic agents, hazardous wastes, and human exposure to these substances through the water supply.

"With the exponential growth of new technologies, and the associated new, potentially toxic substances used, what we do know continues to be far outweighed by what we do not know concerning all of the effects produced by toxic agents," says George Gaines of the Detroit Department of Health. (#210) For example, Bernard Weinstein of Columbia University reports that although it is known that environmental toxins and toxic chemicals contribute to several kinds of cancer, as well as to a variety of reproductive disorders, the mechanisms behind these effects are less well understood. (#456)

Focusing on a particular health risk, Raymond Singer of Mount Sinai School of Medicine is concerned about how little is known of neurotoxicity. Exposure to neurotoxic chemicals, which are present in certain pesticides, solvents, herbicides, metals, polychlorinated biphenyls (PCBs), and other substances found in consumer products, can cause permanent nerve and brain damage, according to Singer. More than 850 chemicals are known to be neurotoxic,[2] and the National Institute for Occupational Safety and Health lists neurotoxicity as one of the 10 leading work-related diseases.[3] However, "the effects of low-level exposure to neurotoxic chemicals to which most of us are exposed remains uncharted," says Singer. He encourages greater public awareness of the signs and symptoms of neurotoxicity, surveillance of workers who are continually exposed to neurotoxic chemicals, labeling of consumer products, and testing of these products under chronic exposure conditions. "Not only the public remains unaware of the widespread and insidious nature of neurotoxic chemicals, but also many health professionals," he states. *(#638)*

Hazardous Wastes

Robert Meeks of the University of Alabama at Birmingham writes that initial steps have been taken to protect the environment and the public from unsafe hazardous waste disposal through legislation. This includes the Toxic Substances Control Act and the Resource Conservation and Recovery Act. It is now up to the scientific community, he claims, "to develop an understanding of the potential and real effects on the health of individuals resulting from their exposure to toxic agents because they live near hazardous waste sites." Meeks proposes comprehensive risk assessment and health monitoring for individuals who are faced with having hazardous waste or toxic agent storage facilities in their communities. *(#622)*

Even with public and private regulatory and control mechanisms, lack of public understanding of the means of disposal and public unwillingness to participate in reducing barriers to safe disposal are hurdles to action, according to Joan Sowinski of the Colorado Department of Health. "If we are to continue to manufacture products in this country, there have got to be ways to safely treat wastes," she says. If regulatory mechanisms are in place, the public must support new waste disposal technologies. Education in the schools is one method of resolving this problem. "I would wager," Sowinski comments, "that elementary school kids know more about the space shuttle than incinerators." Education must outline environmental problems and then provide an awareness of possible solutions. *(#379)*

Water Contamination

Sheldon Murphy of the University of Washington expresses concern about the quality of the nation's water: "Seepage of toxic chemicals into groundwater from toxic waste sites, agricultural applications, and domestic and industrial discharges appears to present a growing problem." *(#357)*

Carl Johnson, representing the American Association of Public Health Physicians, speaks of the contamination of well water in rural areas. He notes that a significant percentage of rural wells in this country are contaminated with nitrate from stockyards, septic tanks, and agricultural chemicals. To prevent infant illness and death from nitrate contamination of well water, management of environmental pollutants must be maintained. Johnson also calls for a reduction in the number of pollutants in water. *(#111)*

Some of the most serious problems with the nation's water quality stem from land and air use practices that have not yielded to regulation, report David Freeman and his colleagues at the Lower Colorado River Authority. Examples of these problems include "an increase in suspended sediments from increased soil erosion; the increasing use of salt on highways in the winter; the increasing use of pesticides; and the increased use of fertilizers causing eutrophication of receiving bodies of water." A specific result of these types of pollution is the nitrification occurring today in the Chesapeake Bay. Identifying and implementing the necessary control measures to mitigate "nonpoint-source" pollution will require multiple strategies, some of which may be expensive, he predicts. *(#067)*

Lead Poisoning

John Strauther of the Detroit Department of Health says that childhood lead poisoning is "the most common preventable pediatric disorder in the U.S. It affects more children than measles, mumps, rubella, and other communicable diseases combined." To prevent its effects he calls for increased professional awareness and screening.

> The medical community needs to be better informed about recent developments in the identification and medical management of lead poisoned children. Although lead poisoning is best handled by public health facilities, it should be part of every physician's responsibility to advise, urge, and refer every parent to have preschool children regularly screened until their sixth birthday. *(#412)*

However, "despite almost 2000 years of experience with the health hazards of lead, we know relatively little about the different forms of lead and their toxicity or even their relative absorption by humans," reports Ellen Mangione of the Colorado Department of Health. The 1990 objective on lead poisoning is one of the four (out of twenty) trackable environmental health objectives, but several testifiers comment that changing knowledge of lead toxicity levels has made the 1990 goal obsolete. *(#362)*

AIR POLLUTION

According to Murphy, indoor air pollution is going to become a more apparent health issue over the next decade. Energy conservation measures have led to tighter buildings which, in turn, prevent the escape of volatile components contained in many new building materials; in addition, there are chemicals that may seep into homes from soil or vaporize from polluted water, fireplaces, stoves, and tobacco smoke. One goal, Murphy argues, should be to better characterize the exposure levels and health risks associated with air contaminants in private and public buildings where people spend most of their lives. *(#357)* Most of those who discussed air pollution, however, were concerned about outdoor pollution, especially that caused by automobiles.

Allen Bell of the Texas Air Control Board suggests a mixture of public and private initiatives to reduce contamination of the environment and keep the public safe from environmental health threats. These include product bans, required or voluntary emission standards, voluntary changes in products to reduce emissions from product manufacture and use, information strategies to promote private behavior that reduces emissions, government subsidies to promote emission reductions, legal sanctions and financial penalties to compensate for past damages, and other economic incentives. *(#017)*

According to Dave Anderson, the American Automobile Association (AAA) believes that auto manufacturers should play a role in reducing harmful car emissions by developing cleaner automobiles that operate efficiently under real-world driving conditions. Anderson, like Bell, underlines the role of public concern in controlling environmental risk. The public wants better air quality, the AAA argues, but has demonstrated concern about the cost of various air quality improvement programs. The AAA concludes, "Officials at all levels of government have an obligation to ensure that costs of such programs are not excessive in relation to proven benefits." *(#008)*

More specifically, the AAA supports the lead phasedown program, already in process, that would permit one-tenth (0.10) of a gram of lead per gallon of leaded gasoline and a method to ensure the availability of additives that would protect engines designed to run on leaded gasoline. *(#008)*

Denver's solution to its air pollution problem, says Beckham, involves a number of major new steps that include year-round daylight saving time to move the afternoon rush out of the central Denver area before the temperature inversion establishes itself; a ban on wood burning during high-pollution days; voluntary driving reduction; expanding mass transit; an enhanced auto inspection program using computerized emission test equipment; and use of high-oxygen gasoline in the winter pollution season. *(#469)* Most of these components could be employed in programs elsewhere.

FOOD-BORNE DISEASE

The Association of Food and Drug Officials (AFDO) reports significant public health problems from food-borne transmission of infectious disease. The total incidence of diarrheal food-borne illness in the United States may be as high as 24 to 81 million cases per year, and the estimated cost of food-borne illnesses is in the range of $1 to $10 billion annually.[4] *(#384)*

James Black of the Oregon Department of Agriculture, representing AFDO, contends that "concern for food-borne pathogens and subsequent illness deserves a higher priority than it has been receiving in the public health system." *(#342)* Pathogens introduced into a community through the food and dairy supply are now recognized to have a potential long-term effect on that community's health. Food-borne pathogens "may lead to such diseases as chronic diarrhea, arthritis, certain types of heart disease, malabsorption of nutrients among the young, and Guillain-Barré syndrome," writes Black. *(#342)*

The AFDO recommendations for addressing the problem of food-borne illness include a reemphasis in schools of the basic sanitation principles that can prevent most of these disease occurrences and a consistent effort by federal, state, and local agencies to address the issues from a research, reporting, and regulatory approach. *(#384)*

Roy Morse, representing the Institute of Food Technologists, offers similar solutions to food poisoning outbreaks: (1) more reporting on the causes of the outbreaks, (2) more research on nutrition by the federal government, (3) increased funding for research and development in the food area, and (4) licensing public health inspectors for restaurant inspection. *(#733)*

Positive identification of the causative agent in a water- or food-borne disease outbreak is the exception rather than the rule, according to Charles Treser, representing the Washington State Public Health

Association. Thus, "it is probably not feasible, or necessarily desirable, to establish objectives for specific causative agents." Instead, he recommends that the Year 2000 Health Objectives include "an explicit objective calling for a 50 percent reduction in the incidence of gastrointestinal illnesses by the year 2000." *(#348)*

IMPLEMENTATION

Public awareness of a range of environmental influences, and the consequent concern, justify the inclusion of environmental health in the Year 2000 Health Objectives, says Bell. The concern of the public "appears to be intensified by the complexity of issues relating to environmental exposure to hazardous substances and the involuntary nature of the health risks." Assessment of the total and relative risks to human health, he argues, could aid tremendously in directing resources and in helping the public evaluate the health impact of environmental conditions. *(#017)*

The rapidity with which new substances are introduced into the market has stymied many attempts to isolate and assess environmental risks to humans. One major restraint in "catching up" with industry output is finance. According to the American Public Health Association's Laboratory Section:

With the exception of the Food and Drug Administration, there is very little monitoring of commercial products on behalf of consumers. The catalogue of drugs and chemicals used for the control of infectious diseases is extensive. If the trend continues of less federal dollars for activities in protection of the consumer, then it is anticipated that the state public health laboratories will have to become more involved in testing consumer products for safety and effectiveness. *(#548)*

Many states and local agencies are given the lion's share of responsibility for managing and maintaining the community's healthful environment, says Larry Kamberg of the Washington State Environmental Health Association. They do not, however, get the lion's share of funds. *(#318)*

For many testifiers, the EPA and the FDA are essential to ensuring environmental public health. For example, William Scheckler of the University of Wisconsin feels that the EPA and FDA strategies should be more public health oriented. "Broader use of epidemiological expertise by the EPA, the FDA, and other federal health agencies should be mandated." Epidemiological evaluation is important in goal setting as well. Scheckler suggests that "all major environmental health protection initiatives undertaken by the federal government be analyzed by appropriate experts in epidemiology and cost benefit and then reviewed in the context of other health promotion and disease prevention priorities before being funded and implemented." *(#194)*

A representative of the Detroit Department of Health feels that the EPA should "have established firm guidelines for acceptable levels of risk for exposure to asbestos and most toxic agents," based on the assumptions that "the focus of safety and health practice will continue to shift toward prevention as opposed to control" and that "technology advances will continue to outgrow data requirements."

This testifier also feels that an expeditious method of controlling potentially harmful chemicals would be to change current EPA regulatory procedures. *(#210)* For example, even though the Toxic Substances Control Act requires the EPA to screen all new chemicals before they enter the marketplace, the agency has been slow in accomplishing its task, according to Paul Rogers of Hogan & Hartson in Washington, D.C. *(#782)* The Detroit official continues, "chemicals are currently regulated one by one. By the year 2000, the EPA must develop a more systematic approach, i.e., regulating chemicals as recognized characteristic groups." *(#210)*

REFERENCES

1. Colorado Department of Health: Health Status in Colorado, 1985. Summary. Denver: June 1986

2. Anger K, Johnson B: Chemicals affecting behavior. Neurotoxicity of Industrial and Commercial Chemicals. Edited by JL O'Donoghue. Boca Raton, Fla.: CRC Press, 1985

3. Centers for Disease Control: Leading work-related diseases and injuries—United States. Morbid Mortal Wkly Rep 32(2):24–26,32, 1983

4. Kvenberg JE, Archer DL: Economic impact of colonization control on foodborne disease. Food Technol, July 1987

TESTIFIERS CITED IN CHAPTER 18

008 Anderson, Dave; American Automobile Association
017 Bell, Allen; Texas Air Control Board
067 Freeman, S. David, et al.; Lower Colorado River Authority
111 Johnson, Carl; South Dakota Department of Health
194 Scheckler, William; University of Wisconsin
210 Gaines, George; Detroit Department of Health
275 Spear, Robert; University of California, Berkeley
318 Kamberg, Larry; Washington State Environmental Health Association
342 Black, James; Oregon Department of Agriculture
348 Treser, Charles; University of Washington
357 Murphy, Sheldon; University of Washington
362 Mangione, Ellen; Colorado Department of Health
379 Sowinski, Joan; Colorado Department of Health
384 Messenger, Tom; Association of Food and Drug Officials
412 Strauther, John; Detroit Department of Health
456 Weinstein, I. Bernard; Columbia University
469 Beckham, Bradley; Colorado Department of Health
548 Blaine, James; American Public Health Association, Laboratory Section
622 Meeks, Robert; University of Alabama at Birmingham
638 Singer, Raymond; Mount Sinai School of Medicine
733 Morse, Roy; Institute of Food Technologists
781 Watts, Malcolm S. M.; University of California, San Francisco
782 Rogers, Paul; Hogan & Hartson (Washington, D.C.)

19. HIV Infection and AIDS

When the health objectives for 1990 were developed, AIDS—acquired immune deficiency syndrome—had not even entered the medical vocabulary. By 1990, however, 128,319 AIDS cases had been reported in the United States,[1] approximately 1 million Americans are infected, and it is projected that more than 400,000 persons will have been diagnosed with AIDS by 1993.[2] Thus, preventing the spread of this fatal disease is seen by witnesses as a top public health priority.

A total of 60 witnesses concentrated on AIDS or infection by human immunodeficiency virus (HIV), the virus that transmits it. Many other witnesses referred to it in the context of drug addiction, reproductive health, occupational safety, and other areas.

The testimony highlighted several important issues. Some of the most dramatic testimony related to the serious problem of HIV infection among intravenous (IV) drug users and the need for aggressive action to combat it. The concern was not only with the drug users themselves, but also with transmission of HIV from them to others through sexual contact. Already, perinatal transmission of AIDS is occurring at alarming rates. Most of these cases are associated with illicit drug use, according to testimony. *(#376)* Many witnesses agree that expanded and improved drug treatment must be a priority in the fight against AIDS.

In addition, some observers predict that as a large number of HIV-positive drug users develop AIDS, the health service delivery system will be overwhelmed. Unlike the homosexual community, where many people with AIDS have private health insurance and support systems, drug users with AIDS tend to be far more dependent on governmental health and welfare programs.

Speakers discussed several populations who, in addition to IV drug users, are at high risk for AIDS or in need of special education, testing, and counseling. They included children and adolescents, minorities, mothers and infants, and at-risk professionals. Several testifiers also emphasized the need to provide these programs for jail and prison inmates. Charles Carpenter of Brown University calls attention to the fact that certain segments of the prison population in some northeastern states have among the highest prevalence rates of seropositivity in North America.

(#789) Kenneth Kizer of the California Department of Health Services recommends "a greater focus on incarcerated populations" as a means of reaching IV drug using populations with information and education about AIDS and HIV infection. *(#591)*

The bulk of the testimony on AIDS and HIV infection focused on expanding education, testing, and counseling programs, with some emphasizing the importance of confidentiality, compassion, and nondiscrimination in these efforts. Witnesses also addressed the role of personal behavior (using condoms, practicing safer sex, not sharing needles), together with preventive services (education, testing, and counseling), as ways to prevent HIV from spreading.

EDUCATION, TESTING, AND COUNSELING

Many witnesses stressed that education and other prevention activities must be tailored to specific target groups: no single approach can reach IV drug users, homosexual/bisexual men, prison inmates, childbearing women, health professionals, minorities, or others at increased risk. Even within these groups, many subgroups exist and require special attention.

Testifiers say that these activities must take place at sites as diverse as the populations they attempt to reach: public schools, sexually transmitted disease (STD) clinics, family planning clinics, drug use "communities," and health professional schools, to name a few. Similarly, a variety of service providers must be involved, including grass roots gay organizations, teachers, health care providers, community groups in minority neighborhoods, outreach workers, and others who can effectively reach a target population.

Charles E. McKinney, education director of the Gay Men's Health Crisis, characterizes AIDS education this way:

Education as a life saving strategy in the fight against AIDS is more than a public service announcement recommending sexual abstinence, saying "No!" to drugs, or using condoms. It is multifaceted, omnidirectional, relentless, and immediate. It is round the clock, in the streets, in recreational facilities, churches and synagogues, social clubs, homes, schools and local supermarkets. It is where the people are, whenever they are there. It is communicating in a common language and level of literacy. It is nonjudgmental. It is sensitive to the cultural differences, patterns of speech, rituals and mores of diverse populations that make up a community. *(#453)*

Many witnesses emphasized the importance of educating people about AIDS, HIV transmission, safer sex, and needle-sharing behavior; but there was also testimony reflecting the gaps in knowledge about *how* to provide education that will result in health-promoting behaviors. Education must be grounded in an understanding of health behavior and attitudes in the high-risk populations, according to witnesses; homosexual men and IV drug users, for example, have different help-seeking behaviors. However, information about the ways to implement educational efforts is incomplete.

Lew Gilchrist of the University of Washington says more knowledge is needed about how to construct effective education messages.

We have a beginning technology. We know, for example, that public response to fear messages is not optimal. It results in short-term behavior change, but no behavior change over the long run. We need to expand our technology for defining and evaluating health education. *(#691)*

Yet regardless of the audience, site, or specific message, all AIDS educational programs should teach "mercy, compassion, and the insidious effects of stigma and prejudice," say Linda Hawes Clever of the Pacific Presbyterian Medical Center. *(#803)*

MANDATORY TESTING, REPORTING, AND CONTACT NOTIFICATION

Most witnesses supported voluntary testing programs to inform individuals about their own HIV status; a few suggested that mandatory testing may be appropriate in certain cases. Glenn Heckmann, Executive Director of the Texas Board of Pardons and Paroles, for example, said that all inmates entering or leaving penal institutions should be tested. He also noted, however, that placement for those that are HIV positive has been very difficult and urged the development of more community resources for these people. *(#093)* Two overriding concerns in both testing and

contact notification among all populations, including prisoners, are confidentiality and documentation. *(#215)* Suggestions were made that the screening of new inmates be forestalled "until civil liberty protection, segregation policy, and housing/medical care issues have been addressed." *(#591)*

Franklyn Judson of the Denver Public Health Department calls for reporting HIV-positive individuals. Noting that Colorado requires such reporting while providing strong guarantees of confidentiality, Judson says that the law has not had the adverse outcomes some feared. There are no indications that human rights violations have occurred and no evidence that reporting has discouraged at-risk individuals from being tested. The importance of confidentiality in reporting was stressed. *(#376)*

The controversial topic of contact notification also came up in testimony. A few witnesses favored mandatory contact of all people named as sex or needle-sharing partners of people with a positive HIV test. According to Charles Mahan of the Florida Department of Health and Rehabilitative Services, an objective for the year 2000 should be the notification of 75 percent of such contacts. *(#138)* Although most witnesses did not include mandatory partner notification in the preventive strategies proposed—due to difficulty in obtaining names, the cost of tracing contacts, and possible negative reaction to a mandatory effort *(#787)*—voluntary identification of partners by HIV-infected individuals was seen as a valid and important objective.

SPECIAL POPULATIONS

Many witnesses addressed education, testing, and counseling needs in the context of specific target populations at risk. The groups discussed most frequently were school children, minorities, drug users, homosexuals, and women of childbearing age.

Children and Adolescents

A large number of witnesses emphasized the importance of comprehensive education programs in the schools. According to Texas Commissioner of Health Robert Bernstein and others, AIDS education should be a part of the regular health education curricula, beginning in the early grades. *(#020; #273)* Education should be explicit and should teach students how to prevent HIV infection, including the role of condoms and abstinence. According to several witnesses, to be effective, this education must be part of a comprehensive health education program that establishes the relationship among personal decision making, self-esteem, behavior, and health. *(#273; #591)* Some witnesses favor standardizing the material so that the quality and uniformity of the information presented are assured. *(#273)* Kizer calls for standardized federal AIDS instructional programs: "This would ensure that any individual presenting information to the public on AIDS has a minimum level of understanding of the AIDS disease, as well as ongoing access to updated information." He also suggests that these programs include ethnically sensitive, targeted subcomponents for specific populations. *(#591)*

Adolescents were identified frequently as a critical target group. Ralph DiClemente of the University of California, San Francisco says that the limited data available indicate that adolescents are not well-informed about the prevention of HIV infection. He recommends required courses in schools, with the following goals, and makes some specific suggestions about their content.

The objective of HIV prevention programs should be to encourage health-promoting behaviors and eliminate or reduce high-risk sexual and drug behaviors. Adolescents cannot be coerced into changing behavior patterns; but, by providing clear and developmentally appropriate information, we can provide an "informational impetus" which, as a direct consequence, may result in the postponement, reduction, or elimination of high-risk behavior. *(#273)*

However, information alone does not change behavior, says Kizer. Programs must "target denial, perceived susceptibility, motivation, self-efficacy, and provide social support for change." *(#591)* Furthermore, they must target those norms that sanction unsafe sex and drug use behavior, including alcohol use and needle sharing. *(#273; #591)*

Some of the suggested objectives for the year 2000 were framed in terms of the proportion of schools that include education about AIDS or the percentage of students informed about the disease and its transmission. In some testimony, witnesses addressed the need for broad-based education about all sexually transmitted diseases, including AIDS. The American School Health Association, for instance, suggests that current federal funding for AIDS education be used for a broader program aimed at all sexually transmitted diseases; that testimony is summarized in

Chapter 20.

Minorities

Minorities have disproportionately high rates of HIV infection and AIDS, and several speakers called for expanded efforts to reach these groups. This issue is discussed further in Chapter 6.

The prevalence of AIDS among Blacks and Hispanics is more than twice that among Whites, according to Frank Marsh of the University of Colorado Health Sciences Center,[3] and if AIDS becomes endemic in the heterosexual community, it will show up in the urban minority community first. *(#677)*

Rudolph Jackson of the Morehouse School of Medicine says that minorities are generally unaware of important information about AIDS, that programs should place a higher priority on providing culturally sensitive information about AIDS to minority communities, and that minority members should be involved at all levels in planning those efforts. Grass roots community organizations can be effective in reaching this population and should get additional funding for that purpose, he added. Jackson also called for research to determine the underlying causes or behaviors that place minorities at greater risk for AIDS. *(#252)* Although some Black and Hispanic preachers are unwilling to become involved in education about sex or the use of sterile needles, Leon Eisenberg of Harvard University suggests that "the goal of minorities *cannot* be achieved" without participation by the church. *(#787)*

Marsh recommends that a central clearinghouse be created for collection and dissemination of culturally relevant materials. *(#677)*

Intravenous Drug Users

The urgent and growing problem of AIDS among IV drug users was raised often. According to statistics from the Centers for Disease Control (CDC) cited in the testimony, an estimated 900,000 Americans inject illicit drugs at least once a week; another 200,000 do so occasionally.[4] The CDC has estimated that as of the end of 1987, 250,000 to 300,000 IV drug users in this country were infected with the HIV virus.[5] *(#609)*

Many witnesses expressed concern about the epidemic spreading from this community into the larger population. *(#442; #609; #677)* Caswell Evans of the Los Angeles County Department of Health

Services emphasizes that preventive measures must be taken immediately if such transmission is to be stemmed.

> We're beginning now to see the presence of the second wave of AIDS patients as represented by the IV drug-using community, which will certainly vastly change our approach to AIDS. If we're going to stop the spread of HIV in the second wave, we've got to target that group of seronegative IV drug users and concentrate on that group now. We've got a limited window of opportunity, and if we're not effective at this point, HIV is going to spread dramatically from that community. *(#286)*

Stephen Joseph, New York City Health Commissioner, and Deborah Prothrow-Stith, Massachusetts Commissioner of Public Health, both cite the extreme shortage of drug treatment services for those who cannot pay as a serious obstacle to halting the continued spread of HIV infection. *(#437; #735)* One of the most frequently mentioned objectives for the year 2000 is that treatment and rehabilitative services be available to all IV drug users. However, even if adequate drug treatments were available, about half of the addicts would probably decline treatment, according to Irma Strantz, Director of the Drug Abuse Program Office at the Los Angeles County Department of Health Services. She says that education and outreach efforts targeted at drug users could increase the demand for treatment. Strantz emphasizes that drug treatment can save society money. *(#609)* Other witnesses note the importance of continued research into better ways to treat drug addiction. *(#442)*

Strantz made many suggestions aimed at aggressively combating illicit drug use and AIDS among IV drug users. Her suggestions include putting outreach/education workers in every area that has a problem with illicit drugs. These workers would distribute vouchers for drug treatment centers as an incentive to obtain treatment quickly and would offer transportation to HIV testing and counseling sites. Risk reduction kits, including condoms and bleach for cleaning needles would be distributed along with culturally relevant material in appropriate languages. Strantz also called for drug use prevention programs in the many settings where youth can be reached before they become addicted. *(#609)* Other techniques suggested for reaching IV drug users included making HIV prevention education and testing available

routinely in all drug and alcohol treatment clinics, as well as in STD clinics *(#591)*; providing sterile "works" to all users *(#787)*; and encouraging "self-organizations" among IV drug users akin to those among gays *(#787)*. However, "the real solution," says Howard Freeman of the University of California, Los Angeles, "is drug control, not cleaning up a few users." *(#792)*

Mothers and Infants

The importance of controlling the spread of HIV infection among drug users also was underscored by witnesses who addressed the growing problem of perinatal transmission of AIDS.

There is not much basis for optimism about the future scope of the problem, says Richard Schwarz of the State University of New York Health Science Center at Brooklyn, who represented the American College of Obstetricians and Gynecologists. *(#442)* According to a 1987 survey, 1 infant in 61 born in New York City tests seropositive for HIV infection.[6]

On the subject of preventing the perinatal transmission of AIDS, witnesses addressed the importance of making education, screening, and counseling available to women of childbearing age. Some witnesses called for routine testing of all pregnant women with risk behaviors for HIV infection. *(#376)* According to others, Medicaid should again finance abortions for low-income women who test positive for AIDS or HIV infection. *(#449)*

At-risk Professionals

Health care providers and other workers such as firemen, morticians, and barbers must also be educated about their own risks and the appropriate precautions. The American Association of Occupational Health Nurses calls for companies to establish policies protecting at-risk workers, particularly health care workers, while also protecting the rights of HIV-positive employees. *(#558)* Others emphasize that the workplace is an important site for education about AIDS. *(#619)*

IMPLEMENTATION

Several testifiers addressed the need for more data on the prevalence of HIV infection in high-risk subgroups and the general population. William Lafferty of the Washington State Department of Public Health, for instance, stresses the need for primary prevention to go beyond data on symptomatic illness; data on HIV prevalence and incidence in both the general and target populations are required as well. Studies of the size, sexual behaviors, drug use patterns, and so on of high-risk populations are seen as essential to prevention efforts. (#698) Studies and more accurate data on the prevalence of homosexual and bisexual behavior also are needed; current Public Health Service estimates are based on data that are decades old. (#787)

Many proposed objectives were expressed in terms of a specific reduction in the prevalence of HIV infection or AIDS, for example, the percentage of IV drug users who would test positive for HIV infection. Some witnesses suggested a percentage of the population that should be practicing safer sex or needle behavior or should be well informed about HIV and its transmission. (#286)

The American Medical Association, for example, says that by the year 2000, the incidence rate of HIV infection should be half of that in the first representative national sampling. Its testimony includes specific goals for subgroups: among sexually active males, the incidence of HIV infection should be reduced to 1 percent of the present rate; among needle-sharing drug users, it should be reduced to 50 percent of the present rate; among sexually active partners of those likely to be infected, it should be reduced to 10 percent of the present rate; and among newborns of high-risk parents, it should also be reduced to 10 percent of the present rate. (#095)

However, as many testifiers noted, setting quantifiable goals for limiting the spread of HIV infection and AIDS in the next decade is a tricky business. Much depends on the path this epidemic takes and whether preventive vaccines, cures, or other events could drastically alter its course. Witnesses proposed continued research aimed at vaccines and better therapeutic agents, and noted that soon treatment will be provided for those who are HIV positive but asymptomatic. In the meantime, however, if progress is to be made in halting the spread of HIV infection and AIDS, it will have to come from preventive strategies, according to witnesses.

REFERENCES

1. Centers for Disease Control: HIV/AIDS Surveillance, Atlanta: April 1990

2. Centers for Disease Control: Estimates of HIV prevalence and projected AIDS cases: Summary of a workshop, October 31–November 1, 1989. Morbid Mortal Wkly Rep 39(7):110–119, 1990

3. Centers for Disease Control: Human immunodeficiency virus infection in the United States: A review of current knowledge. Morbid Mortal Wkly Rep Supplement 36(S6):1–48, 1987

4. Centers for Disease Control: op. cit., reference 2

5. Ibid.

6. Lambert B: "One in 61 babies in New York City has AIDS antibodies study says." New York Times: A1, January 13, 1988

TESTIFIERS CITED IN CHAPTER 19

020 Bernstein, Robert; Texas Department of Health
093 Heckmann, Glenn; Texas Board of Pardons and Paroles
095 Hendee, William; American Medical Association
138 Mahan, Charles; Florida Department of Health and Rehabilitative Services
215 Turnock, Bernard; Illinois Department of Public Health
252 Jackson, Rudolph; Morehouse School of Medicine
273 DiClemente, Ralph; University of California, San Francisco
286 Evans, Caswell; Los Angeles County Department of Health Services
376 Judson, Franklyn; Denver Public Health Department
437 Joseph, Stephen; New York City Department of Health

442 Schwarz, Richard; State University of New York Health Center at Brooklyn
449 Santee, Barbara; Women and AIDS Resource Network
453 McKinney, Charles; Gay Men's Health Crisis (New York)
558 Babbitz, Matilda; American Association of Occupational Health Nurses
591 Kizer, Kenneth; California Department of Health Services
609 Strantz, Irma; Los Angeles County Department of Health Services
619 Schramm, Carl; Health Insurance Association of America
677 Marsh, Frank; University of Colorado Health Sciences Center
691 Gilchrist, Lew; University of Washington
698 Lafferty, William; Washington State Department of Public Health
735 Prothrow-Stith, Deborah; Massachusetts Department of Public Health
787 Eisenberg, Leon; Harvard University
789 Carpenter, Charles C. J.; Brown University
792 Freeman, Howard; University of California, Los Angeles
803 Clever, Linda Hawes; Pacific Presbyterian Medical Center (San Francisco)

20. Sexually Transmitted Diseases

Although AIDS is the sexually transmitted disease (STD) that has received most attention lately, the hearings highlighted the serious health problems associated with other STDs as well. Thirty-eight witnesses focused on such sexually transmitted diseases as syphilis, gonorrhea, herpes simplex virus, hepatitis B, human papilloma virus, and chlamydia in their testimony.

Chlamydia, in particular, was cited repeatedly as a serious public health problem. Twenty-five years ago it was virtually unheard of; now it is the most prevalent STD in the United States. An estimated 3 to 4 million new cases occur among adults and infants each year.[1] Reporting of chlamydia is incomplete, but the condition is thought to be much more prevalent than gonorrhea. (#591)

The incidence of STDs is rising for some conditions and falling for others. For example, the incidence of syphilis increased 26 percent between 1986 and 1987.[2] (#177) Testimony linked the incidence to an increase in unprotected sexual activity. (#413; #414) Some critics have attributed it in part to lagging public health prevention and control efforts, as a result of transferring resources from STDs to AIDS. (#032; #413; #694) Albert Brunwasser of the Allegheny County Health Department in Pennsylvania summarized the concerns of many when he stated that "AIDS should be incorporated into the national objectives for sexually transmitted diseases, but should not be allowed to use resources at the expense of other parts of the program. That is, increases in other sexually transmitted diseases should not be allowed to occur because all time and effort is expended on HIV infection." (#032)

As with AIDS, education and testing were viewed as important components of any effort to reduce the incidence of STDs. Unlike AIDS, however, some STDs can be treated successfully. Expanded diagnosis and treatment services, therefore, also were identified as important means of decreasing the number of carriers and halting the spread of these diseases.

The American Academy of Pediatrics identifies four elements necessary to reduce STDs: public awareness and education, access to health care, treatment by professionals who can detect the diseases in their early stages, and reduction in the number of carriers in the general population. (#115)

Although STDs were a serious public health problem long before AIDS appeared, several witnesses made reference to some important links between AIDS and other STDs. First, there is apparently an increased susceptibility to HIV infection if another STD is present; this is especially alarming in light of the increased incidence of some STDs in certain populations. Second, successful AIDS education programs encouraging the use of condoms also decrease the rate of STDs. This has occurred in the gay community, in particular. Finally, the fight against AIDS initially drained resources from the fight against other STDs. Many witnesses believe that resources are still being diverted away from STDs, which poorly serves both causes. (#032, #413, #695)

Another important issue raised again and again in the testimony on STDs is the urgency of the problem among teenagers and young adults. C. M. G. Buttery, Commissioner of the Virginia Department of Health, points out that "sexually transmitted diseases predominantly affect the young, therefore this age group must be educated about preventive measures before they become sexually active." (#034) Much of the testimony noted the importance of developing effective education, screening, diagnosis, treatment, and follow-up services for them. A final point from the hearings worth emphasizing is concern about congenital STDs. Infected mothers can pass on disease to their offspring; reducing the rate of infection in newborns was a goal identified by several witnesses.

TARGETING YOUTH

Every year 2.5 million teenagers become infected with an STD, according to testimony from the American School Health Association (ASHA).[3] It is estimated that a teen's risk of contracting an STD is two or three times higher than that of someone age 20 or older.[4] (#232)

The ASHA cites a 1983 national survey which found that only one-third of adolescents consider themselves "very informed" about STDs.[5] Education and prevention programs must be expanded, according to the ASHA, and community health and social service agencies, as well as schools, should be part of the effort. As models, the ASHA points to school-linked clinics, school-based clinics, and school or community-based education programs that have been effective in preventing teenage pregnancy: "For an STD education program to have an impact, more than one lesson that may be typical at most schools is needed. A study of various health curriculums demonstrated that behavior change occurred after 40-50 hours of instruction."[6] (#232)

The ASHA recommends that STD instruction be part of the health education curriculum from kindergarten through the twelfth grade in 90 percent of all school districts by the year 2000. It argued that to wait until the junior or senior year for such instruction—as called for in the 1990 Objectives—is not prudent because many adolescents become sexually active before that time. Others propose similar goals. The ASHA notes that very few states now mandate that venereal disease instruction be part of the health education program. (#232) Although the value and importance of STD education were emphasized by many, "the difficulty of 'educating' away our society's ills" also was underscored; teachers should not be expected to be "agents of social control," according to Thomas Bell of the University of Washington. (#329)

The ASHA also proposes that a goal for the year 2000 be implementation of STD prevention programs for adolescents in 40 percent of U.S. communities. Funds should come from both public and private sources. The federal government should fund STD prevention programs through state and local education agencies, much as it funds drug abuse and AIDS prevention efforts. (#232)

The importance of reaching teenagers and young adults was echoed in hearings held by the American College Health Association. When asked to name the top health issues on college campuses, college health officials consistently named STDs among the top three. Among the reasons cited for the high level of concern were college students' inadequate health/sexuality education in high school and at home; their sexual inexperience, coupled with a desire to experiment and explore; and their casual attitudes about sex and life in general. At least one witness saw this as an opportunity as well as a problem.

> The young adult population in undergraduate and graduate schools are extremely inquisitive and eager to learn. Now that health care in our country has shifted to health promotion, disease prevention, and disease protection, college health services have a unique opportunity to help students look at their lives in a preventive manner. (#759)

College administrators share the view of many other witnesses that young people should be well informed about STD transmission before they reach college age, because sexual activity often already has begun by that time. Such education must start even before the junior or senior year in high school—the target group for some efforts—according to several witnesses. For example, Diane Allensworth of ASHA noted that in 1983 there were almost 30,000 pregnancies in girls less than 15 years old.[7] (#232)

Other witnesses addressing the STD problem among young people focus on the hard-to-reach teens. Marlin Johnston of the Texas Department of Human Services says that teenage runaways are at high risk for STDs: many girls have been raped or are pregnant, and many boys even less than 14 years old are sexually active. (#112) Herbert Rader, representing the Salvation Army, reports that "children are selling themselves for drugs without any regard to the risks they are taking." His organization attempts to reach these children with programs aimed at improving their self-image. Rader also says that preventive programs which do not pay adequate attention to moral strength and character issues will not solve the STD problem. (#432)

REDUCING CONGENITAL SEXUALLY TRANSMITTED DISEASES

Reaching teenagers is all the more important because STDs can cause disease in the infants of affected mothers. With the high rate of teenage pregnancy, reduction in the number of teenage carriers can significantly decrease the number of congenital STD cases.

A mother with chlamydia, for example, can pass on conjunctivitis, pneumonia, and other respiratory infections to her baby. Congenital syphilis can cause death. Thomas Weller of Harvard University says that congenital cytomegalovirus (CMV) infections can also severely damage infants; but unlike syphilis, which can be treated with penicillin, there is no treatment for congenital CMV.[8] (#790)

Several witnesses proposed specific goals for reducing the rate of congenital STDs. The American Academy of Pediatrics (AAP), for example, says that by the year 2000 the rate of congenital syphilis should be no more than 3.5 per 100,000 live births. This represents approximately a 50 percent reduction from the 1985 rate of 7.1 per 100,000. The AAP also proposes targets for herpes (5 per 100,000 live births compared to 16.8 per 100,000 in 1979) and chlamydial pneumonia (250 per 100,000 live births, down from 720 per 100,000 in 1979) contracted from the mother.[9] (#115) Many mothers giving birth to babies with congenital STDs have had little or no prenatal care, and some have been involved with drugs, according to John Parker of the Detroit Department of Health. Programs aimed at producing healthy babies must address all these things and more because "everything seems to be dovetailing," he says. *(#413)*

IMPLEMENTATION

Much of the testimony on STDs focused on implementation issues: the provision of high-quality laboratory and clinical services; the need for more surveillance systems and more research; and the difficulty of setting quantitative objectives for STDs, especially because of interactions with AIDS.

Improving Services

Achieving the desired reductions in STDs will require improvements in the quality and availability of health services, according to witnesses.

Laboratory services, in particular, were discussed by several testifiers. Many facilities lack adequate laboratory services to establish the diagnosis of STDs, according to Berttina Wentworth of the American Public Health Association's Laboratory Section. She says that at these places, STDs must be diagnosed on the basis of clinical signs, which is an inadequate approach. Asymptomatic and subclinical conditions are missed, and some symptomatic disease also goes undetected; she proposes that "by the year 2000 at least 90 percent of medical facilities responsible for the diagnosis and treatment of STDs shall have sufficient laboratory services available to them for the detection of the etiologic agents or for serological diagnosis of such diseases as gonorrhea, syphilis, herpes virus, chlamydia, *Trichomonas vaginalis* and *Candida albicans* infections." *(#754)*

Henry Isenberg of the Long Island Jewish Medical Center also emphasizes the importance of improving laboratory capability to diagnose STDs.

More rapid, simple and accurate diagnostic tools for the detection of gonorrhea, chlamydia, and herpes virus, especially in women, directly in specimens are required and a development of such agents should be supported. The ability to discern the antibiotic susceptibility, especially of the gonococcus directly in the specimen, is also a very desirable objective for the year 2000. *(#438)*

Some witnesses also addressed the need to expand the capacity and improve the performance of clinical services. According to Parker, at the local level this would mean renovating facilities to meet the demands of more people per day; getting private clinics more involved in treatment; continuing the emphasis on follow-up; improving physician education; and hiring additional personnel. *(#413)* Parker's testimony illustrates the kind of commitment and resources required to aggressively combat STDs. Bell says the STD control effort has lacked that aggressive approach, and contrasts it with the more vigorous campaign to eliminate smallpox. *(#329)*

Bell notes that gonorrhea can be treated simply, usually with a single dose of antibiotic. Yet, he says, incidence rates are essentially unchanged. According to a mathematical model he describes, curing a relatively small number of carriers could interrupt transmission of the disease.[10] "If the model is correct, then we're really missing a great opportunity," he says. Based on this, Bell calls for mass screening in the military, adult and juvenile correctional facilities, and perhaps in high schools, although he acknowledges that the last would be controversial. *(#329)* Other witnesses identified pregnant women or immigrants as groups that should be screened routinely.

Making sure that those with treatable conditions complete therapy is an important goal, witnesses agreed. Follow-up to make sure the course of therapy is completed is critical. However, the limitations of relying on therapy also were underscored. First, only some diseases are treatable. Moreover, the development of resistant strains of causative agents poses a constant challenge to effective treatment of conditions that have been controllable. Steven Blum of the American College Health Association cites a 1980 outbreak of resistant strains of gonorrhea as an example. *(#759)*

Expanding Research and Reporting

Several witnesses mentioned the need to expand knowledge about STDs so that they can be more effectively prevented. Among the topics discussed was the need for additional research into the development of vaccines to prevent sexually transmitted diseases. Research into better and more extensive screening tests to identify them also was urged.

The importance of better reporting and surveillance also arose during the testimony. More comprehensive reporting of chlamydia was mentioned by several witnesses. *(#137; #259)*

A few witnesses called for increased focus on the human papilloma virus (HPV). Hunter Handsfield of the Seattle-King County Department of Public Health says it is probably too soon to recommend control of the HPV; effective surveillance is needed at this stage. *(#695)* However, by the year 2000, prevention and treatment of HPV infections of the genitalia and perineum should be an integral part of every STD control program, according to Robert Bernstein, Commissioner of the Texas Department of Health. *(#020)* Isenberg calls for continued research into the cause of the virus and its relationship to cancer. *(#438)*

Setting Quantifiable Goals

In addition to the goals for congenital STDs identified above, a variety of targets were suggested for specific conditions in the general population. However, Handsfield emphasizes that these numeric goals should be stated for population subgroups. He notes, for example, that the overall incidence of gonorrhea in Seattle-King County, Washington, is decreasing, but in some groups, such as inner-city Blacks, it is increasing. The decrease is due largely to the decline in disease among gay men who are practicing safe sex in response to the AIDS epidemic. *(#695)*

Although the AIDS epidemic is associated with some reduction in other STDs, testimony also indicated that the fight against AIDS has diverted attention from, or decreased funding for, other STDs. Handsfield comments, "Funding for AIDS control was initially largely taken from the coffers of sexually transmitted disease control programs. This must not be permitted to continue and it must in fact be reversed." *(#695)*

Witnesses also cited evidence that the presence of an STD may make transmission of AIDS more likely, which means that a coordinated effort at combatting AIDS and other STDs is essential. *(#695)* The ASHA calls for STD prevention programs for adolescents that "combine and coordinate the multiple health/social services of the community with those of the schools in 40 percent of U.S. communities." *(#232)* Although some health jurisdictions may be unable to expand, the concept of combining local resources into a total communicable disease clinic makes sense because, as Kizer says, "the same groups being seen in STD facilities are those who are at high risk for HIV, as well as other diseases." *(#591)*

REFERENCES

1. Centers for Disease Control: *Chlamydia trachomatis* infections: Policy guidelines for prevention and control. Morbid Mortal Wkly Rep Supplement 34(3S):53s−74s, 1985

2. Centers for Disease Control: Summary of notifiable disease: 1987. Morbid Mortal Wkly Rep 36(54), 1988

3. U.S. Department of Health, Education and Welfare: Healthy People: The Surgeon General's Report on Health Promotion and Disease Prevention (DHEW Publication No. [PHS] 79-55071), 1979

4. Children's Defense Fund: A Children's Defense Budget. Washington, D.C.: 1986

5. Parra WC, Cates W: Progress toward the 1990 objectives for sexually transmitted disease: Good news and bad. Public Health Rep 100(3):261−269, 1985

6. Connell DB, Turner RR, Mason EF: Summary of findings of the school health education evaluation: Health promotion effectiveness, implementation and costs. J Sch Health 55(8):316−321, 1985

7. Children's Defense Fund: Adolescent Pregnancy: Whose Problem Is It? Washington, D.C.: 1986

8. Yow MD: Congenital cytomegalovirus disease: A NOW problem. J Infect Dis 159:163−167, 1989

9. U.S. Department of Health and Human Services: The 1990 Health Objectives for the Nation: A Midcourse Review. Washington, D.C.: U.S. Government Printing Office, 1986

10. Yorke JA, Hethcote HW, Nold A: Dynamics and control of the transmission of gonorrhea. Sex Trans Dis 5:51–56, 1978

TESTIFIERS CITED IN CHAPTER 20

020 Bernstein, Robert; Texas Department of Health
032 Brunwasser, Albert; Allegheny County Health Department (Pennsylvania)
034 Buttery, C. M. G.; Virginia Department of Health
112 Johnston, Marlin; Texas Department of Human Services
115 King, Carole; American Academy of Pediatrics
137 Mack, Douglas; Kent County Health Department (Michigan)
177 Randolph, Linda; New York State Department of Health
232 Allensworth, Diane; American School Health Association
259 Hunter, Katherine; Baptist Medical Center, Montclair (Alabama)
329 Bell, Thomas; University of Washington
413 Parker, John; Detroit Department of Health
414 Love, Melinda; Detroit Department of Health
432 Rader, Herbert; The Salvation Army in the United States
438 Isenberg, Henry; Long Island Jewish Medical Center
591 Kizer, Kenneth; California Department of Health Services
694 Hagens, William; Washington State House of Representatives
695 Handsfield, H. Hunter; Seattle-King County Department of Public Health
754 Wentworth, Berttina; American Public Health Association, Laboratory Section
759 Blum, Steven; American College Health Association
790 Weller, Thomas; Harvard University

21. Infectious Disease

Under the rubric of infectious disease, witnesses gave testimony on several different conditions, each with its own strategy for prevention. Forty-four witnesses addressed infectious disease as a primary or secondary area of concentration in their testimony. Several others, particularly health department representatives, identified needs or objectives in infectious disease as part of more extensive statements. Infectious diseases result in approximately 2 million years of life lost before age 65; 52 million hospital days; and nearly 2 billion days lost from work, school, and other major activities each year. The estimated direct cost is more than $17 billion annually, in addition to lost workdays and other indirect costs.[1]

Testimony made clear that although much of the nation's public health focus is on prevention of chronic disease, there are important targets to meet in reducing the incidence of infectious disease. Some conditions that received more attention in the past because of epidemic rates or outbreaks, such as tuberculosis and legionnaires' disease, require sustained or renewed attention. One important issue that emerged, for example, is the recent increase in tuberculosis after a long period of decline. It is especially important to address this because of the widespread view among the public and some health professionals that it is a disease of the past. Several witnesses attribute at least a part of the increased rate of tuberculosis to the spread of AIDS and human immunodeficiency virus (HIV) infection, which depress the immune system. *(#034; #177; #201; #580)*

Although campaigns to immunize all school children have done a considerable amount to reduce childhood communicable diseases—and continuation and expansion of these campaigns are viewed as vital to future success—efforts to immunize very young children, some targeted groups of adults, and the elderly have been much less effective. The influenza vaccine costs only $2.50 per dose and is "very cost effective," yet rates are far below the 1990 objective of vaccinating 60 percent of older adults annually. *(#247)* To reach the target audience, "outreach programs will be required," says William Carter of the Seattle Veterans Administration Medical Center, and "these programs will have to address the motivational issues underlying people's reluctance to obtain flu vaccine." *(#247)* The hepatitis B vaccine, too, is widely available, yet many in high-risk groups do not avail themselves of the opportunities for immunization.

Testimony also made clear that continued, sustained efforts are needed to combat infectious diseases posing persistent public health problems. For example, the country has yet to achieve the reduction in hospital-acquired (nosocomial) infections that officials say is possible through preventive strategies. According to Michael Jarrett, Commissioner of the South Carolina Department of Health and Environmental Control:

> Due to change in reimbursement and in practice patterns, only the sickest of patients are now in the hospitals. There are fewer patients in the hospital but their severity of illness has increased. These patients are individually more vulnerable to infection than the typical patient of 5–10 years ago. However, this is due as much to reimbursement changes as it is due to the increased sophistication of medical technology. *(#108)*

Another recurrent theme in the testimony worth emphasizing is the need to improve reporting and data collection. Suggestions in this area were diverse, but all pointed to the important role of surveillance and dissemination of data in preventing infectious disease.

IMMUNIZABLE DISEASES

Several witnesses addressed goals related to increased immunizations. For both older adults and very young children, immunization rates generally fall below desired levels. Immunization rates for adults also are low, generally less than 5 percent for targeted groups for hepatitis B and influenza.[2] *(#298)* Educational campaigns, improved strategies to encourage individuals to choose to be vaccinated, research on vaccines with fewer side effects, free or subsidized immunizations, and mass immunization programs are among the strategies recommended to increase the immunization rates.

Linda Randolph of the New York State Department of Health identifies several immunization goals for adults: ensuring that all women of childbearing age are immunized against rubella; ensuring that all high-risk groups are informed of the importance of vaccination against hepatitis; and ensuring that all those at special risk of contracting pneumococcal pneumonia, and most of those at risk of becoming severely ill from influenza (i.e., the elderly, the disabled, and the chronically ill), will be fully immunized. Randolph also wants all pregnant women to be screened for current hepatitis B infection so that if they test positive, their newborn infants can be immunized to prevent acquisition of the disease. (#177) Much of the testimony reinforced the need to reach these goals.

Several witnesses expressed concern about the low influenza immunization rates among the elderly. Carter notes that only about 20 percent of persons aged 65 and older receive the influenza vaccine in any given year.[3] He reports that a pilot program at several Veterans Administration hospitals and health maintenance organizations succeeded in increasing the immunization rate to more than 50 percent during the first year. Such an intervention could be initiated at most, if not all, medical centers. (#247)

Influenza vaccines are very cost-effective, witnesses emphasized. Steven Mostow of the Rose Medical Center in Denver, comments that although Medicare policies have been liberalized somewhat to cover vaccinations, insufficient funds are available to provide vaccinations for all those at risk. (#380)

Others noted the rise in hepatitis B from approximately 45 cases per 100,000 population in 1978 to approximately 69 per 100,000 in 1985,[4] and the consequent importance of immunizing those at risk for the disease. Hepatitis can be transmitted through contact with infected blood or through sexual contact. High-risk groups include health professionals, intravenous drug users, mentally ill or retarded patients in institutions, and recipients of blood transfusions. (#414) The American Association of Occupational Health Nurses says that "hepatitis B is the major infectious occupational health hazard in the health care industry." (#558)

Several witnesses proposed subsidizing hepatitis B vaccine so that it could be available at low cost or without charge. (#084; #414; #558) One study was mentioned, however, which found that many health professionals failed to be immunized even when it was readily available at no cost. (#558; #576; #580)

The American Medical Association says that 90 percent of both those at intermediate risk (e.g., prisoners, staff at institutions for the mentally retarded, and health care workers) and those at high risk (e.g., drug users, hemodialysis patients, immigrants or refugees from countries where hepatitis B is endemic, and household contacts with hepatitis B carriers) should be immunized by the year 2000. The institutionalized mentally retarded, who also are at high risk, should be immunized routinely according to the American Medical Association (AMA). (#095) Robert Bernstein, Commissioner of the Texas Department of Health, proposes as an objective that hepatitis B cases be reduced about half to fewer than 12,000 per year by the year 2000. (#020)

Targets also were proposed for childhood immunizations. The American Academy of Pediatrics (AAP) says that 95 percent of children should be fully immunized by the age of two for measles, rubella, mumps, polio, and diphtheria. This would amount to a 14–24 percent increase over 1985 immunization rates.[5] The AAP feels that achievement of this goal will depend on public awareness of the need for full immunization, vaccine cost, the development of new vaccines, and federal and state support for a vaccine program. (#115) Witnesses stressed the importance of providing information and referrals about immunizations to all mothers of newborns. (#020)

The AAP also proposes as an objective for the year 2000, the eradication of measles throughout the world. According to its testimony, there were 2,700 cases in 1985 in the United States.[6] The cooperation of all countries is required to meet this goal. (#115)

A proposed target for older children is that at least 97 percent of all children attending child-care facilities and schools (kindergarten through twelfth grade) should be fully immunized and should be in compliance with state laws or regulations. (#020) Through a rigorous program of immunization record checks and parental notification of noncompliance, Detroit schools increased the number of entering students who were completely immunized from 70–72 percent in the fall to 90–91 percent at the end of the year, with 96–97 percent immunized against measles, mumps, and rubella. A representative of the Detroit Department of Health says, "Strict enforcement of school immunization requirements is the only opportunity to change immunization from parental option to legal mandate. It is the single greatest force in raising the immunization levels of the community to the extent necessary to control and prevent vaccine preventable disease." (#393)

The AMA recommends that routine pediatric vaccines be given to adults to raise their level of immunity by at least a factor of three. (#095)

Witnesses also called for more attention to immunizations against diphtheria, tetanus, and poliomyelitis. *(#298, #791)*

NOSOCOMIAL INFECTIONS

Another area of infectious disease control that received considerable attention is nosocomial (hospital-acquired) infections. Several witnesses cited data from the Centers for Disease Control (CDC) on the scope of the problem. Those figures show that 5 percent of hospital patients acquire a nosocomial infection, resulting directly or indirectly in 80,000 to 100,000 deaths a year. According to the CDC figures cited, about 32 percent of these infections are preventable.[7] *(#575; #619)*

Lorraine Harkavy, a former president of the Association for Practitioners in Infection Control, tells of the needless suffering and high cost of nosocomial disease. She says that more than $2.8 billion is spent each year to treat it.[8] Like several other witnesses, she recognizes that "infection is often a consequence of a highly technological medical equation" whereby "important and life saving invasive procedures" such as surgery, catheters, immunosuppressive drugs, and sophisticated antibiotics "expose the patient to the risk of acquiring a nosocomial infection." Yet simple procedures—such as care providers' washing their hands—could help reduce the rate of infection. Nevertheless, "we are far from our goal of minimizing and preventing what has become a major public health problem and one of the leading causes of death," and, she says research into nosocomial infections should be given a top priority for government funding by the year 2000. *(#084)*

The American Hospital Association (AHA) says that infection control is a high priority for hospitals. The AHA says that the "greatest challenge" to institutions seeking to reduce the incidence of infections is ensuring that health care providers comply with standards of care that reduce the risk of nosocomial infection. *(#576)*

An approach favored by the Health Insurance Association of America is setting specific targets for reducing the rates of nosocomial infection associated with the urinary tract, surgical wounds, the respiratory tract, and intravenous-related bacteremia. Most hospitals track these rates, and CDC statistics provide baseline figures. Each institution should meet goals reflecting reductions in the percent of patients who acquire nosocomial infections, according to the association. *(#619)*

The AHA points out, however, that it is often difficult for hospitals to measure accurately the progress toward infection control goals. The number of infections at the average hospital may be too small to see a statistically significant change in rates after implementation of a control program. The reliability of infection rates may also have to be evaluated because of weaknesses in even sophisticated surveillance systems. Jarrett suggests that requiring public disclosure of rates at individual hospitals might lead to swifter reductions in infection rates. *(#108)*

Nursing homes, too, must improve their infection control procedures, witnesses say. Katherine Hunter, a clinical microbiologist in Birmingham, Alabama, suggests that a 1990 objective stating that all nursing homes should have a results-oriented infection control committee analogous to those in hospitals must be continued for the year 2000. She identified three strategies to reduce nursing home infections: upgrade inspection criteria by agencies to be more clinically relevant; increase the training level of nursing home employees to at least 85 percent skilled level; and initiate one-on-one working relationships between nursing home and infection control personnel or organizations, such as the Association for Practitioners in Infection Control. *(#259)*

Recognizing the complex nature of nosocomial infections, along with the universally felt need to do more to combat them, Henry Isenberg of the Long Island Jewish Medical Center says that "perhaps by the year 2000 some real understanding of this very costly problem may be gained." *(#438)*

TUBERCULOSIS

The rise in incidence of tuberculosis, following its steady decline, was an area of concern for several witnesses. Poverty, overcrowded urban areas, homelessness, and the AIDS epidemic may all be contributing to the sudden upsurge in cases, they say. Tuberculosis has become a nosocomial infection of nursing homes and homeless shelters, according to testimony. *(#259)*

Kathy Harris of the Detroit Department of Health described the tuberculosis epidemic in her city, adding that the number of cases will increase "until the public is made aware of the transmission of tuberculosis and available treatment." She believes that an all-out effort to educate the public and professionals about the disease is needed.

The majority of people in Detroit believe tuberculosis no longer exists, that it was "cured" years ago. Those who are aware of tuberculosis do not believe the documented statistics regarding the rise of the disease or that tuberculosis can kill. Tuberculosis is still considered a "poor man's disease," and this stigma prevents some individuals from even seeking testing, along with the misconception that "you must be locked up" to be treated. (#417)

Harris is especially concerned about counteracting the disease among the hidden—the homeless, drug users, and others who are at high risk but who do not understand the importance of preventive health measures or who refuse to be tested. She also includes families that do not receive regular medical care in this group. (#417) Dieter Groschel of the American Society for Microbiology sees two other populations that require special attention in the fight against tuberculosis: "Aside from the immunosuppressed person, tuberculosis is still mainly borne by minorities (62 percent in 1982) and foreign-born poor (26 percent)." (#580) Responding to similar concerns, Bernstein proposes that by 2000, the incidence of tuberculosis in the United States be reduced to 6 cases per 100,000 population, but that in counties bordering Mexico the goal should be 12 cases per 100,000. (#020)

OTHER INFECTIOUS DISEASES

Although immunizations, nosocomial infections, and tuberculosis received the most attention from witnesses, other topics were also mentioned. Some noted that food-borne disease is an important, often overlooked problem. (#259; #348) Hunter emphasizes the importance of reducing the incidence of food-borne disease: "Even though enteric infections may not present the morbidity and mortality of other infections, there can be considerable costs, ranging from the costs of medication to the man-hours lost." (#259)

Charles Treser, representing the Washington State Public Health Association, is also concerned about food-borne disease and infectious diseases with an environmental component, such as water-borne (legionnaires' disease) and vector-borne (diarrhea) diseases. He says that "as we address new and emerging problems like toxic substances and hazardous waste, we [must] not lose sight of the problems of infectious diseases that are still there and require

some kind of a maintenance effort." (#348)

Isenberg recommends that attention be given to the increase in acute rheumatic fever in a number of states and a possible increase in hospital- or community-acquired pneumococcal disease. (#438) Thomas Grayston of the University of Washington echoes Isenberg's concern, especially as it applies to pneumonia, which ranks as the sixth leading cause of death in the United States.[9] It is especially devastating to older persons and those with chronic illnesses. (#693)

Grayston also calls for a major research effort to help prevent the common cold. The tremendous amount of research into the cause and cure of AIDS has resulted in "much more sophisticated ways to produce vaccines," he says, although he believes that the ultimate answer "probably is going to have to be prevention." (#693) Other nonimmunizable diseases, including chicken pox, typhus, giardiasis, bacterial meningitis, legionellosis, and Lyme disease also were addressed. (#312)

Various reviewers brought up several "sources" of infectious diseases that command attention in any attempt to control their spread. For example, child care centers serve as transmission conduits for children's diseases including giardiasis, cryptosporidiasis, and cytomegalovirus. (#790) The problems associated with control of diseases imported by both immigrants and travelers must be addressed if infectious diseases such as measles and poliomyelitis are ever to be eradicated. (#789; #791)

IMPLEMENTATION

Despite the diversity of testimony on infectious diseases, some issues were raised that relate to preventive strategies for several different conditions.

One such overarching issue is the need for better surveillance, reporting, and data collection. A number of needs were identified. Examples include broadening participation in the CDC's National Nosocomial Infection Survey (#438); increasing uniformity in the definition and calculation of nosocomial infection rates (#619); monitoring illnesses brought in by immigrants or foreign travelers (#177; #201); improving data collection on conditions associated with environmental factors and disseminating data to health officials in a useful form (#348); and establishing a standardized reporting system for infectious diseases throughout the United States that is compatible with the health objectives. (#259) Witnesses emphasized that obtaining and disseminating data are essential in the fight against infectious disease.

Improving laboratory capability is another overarching issue. The objectives proposed in this area relate, for example, to reducing the time from receipt of a sample in the laboratory to communicating useful information to the physician. Some of the suggestions for improved laboratory performance also relate to expanded surveillance and reporting. *(#438)*

Many of the goals identified in this category are extensions of goals established for 1990. Witnesses noted that achieving them is equally or more urgent now. Harkavy, observing how many 1990 goals remain relevant for the year 2000, offered the following perspective on the effort to make gains in infectious disease control: "Perhaps it is not so much a need for new objectives, but rather a recognition that reaching these goals requires vigilance, manpower, resources, and money, much of which is not being directed to the achievement of these current needs, let alone future ones." *(#084)*

REFERENCES

1. Amler RW, Dull HB (Eds.): Closing the Gap: The Burden of Unnecessary Illness. New York: Oxford University Press, 1987

2. William WW, Hickson MA, Kane MA, et al.: Immunization policies and vaccine coverage among adults: The risk for missed opportunities. Ann Intern Med 108:616–625, 1988

3. Fedson DS: Influenza and pneumococcal immunization strategies for physicians. Chest 91(3):436–443, 1987

4. Centers for Disease Control: Hepatitis Surveillance Report No. 50. Atlanta: 1986

5. National Center for Health Statistics: Health United States, 1986 (DHHS Publication No. [PHS] 88-1232), 1987

6. Centers for Disease Control: Summary of notifiable diseases in the United States, 1985. Morbid Mortal Wkly Rep 34(54):1–21, 1987

7. Centers for Disease Control: National Nosocomial Infections Study. Atlanta: 1984

8. Dixon RE: Cost of nosocomial infection and benefits of infection control programs. Prevention and Control of Nosocomial Infections. Edited by RP Wenzel. Baltimore: Williams and Wilkins, 1987

9. National Center for Health Statistics: Health United States, 1989. (DHHS Publication No. [PHS] 90-1232), 1990

TESTIFIERS CITED IN CHAPTER 21

020 Bernstein, Robert; Texas Department of Health
034 Buttery, C. M. G.; Virginia Department of Health
084 Harkavy, Lorraine; LMH Health Associates (Potomac, Maryland)
095 Hendee, William; American Medical Association
108 Jarrett, Michael; South Carolina Department of Health and Environmental Control
115 King, Carole; American Academy of Pediatrics
177 Randolph, Linda; New York State Department of Health
201 Smith, George; Tennessee Department of Health and Environment
247 Carter, William; Seattle Veterans Administration Medical Center
259 Hunter, Katherine; Baptist Medical Centers, Montclair (Alabama)
298 Williams, Robert; Baylor College of Medicine
312 Dickson, Bob; Texas Commission on Alcohol and Drug Abuse

348 Treser, Charles; University of Washington
380 Mostow, Steven; Rose Medical Center (Denver)
393 Gaines, George; Detroit Department of Health
414 Love, Melinda; Detroit Department of Health
417 Harris, Kathy; Detroit Department of Health
438 Isenberg, Henry; Long Island Jewish Medical Center
558 Babbitz, Matilda; American Association of Occupational Health Nurses
575 Reveal, Marge; American Dental Hygienists' Association
576 Owen, Jack; American Hospital Association
580 Groschel, Dieter; American Society for Microbiology
619 Schramm, Carl; Health Insurance Association of America
693 Grayston, J. Thomas; University of Washington
789 Carpenter, Charles C. J.; Brown University
790 Weller, Thomas; Harvard University
791 Lucas, Adetokunbo; Carnegie Corporation of New York

22. Maternal and Infant Health

A nation's infant mortality rate is often regarded as an indicator of a country's effectiveness in addressing health needs. By that measure, the United States is ailing. Primarily because of relatively high rates among the poor, minorities, and adolescents, the United States falls toward the bottom of the list when the infant mortality rates of industrialized nations are ranked.

Yet behind that grim fact lies a tremendous opportunity. The 133 witnesses who concentrated on maternal and infant health emphasized that biological breakthroughs or technological miracles are not required to improve those statistics—the knowledge necessary to make progress is already at hand. Preventive measures, primarily adequate prenatal care, can improve pregnancy outcome. Cessation of tobacco, alcohol, or drug use during pregnancy is also an important means of reducing the infant mortality rate and morbidity in newborns.

These preventive strategies have not changed much since the 1990 Objectives were formulated. If objectives for the year 2000 are to be met, the national commitment to making those strategies available must change, according to many witnesses.

Although there has been some overall decline in the infant mortality rate in the past decade, many of the 1990 Objectives pertaining to infant mortality will not be met, especially those relating to minorities. In addition, there is now concern that progress is slowing and infant mortality rates for some subpopulations may actually be increasing. A witness for the March of Dimes Birth Defects Foundation sets the scene this way:

> Ensuring all infants a healthy start in life and enhancing the health of their mothers must be a top priority in the 1990s if we are to ensure the future health of our nation. Progress on infant mortality is slowing; maternal mortality among Black and non-White mothers is increasing; low birth weight may be on the rise; and not enough women are getting early prenatal care. It is a situation that raises great concern about the health of America's future generations. *(#044)*

Much of the testimony on maternal and infant care echoed this view that the United States must make maternal and infant health a national priority. Several witnesses called for a policy to ensure that pregnant women and their infants have access to adequate care; the United States is one of the few industrialized nations without such a policy.

The objectives proposed for the year 2000, many of them carryovers from the 1990 Objectives, are related to both process and outcome. In the first category, there is emphasis on adequate prenatal care and reducing risk factors in pregnant women; in the second category, there are reductions in the proportion of low-birth-weight babies and in infant mortality rates.

Witnesses noted that adolescents, Blacks, and Hispanics should be targeted for intervention. One witness said that the 1990 objectives calling for reductions in the number of women who get *no* prenatal care should be replaced with measures of *inadequate* prenatal care. *(#044; #108; #316)*

Yet over and over again, the testimony made clear that well-laid plans can go only so far. Commitment and the resources to back it up are required if the strategies are to translate into improvements in maternal and infant health.

PRENATAL CARE

Research has clarified the link between early and regular prenatal care and improved pregnancy outcome. Low birth weight, for example, has been shown to occur more often when prenatal care is inadequate. Yet witnesses repeatedly commented that too many mothers, particularly in minority and adolescent populations, are not receiving such care.

According to testimony from the American College of Obstetricians and Gynecologists (ACOG), 76 percent of pregnant women receive prenatal care in the first trimester; 6 percent have their first visit during the third trimester. Among Blacks, however, only 62 percent begin prenatal care in the first trimester, and 10 percent do not begin until the third trimester. Only about 60 percent of Hispanic women receive prenatal care during their first trimester, and 12 percent of Hispanic mothers who delivered in 1980 received no prenatal care until the third trimester.[1] *(#279; #308)* Medicaid patients and the uninsured are more likely to get insufficient care, defined as eight or fewer visits or care that begins in the second or third trimester.[2] (#279)

According to the ACOG, the percentages of pregnant adolescents who receive first trimester care are even lower: 36 percent of mothers younger than 15, and 34 percent of mothers 15–19 years old.[3] Even those adolescents who start early do not necessarily maintain an appropriate care schedule throughout their pregnancy.[3] (#279)

Yet although many testifiers discussed "adequate" prenatal care as the ideal to be attained, agreement could not be reached on how much care, provided when, and of what kind or quality equates with "adequate." For example, the ACOG refers to a 1987 General Accounting Office (GAO) report on prenatal care among Medicaid recipients and uninsured women that offers one definition:

There is a need to adopt a simple, straightforward definition of adequate prenatal care. In the GAO report, insufficient care was defined as either eight or fewer visits or beginning care in the second or third trimester. There is a clear need for standard definitions of a prenatal visit to provide a basis for national consistency in future assessment of trends in this area.[4] (#279)

After testimony was submitted, the Public Health Service published a report on the appropriate content of prenatal care. The report made specific recommendations about enriching care and changing the visit schedule according to presenting risk factors and previous pregnancies. In outline, the study suggests a preconception visit, followed by at least nine other visits. The first visit should be within the first trimester (six to eight weeks).[5]

Prenatal care and other public education efforts should be used to alert pregnant women to preventable risk factors for low birth weight and poor pregnancy outcome. Risk factors cited in the testimony include smoking, alcohol use, drug abuse, sexually transmitted disease, poor nutrition, and psychosocial factors. Smoking and poor nutrition are associated with low birth weight and other problems in the neonate. Several witnesses addressed the need to reduce smoking and improve nutrition among pregnant women. Excessive alcohol intake can cause fetal alcohol syndrome. Lyn Weiner and Barbara Morse of Boston University School of Medicine say that the condition is underdiagnosed and this is hindering

early intervention and appropriate treatment. (#542) Congenital syphilis is on the increase, according to witnesses; Michael Jarrett, Commissioner of the South Carolina Department of Health and Environmental Control, proposes that efforts be made to identify and treat women with syphilis during pregnancy. (#108)

Many of these risk factors were addressed in the 1990 Objectives. Some witnesses say that more attention should be paid to reducing cocaine use among pregnant women and to the importance of psychosocial evaluation and care during pregnancy in the Year 2000 Health Objectives. (#418; #421)

Modern technology, although admittedly expensive, has been extremely useful in detecting high-risk pregnancies. According to Robert Welch and Robert Sokol of the Hutzel Hospital in Detroit and Wayne State University, one "major difference between our prenatal outcome in the U.S. versus European countries is that patients in many European countries have universal ultrasound screening early in pregnancy." Welch and Sokol suggest that uniform ultrasound testing be performed during pregnancy and that maternal serum alpha-fetoprotein testing be done in 100 percent of pregnancies. (#421)

Other important issues in prenatal care, including availability of providers, financial constraints, and outreach programs, are treated in the implementation section of this chapter.

MATERNAL MORTALITY AND COMPLICATIONS

Delivery has its own set of preventive strategies. Several witnesses expressed concern about maternal mortality rates, particularly among non-White and poor mothers. (#044; #199; #383) Black and other non-White mothers are more than three times as likely to die as White mothers, according to figures cited by the Children's Defense Fund.[6]

In its testimony, the March of Dimes Birth Defects Foundation notes that up to 75 percent of maternal mortality may be preventable and suggests that the disparity in rates may be due to minority women's lack of access to, or underutilization of, obstetrical services.[7] The March of Dimes recommends expanding access to early prenatal care by expanding funding for the Maternal and Child Health Block Grant, and by expanding Medicaid to provide services for more pregnant women, infants, and children. (#044) Kristine Siefert, representing the National Association of Social Workers, agrees that much maternal mortality can be prevented. She also says that maternal mortality review committees should be reinstated where they have been discontinued. These committees should address social as well as medical factors when they assess whether a death could have been prevented. By the year 2000, according to Siefert, the maternal mortality rate should not exceed 3 per 100,000 live births, half of the current rate. *(#199)*

NEWBORN CARE

Eunice Ernst, representing the National Association of Childbearing Centers, calls for the expansion of childbirthing centers outside of hospitals. *(#060)* On the other hand, delivering high-risk babies at centers where special needs can be met is also important; an objective proposed by Roger Rosenblatt of the University of Washington is that 75 percent of all births involving newborns weighing less than 1,500 grams occur at Level III perinatal referral centers. *(#316)*

Several witnesses called for more screening of newborns. Richard Schwarz of the State University of New York Health Science Center at Brooklyn proposes as a goal the development of an accurate antigen test to identify infants infected with the human immunodeficiency virus so that early intervention is possible. *(#442)* The value of newborn screening for metabolic disorders, as identified in the 1990 Objectives, was underscored. Jarrett says that newborns also should be screened for sickle cell anemia and other hemoglobinopathies. *(#108)*

David Wirtschafter of Southern California Kaiser Permanente says that better communication is needed between parents and providers about "rescue" technologies for seriously ill newborns. *(#582)* Several statements note the need for follow-up of infants with special needs. *(#324; #371)* The importance of genetic counseling for parents of affected infants or for those at risk of bearing affected children is noted by William Montgomery of the American Academy of Pediatrics and others. *(#722)* Improved parenting education, also mentioned in this connection, is discussed in detail in Chapter 14.

Many witnesses representing breast-feeding organizations, such as the La Leche League or the International Lactation Consultant Association, focused their testimony entirely on breast-feeding. They testified that it is healthier and less expensive than bottle feeding. Allan Cunningham, of Columbia University College of Physicians and Surgeons and the Mary Imogene Bassett Hospital, and others say research suggests that it may have long-term as well as short-term medical and psychological benefits.

(#046)

Many of these testifiers proposed that by the year 2000, 85 percent of women be breast-feeding when they leave the hospital, and 50 percent after six months. This is a slight increase over the 1990 targets, which they said would not be met. Some testifiers suggested that the year 2000 goals be stated such that no ethnic group or region falls below a given percentage. *(#158)*

Increased public and professional awareness is needed to meet this goal. Witnesses urge increased emphasis in medical schools and continuing medical education about the benefits of breast-feeding. Deborah Bublitz, representing La Leche League, says it is also essential to get hospitals to endorse breast-feeding as the feeding method of choice among new mothers.

Establish breastfeeding as the primary house formula in all hospitals, with formula only as a supplement. To provide this, a support network that works both in the hospital and an outreach program after the hospital must be actively implemented. *(#033)*

Media messages and other techniques to educate the public also are needed. Many feel that employer policies should make breast-feeding easier, and they call for special areas for breast-feeding in the workplace and in public settings. They also raise the issues of marketing practices of infant formula companies and company grants to hospitals linked to use of their products. *(#010; #049)*

IMPLEMENTATION

According to witnesses, if our nation's infant mortality rates, maternal mortality rates, and percentage of low-birth-weight infants are to improve, a variety of barriers must be overcome so that all can have easy, affordable access to care. A need for better and more consistent data also was expressed.

Availability of Providers

Several witnesses expressed concern that the malpractice environment is causing obstetricians and other providers to discontinue or limit their obstetrical practices. This makes it more difficult for some women—particularly low-income women and those in rural areas—to obtain needed services. *(#215; #244; #360; #726)* These witnesses recommended capping malpractice awards and using alternative practitioners such as rural midwives.

The closure of many community hospitals also has affected access. Many hospitals that are closing are in rural or indigent areas where services already are limited. (#003)

In addition, testifiers reported that some physicians are refusing to treat Medicaid patients because of what they consider inadequate reimbursement rates. One witness suggested that the Year 2000 Health Objectives include a goal about physicians accepting Medicaid patients. (#316)

According to numerous witnesses, licensed, qualified midwives and nurse midwives can do much to alleviate the problems related to a poor supply of providers. The American College of Nurse-Midwives (ACNM) says that studies have demonstrated that nurse midwives have reduced infant mortality rates significantly.[8] (#003) Katherine Carr, who represented ACNM at a hearing, identifies several reasons why they may be especially effective in providing prenatal care.

Midwives are experts in the psychosocial, as well as the physical assessment, aspects of prenatal care. Midwives provide nutritional and other educational counseling and communicate caring to their clients. It has been found that the amount of caring perceived by the woman in the services provided may actually influence her outcomes. It's also been hypothesized that perception of caring influences the rate of litigation. (#690)

Carr also says that increasing the use of qualified midwives as part of the health care team in deliveries, especially for high-risk populations, could lead to reductions in infant mortality rates. Currently, midwives attend less than 4 percent of births in the United States. Carr suggests that by the year 2000, 10 percent of U.S. births be attended by midwives. Restrictions on the practice of qualified, licensed midwives and certified nurse midwives keep them from realizing their potential, she says. (#690)

Many in the medical community, especially, expressed reservations about this recommendation. Although most agreed that these certified nurse midwives and other licensed, qualified midwives can contribute significantly to providing prenatal care, concern was expressed about their effectiveness in performing solo deliveries; however, there was support for their role in deliveries when they are backed up by an obstetrician. (#421) Several testifiers also felt strongly that there is no role for "lay" midwives. This latter group has no formal training and should not be confused or equated with licensed or certified midwives. (#421; #801)

Even among those who were optimistic about the potential of licensed and certified midwives to supplement physicians in prenatal and delivery care, especially among the underserved, there was recognition that the existing pool of these professionals is relatively small; there are approximately 2,500 certified nurse midwives in the United States today. (#268; #316) Roger Rosenblatt of the University of Washington reports that studies in that state show that midwives are less likely to take care of underserved population groups than general and family physicians, while costing about the same. (#316)

Financial Constraints

To a large extent, states have been unable to close gaps in access because their public health budgets have been tightened. Many witnesses say that increased funding of maternal and child health block grants and of the Women, Infants, and Children supplemental feeding program, as well as extension of Medicaid benefits to more women and infants, is critical to the effort to provide adequate prenatal care. Prenatal care is a cost-effective investment, they emphasize. The Michigan Department of Public Health estimates that for every dollar spent to provide prenatal care to uninsured women, more than $6 is saved in expenditures for neonatal intensive care. The average Michigan Medicaid hospital payment for normal newborns in 1986 was $813; for newborns with health problems the cost ranged from $1,940 for full-term to $7,503 for premature newborns with major problems. (#397)

Nurse midwives, nurse practitioners, visiting nurses, and other qualified, licensed midwives can provide effective prenatal care at a lower cost than physicians and should be used more to address unmet needs, according to representatives of those groups. (#003; #074; #268; #383; #444; #690)

However, state financing mechanisms often do not pay enough to cover even basic care and delivery costs. In Colorado, for example, reimbursement rates for Medicaid patients (vaginal delivery, including prenatal care) for 1987–1988 were $510; fees for patients covered by another state program are $309 per delivery. In looking at these figures, Ned Calonge of the University of Colorado Health Sciences Center believes that "family physicians could have strong economic incentives for stopping obstetrical services, especially to Medicaid and indigent patients, and obstetricians already face similar economic pressures." *(#244)*

Need for Outreach Programs

Not all the barriers to obtaining prenatal care involve the availability of services, however. Sociocultural barriers also keep pregnant women from using available services and require special outreach efforts to encourage women to take advantage of services.

Edna Batiste describes how the Primary Care Network of the Detroit Department of Health is attempting to provide prenatal services to those who need them. However, it is not easy, she says. The recommendation of the American College of Obstetricians and Gynecologists for 12 or more prenatal visits, beginning in the first trimester, "is not only difficult but almost impossible to accomplish" in the inner-city population she serves. "Their lifestyles and multiplicity of problems simply will not allow this." There are intrinsic barriers of lifestyle, life experience or lack of it, educational levels, attitudes, and beliefs. *(#016)*

Batiste and others emphasize the importance of outreach efforts to adolescent, minority, and low-income groups who are not obtaining prenatal care. Culturally sensitive material and providers are required. Jo McNeil representing the American Nurses' Association says that one way to reduce poor outcomes among low-income pregnant women is to work with public assistance agencies already serving that population.

These women usually request financial help and can be identified and given health care assistance as quickly as they can be given funds for housing and food, if the agencies had a system of working this out together. By asking the client to come in and get her check, at least a monthly opportunity would be available for group education. *(#359)*

Outreach programs also need to be designed so that pregnant women and new mothers are motivated to take advantage of them. The ACOG says, "We have to develop innovative methods of education" if we are to reach lower socioeconomic women with information about nutrition. *(#279)* The National Mental Health Association calls for "psycho-social support and intervention to pregnant women and to families with infants." *(#418)*

Data Needs

In addition to concerns expressed about the need for a widely accepted and practical definition of "adequate" prenatal care, several witnesses pointed out other data needs.

Miriam Orleans of the University of Colorado School of Medicine asks, "What goes on in prenatal care? What works, what doesn't?" She suggests that "by 1990 we increase our efforts to conduct randomized controlled trials in order to evaluate our interventions. We increasingly demand trials of obstetrical interventions, but are far less rigorous about programs and social interventions." *(#168)* An example of a specific type of data need is identified by Weiner and Morse, who propose the establishment at the Centers for Disease Control of a national registry to measure the incidence of fetal alcohol syndrome. *(#542)*

REFERENCES

1. National Center for Health Statistics: Health United States, 1989 (DHHS Publication No. [PHS] 90-1232), 1990

2. U.S. General Accounting Office: Prenatal care: Medicaid recipients and uninsured women obtain insufficient care. Report to the Chairman, Subcommittee on Human Resources and Intergovernmental Relations, Committee on Government Operations, House of Representatives. GAO/HRD 87-137, September 1987

3. Hughes D, Johnson K, Rosenbaum S, et al.: The Health of America's Children: Maternal and Child Health Data Book. Washington, D.C.: Children's Defense Fund, 1988

5. Public Health Service: Caring for Our Future: The Content of Prenatal Care. A Report of the PHS Expert Panel on the Content of Prenatal Care. Washington, D.C.: U.S. Government Printing Office, 1989

6. Hughes D et al.: op. cit., reference 3

7. Ibid.

8. Thompson, J: Nurse midwifery care 1925 to 1984. Annual Review of Nursing Research, vol. 4. Edited by HH Werley, JJ Fitzpatrick, R Taunton. New York: Springer-Verlag, 1986

TESTIFIERS CITED IN CHAPTER 22

003 Alden, John; American College of Nurse-Midwives
010 Auerbach, Kathleen; University of Chicago, Wyler Children's Hospital
016 Batiste, Edna; Detroit Department of Health
033 Bublitz, Deborah; University of Colorado Health Sciences Center
044 Corry, Maureen; March of Dimes Birth Defects Foundation
046 Cunningham, Allan; Columbia University
049 Desmarais, Linda; International Lactation Consultant Association
060 Ernst, Eunice K. M.; National Association of Childbearing Centers
074 Grigsby, Sharon; The Visiting Nurse Foundation
108 Jarrett, Michael; South Carolina Department of Health and Environmental Control
158 Mulford, Christine; International Lactation Consultant Association of Eastern Pennslvania
168 Orleans, Miriam; University of Colorado Health Sciences Center
199 Siefert, Kristine; University of Michigan
215 Turnock, Bernard; Illinois Department of Public Health
244 Calonge, Ned; University of Colorado Health Sciences Center
268 Work, Rebecca; University of Alabama at Birmingham
279 Davidson, Ezra; King-Drew Medical Center (Los Angeles)
308 Smith, Peggy B.; Baylor College of Medicine
316 Rosenblatt, Roger; University of Washington
324 Hill, L. Leighton; University of Texas Health Science Center at Houston
359 McNeil, Jo; South Puget Sound Community College
360 Kopelman, J. Joshua; The OB-GYN Associates (Denver)
371 Schiff, Donald; American Academy of Pediatrics
383 Demmin, Tish; Midwives' Alliance of North America
397 Gaines, George; Detroit Department of Health
418 Tableman, Betty; Michigan Department of Mental Health
421 Welch, Robert and Sokol, Robert; Wayne State University/Hutzel Hospital (Detroit)
442 Schwarz, Richard; State University of New York, Health Science Center at Brooklyn
444 Mendelsohn, Sally; Midwives' Alliance of North America
542 Weiner, Lyn and Morse, Barbara; Boston University
582 Wirtschafter, David; Southern California Kaiser Permanente
690 Carr, Katherine; American College of Nurse-Midwives
722 Montgomery, William; Mount Carmel Mercy Hospital (Detroit)
726 Wright, Terri; Detroit/Wayne County Infant Health Promotion Coalition
801 Schlotfeldt, Rozella; Cleveland Heights, Ohio

23. Adolescent Pregnancy

Approximately 1 million teenagers become pregnant each year; about half of them give birth. Although the birthrate for teenagers has been declining for many years, adolescent pregnancy, abortion, and childbearing are considerably higher in the United States than in most developed countries.[1]

There are serious health and social consequences for both teen mothers and their children. Infants of adolescent mothers under age 15 are twice as likely to have low birth weight, according to Richard Smith of the March of Dimes Birth Defects Foundation.[2] (#203) These mothers are more likely to experience toxemia, anemia, and other complications during pregnancy, says the American School Health Association (ASHA). (#006) For young teen mothers (15 and younger), the risk of maternal death is three times as high as for mothers aged 20 to 24, according to Walter Ostergren of Life Planning/Health Services in Dallas.[3] (#640) In addition, Smith, Ostergren, and others report that teenage mothers do not achieve income or educational levels as high as those who become mothers later.[4] (#006; #640)

However, the problems associated with adolescent pregnancies and births must be examined in the social and economic climates in which most of these pregnancies occur. Research has established a strong link between poor socioeconomic status and early, sometimes socially accepted, sexual activity. In addition, many witnesses point to the fact that for some teenagers, pregnancy is intentional. Thus, to have an impact on the adolescent pregnancy rate, public health efforts must look beyond the obvious and dramatic statistics to the broader and deeper social issues that weigh heavily on this problem.

The 44 witnesses who focused on adolescent pregnancy and reproductive health highlighted efforts in several locales—Texas, Detroit, Rhode Island, Colorado, Los Angeles County, and elsewhere—that are aggressively combating teenage pregnancy and its adverse outcomes. They also identified additional measures that still must be taken or expanded if targets are to be met. The 1990 goals for reductions in teenage fertility will not be met, witnesses say. (#218; #279; #360)

Testimony provided evidence that preventive strategies can reduce teenage pregnancy rates and adverse pregnancy outcomes. Smith, for example,

reports that a program sponsored by the March of Dimes Birth Defects Foundation at Henry Ford Hospital in Detroit reduced the neonatal mortality rate among infants of adolescent mothers from 25.6 per 1,000 to 8.4 per 1,000 over a six-year period. (#203)

However, Denman Scott, Director of the Rhode Island Department of Health, notes that teenage pregnancy rates are lower in 32 developed countries than they are in the United States, despite the fact that teens begin sexual activity equally as early.[5] (#461) Deborah Bastien of Galveston, Texas, adds that in those countries, family planning services and sex education are more widely available.[6] (#236)

CONTRIBUTING CAUSES

Availability and Use of Contraception

According to Ostergren, there are about 5 million sexually active teenagers in the United States who need contraceptives, but family planning clinics serve only about half of them.[7] (#640)

Witnesses note that by the time most teenagers seek contraceptives, they have been sexually active for at least a year. Reasons given for failing to obtain contraceptives include economic barriers and inadequate education about contraception and pregnancy. (#006; #236) For some Hispanic teenagers, especially those using public clinics, there are additional barriers; often, they are asked questions about their legal status, which discourages them from going to clinics, according to Peggy Smith of Baylor College of Medicine.[8] (#308) Another problem is that teenagers may fear visiting a private physician because of confidentiality concerns. An American College of Obstetricians and Gynecologists (ACOG) spokesperson pointed out that his organization is working to assure teenagers that they are entitled to guarantees of patient-physician confidentiality, except in extraordinary circumstances. (#279)

For most teenagers, pregnancy reflects a failure to use contraceptives or contraceptive failure. Yet for some, it represents a conscious decision about how to proceed with their lives. (#003; #308; #640) For example, among adolescent Hispanic teens in Texas, Smith says that from 22 to 63 percent of pregnancies are intended. The consequences of out-of-wedlock pregnancy are seen as "negligible," she says.[9] *(#308)* Similarly, in the Black culture in Texas, childbearing is seen as a right of passage into womanhood and the child is often a source of pride to the grandmother. Marriage for Blacks was forbidden during slavery and still is not a social norm. *(#797)* Unintended pregnancies are related both to the unavailability of family planning services and to a reluctance on the part of teenagers to obtain or use contraceptives, according to witnesses. However, teenagers do not always continue the use of contraceptives once they have been obtained, according to testimony, and this matter should be targeted in education and outreach efforts. Low-income women are more likely to discontinue contraceptive use than higher-income women, according to Diana Bonta of the Los Angeles Regional Family Planning Council. *(#024)*

Socioeconomic Factors

The testimony of several witnesses makes clear, however, that the issue of teenage pregnancy often goes beyond contraceptives. What also must be considered is the social environment and the resultant self-image and outlook on life.

A number of studies have looked at the relationship between socioeconomic status and teenage pregnancy or early sexual activity. Although studies differ in methodologies, populations studied, study objectives, and so on, many point to the fact that chronic economic disadvantage may give rise to outlooks on marriage and family that make early sexual behaviors acceptable. A number of studies also suggest a strong association between low intellectual ability, low academic achievement, lack of educational goals, and early sexual experience among both Black and White students. Religiousness, on the other hand, regardless of the faith, appears to lead to initiating sexual activity at a later age.[10]

Edna Batiste of the Primary Care Network of the Detroit Department of Health describes a syndrome that characterizes many pregnant Black teenagers that she sees. The girl's environment involves poverty, single-parent homes, increasing high school dropout rates (now 40 percent in Detroit), and unemployment. She has a baby, drops out of school, and gets a low-paying job, if she can get a job. She does not want to marry the father because he has no job, is on drugs, does not care, or disappears. Welfare becomes necessary and self-esteem is low. *(#016)*

Other testifiers agree. Mary Lou Balassone of

Seattle, Washington, states her belief that just like teen pregnancies, the high rate of repeat pregnancies "is tied to economic and social factors." *(#246)* When a teen becomes pregnant, education is the first "luxury" to be dismissed, followed closely by youthful dreams and aspirations, according to Cathy Trostmann of Houston. *(#302)* Devising strategies for keeping teens in school is a priority for Jackie Rose of the Clackamas County Department of Human Services in Oregon. As an example, she suggests "teaching teens and their families techniques for success." *(#343)* Bernard Turnock of the Illinois Department of Public Health calls for "increased education and job training opportunities to impact the social and economic factors" contributing to a higher rate of pregnancy among non-White adolescents. *(#215)*

PREVENTION STRATEGIES

One approach to preventing teenage pregnancy is sex education in the schools. Although this topic has prompted considerable public debate, witnesses did not reflect the polar views sometimes heard. No one argued against sex education in schools. Many witnesses, including some who testified specifically about AIDS or sexually transmitted disease, proposed objectives aimed at including sex education in the health curriculum beginning in the early grades.

The American School Health Association (ASHA) says that mandatory school-based sex education has not been pursued as aggressively as it should because of the controversy surrounding the timing and content of such programs. Yet the ASHA notes that Gallup polls show increasing support for school-based sex education; recent polls indicate that 80 percent now favor it with parental consent.[11] The ASHA recommends that agencies receiving federal funds for AIDS education be required to expand their programs to include pregnancy prevention. *(#006)* Conversely, others suggest that information about AIDS and other sexually transmitted diseases also be included in education efforts aimed at preventing adolescent pregnancies.

Some witnesses suggest that the benefits of delaying sexual activity be stressed in adolescent education programs, but others feel that relying on this message is not sound. Ezra Davidson, representing the American College of Obstetricians and Gynecologists (ACOG), comments: "If we adopt an unrealistic and unbelievable line of reasoning that the only acceptable behavior is abstinence, we can probably not expect to see continued progress in reducing unintended teenage pregnancies." (#279) Davidson describes arrangements that ACOG has made with the national television networks to broadcast public service announcements. These announcements carry two messages: (1) sex before you can accept responsibility for it is not desirable; and (2) if you have sex, the responsible thing is to protect yourself against unintended pregnancy. (#279)

Several studies have documented the success of school-based clinics—that is, primary health care centers located on school grounds—in helping reduce adolescent pregnancies. The ASHA cites several school-based clinics in St. Paul in which birth rates dropped 40–50 percent, with about 80 percent of those having babies remaining in school.[12] (#021) In another inner-city study, junior and senior high school students received sexuality and contraceptive education, counseling, and medical and contraceptive services at a clinic several blocks from the school. Among students exposed to the program, pregnancies increased 13 percent after 16 months; among non-program students, the increase was 50 percent. After 28 months, pregnancies declined 30 percent for those in the program and increased 58 percent for non-program students.[13] (#006)

Bonta says that although the typical client at the Los Angeles Regional Family Planning Council is between 20 and 34 years of age, the council has several goals designed to enhance life options for adolescents, particularly low-income ones. Its services to teens include providing incentives to defer sexual activity, programs to reduce unintended pregnancies, and programs to improve the availability of contraceptives. She identifies several components of the program: upgraded family life planning courses, including male responsibility; programs to improve school performance and staying in school; afterschool programs; programs to improve family relationships or develop positive adult role models; employment programs; teen peer counseling programs for the 9 to 12 age group; outreach efforts to high school dropouts; and school-based programs to set individual goals, because pregnant teens have lower educational and occupational goals. (#024)

Other witnesses emphasize the importance of addressing the larger social context of adolescent pregnancy. They mention community-wide efforts involving employment and other programs to combat the problem. (#006; #016; #215) Batiste says that the classic public health approach, involving teams of professional community health workers who work face to face with teens in selected districts, is needed. These efforts can reach teens who have dropped out of school, as well as those still enrolled. (#016) George Flores of San Antonio's Metropolitan Health District emphasizes the need to involve schools, churches, and parents in community programs. (#745)

Prevention strategies should focus not only on preventing the first pregnancy but also on avoiding repeat pregnancy, says Balassone. For example, in a group of teenagers interviewed in 1979, 17.5 percent of those who had had a premarital pregnancy were pregnant again within a year. Within two years, 31 percent had a repeat pregnancy.[14] (#246) Donnie Hanson and Peter Vennewitz of the Washington State Department of Social and Health Services recommend adding an objective that the number of adolescents experiencing second or subsequent births be no more than 10 percent of those giving birth. (#218)

Other strategies identified by witnesses include increased availability of family planning services and contraceptives; increased use of nurse midwives to provide contraceptive information, because they can do it effectively and at a lower cost than physicians (#003); and enclosing educational material about preventing pregnancy in tampon and sanitary pad boxes, as is done for toxic shock syndrome (#360).

A few witnesses note that recent research suggests a link between sexual abuse and pregnancy among young teenagers, and suggest that increased efforts aimed at preventing sexual abuse of children could affect the pregnancy rate among young teens. (#215; #218)

REFERENCES

1. Hayes CD (Ed.): Risking the Future: Adolescent Sexuality, Pregnancy, and Childbearing, vol. I. Washington, D.C.: National Academy Press, 1987

2. Friede A, Baldwin W, Rhodes PH, et al.: Young maternal age and infant mortality: The role of low birthweight. Pub Health Rep 102(2):192–199, 1987

3. Hughes D, Johnson K, Rosenbaum S, et al.: The Health of America's Children: Maternal and Child Health Data Book. Washington, D.C.: Children's Defense Fund, 1988

4. Makinson C: The health consequences of teenage fertility. Fam Plann Perspect 17(3):132–139, 1985

5. Westoff CF, Calot G, Foster AD: Teenage delivery in developed nations. Fam Plann Perspect 15:105–110, 1983

6. Edelman ED, Pittman KJ: Adolescent pregnancy: Black and White. J Commun Health 11(1): 63–69, 1986

7. The Alan Guttmacher Institute: Public concerns about family planning programs in teens. Issues in Brief 5(4), January 1985

8. Smith PB: Sociologic aspects of adolescent fertility and childbearing among Hispanics. J Dev Behav Ped 7(6):346–349, 1986

9. Smith PB, Weinman ML, Mumford DM: Social and affective factors associated with adolescent pregnancy. J Sch Health 90–93, 1982

10. Hayes CD: op. cit., reference 1

11. Louis Harris and Associates, Inc.: Public attitudes about sex education, family planning, and abortion in the United States. New York: Planned Parenthood Federation of America, 1985

12. Lovick SR, Wesson WF: School-Based Clinics: Update. Washington, D.C.: Center for Population Options, 1987

13. Zabin LS, Hirsch MB, Smith EA, et al.: Evaluation of a pregnancy prevention program for urban teenagers. Fam Plann Perspect 18(3):119–126, 1986

14. Hayes CD: op. cit., reference 1

TESTIFIERS CITED IN CHAPTER 23

003 Alden, John; American College of Nurse-Midwives
006 Allensworth, Diane; American School Health Association
016 Batiste, Edna; Detroit Department of Health
021 Blair, Steven; Institute for Aerobics Research (Dallas)
024 Bonta, Diana; Los Angeles Regional Family Planning Council
203 Smith, Richard; Henry Ford Hospital (Detroit)
215 Turnock, Bernard; Illinois Department of Public Health
218 Hanson, Donnie and Vennewitz, Peter; Washington State Department of Social and Health Services
236 Bastien, Deborah; Galveston, Texas
246 Balassone, Mary Lou; University of Washington
279 Davidson, Ezra; King-Drew Medical Center (Los Angeles)
302 Trostmann, Cathy; Houston, Texas
308 Smith, Peggy B.; Baylor College of Medicine
343 Rose, Jackie; Clackamas County Department of Human Services (Oregon)
360 Kopelman, J. Joshua; The OB-GYN Associates (Denver)
461 Scott, H. Denman; Rhode Island Department of Health
640 Ostergren, Walter; Life Planning/Health Services, Inc. (Dallas)

745 Flores, George; Metropolitan Health District, San Antonio
797 Chater, Shirley; Texas Woman's University

24. Cardiovascular Disease

Heart disease and stroke are the first and fourth leading killers of Americans. Since 1950, death rates for these two cardiovascular diseases have declined substantially: 47 percent for heart disease and 69 percent for stroke. As a result, stroke has dropped from the third to the fourth leading cause of death.[1]

To maintain these impressive improvements, however, 42 witnesses called for continued efforts aimed at reducing the primary risk factors associated with cardiovascular disease (CVD), high blood pressure (hypertension), high serum cholesterol level (hypercholesterolemia), and smoking—as well as the secondary risk factors of sedentary lifestyles and obesity. Because three of these five risks are treated in some depth in separate chapters within this document (tobacco, Chapter 10; nutrition, Chapter 12; and physical activity, Chapter 13), the focus here is primarily on hypertension and high cholesterol.

Although these two risks are associated with separate genetic and environmental factors, several common approaches to their control are identified, as are several common populations that require special attention. Dietary change is the strategy raised most often for combating both high blood pressure and high cholesterol; food labeling also is mentioned repeatedly as a way to help individuals adopt healthy diets. Other strategies to prevent both hypertension and high cholesterol include public and professional awareness, screening, follow-up, and compliance, according to witnesses.

Minorities, especially Hispanics and Blacks, are seen as particularly vulnerable to CVD. For example, Michael Crawford of the University of Texas Health Science Center at San Antonio says that from 1970 to 1980 in San Antonio, among males aged 35 to 44, non-Hispanic Whites experienced an 8 percent decline in heart disease mortality, whereas Hispanic males experienced a 62 percent rise. He states, "across all age categories we see the same trend; that the Hispanic male is not experiencing this decline to the extent that the non-Hispanic White is, and in some age categories, the younger men have increased in this mortality." Crawford calls for education designed especially to encourage Hispanic men to alter their lifestyles. *(#743)*

Also singled out as needing special attention are the elderly, the medically or economically disad-

vantaged, and males. Although some risk factors for CVD can be found in young children and teenagers *(#182; #261)*, disagreement exists on how rigorously and how early interventions should be started. A number of testifiers see funding for research and for surveillance as a problem in need of attention between now and the year 2000.

HYPERTENSION

Several witnesses noted that when the 1990 Objectives were written, high blood pressure was defined as 160/95 mm/Hg or higher. Since then, however, studies have demonstrated the value of treating mild hypertension, and the definition of high blood pressure has changed to 140/90. The objectives should reflect that change, according to witnesses. *(#591)*

To help prevent hypertension, the American Heart Association (AHA) dietary guidelines call for efforts to reduce sodium intake.

> Sodium intake currently far exceeds the physiological needs of healthy Americans. The body can function quite normally and indefinitely with sodium intakes of less than 0.2 gram per day. Present consumption has been estimated at 4 to 5 grams per day. Cross-cultural studies show a clear relationship between the incidence of high blood pressure and the sodium content of the habitual diet. The AHA believes that the epidemiologic evidence is compelling and that a reduction of sodium intake to 1 gram per 1,000 calories, not to exceed 3 grams, is safe, feasible, and likely useful in prevention of high blood pressure in many Americans. This represents 2 grams of sodium per day for the average person consuming 2,000 calories.[2] *(#636)*

The Salt Institute, however, says that new data about the relationship between sodium or salt intake and hypertension also argue for changing the 1990 Objectives on that subject. On the basis of these studies, researchers concluded that for two-thirds of the population a general recommendation to reduce sodium chloride intake would have no benefit and could be harmful. *(#082)* "It seems clear that the question of diet and hypertension is so complicated and dependent on individual (probably genetic) factors that a general population dietary guideline is inappropriate," according to Richard Hanneman. *(#082)*

Although only one-third of the population is thought to be salt sensitive, a reviewer points out that no one knows who those 80 million Americans are. Because there is no known benefit from consuming large amounts of salt, and substantial benefit can be gained by a large number of people from cutting down, many believe that a general recommendation to cut down salt intake makes sense. *(#800)*

California Department of Health Services Director Kenneth Kizer underscores the point that follow-up is an essential component of screening programs. He cites 1983 data that 90 percent of California adults had their blood pressure measured in the previous two-year period, but of those referred for evaluation and diagnosis, many do not complete the referral. Among those diagnosed and under treatment, many do not adhere strictly to the treatment plan and remain uncontrolled. Only a small fraction of hypertensive adults are achieving and maintaining control of their blood pressure levels, according to Kizer. As a result of these figures, the thrust of California's hypertension control program is enrolling and maintaining hypertensive individuals in a health care setting that promotes adherence to control programs. *(#591)*

The American Association of Occupational Health Nurses emphasizes worksite intervention and cites more optimistic figures.

> The worksite is an ideal place for screening, education, intervention and prevention services. Employers benefit from decreased incidence or early detection of chronic health problems through reduced health insurance and disability costs and reduced absenteeism. Providing services at the worksite is cost effective and offers opportunities for increased compliance and better treatment outcomes. A recent review of several worksite hypertension control programs documented that 88 to 90 percent of hypertension employees treated at the worksite controlled their blood pressure. The success of these programs, which included detection, referral, treatment and follow-up, rested strongly upon the skills of the health care providers—primarily nurses. *(#558)*

HIGH BLOOD CHOLESTEROL

Additional testimony on reducing serum cholesterol focused on limiting the intake of both dietary fat and dietary cholesterol, and as a secondary preventive measure, on expanding screening programs to identify individuals with high cholesterol or specific dietary goals.

The American Heart Association reports that a certain amount of cholesterol is necessary in the body for building cell walls and other functions, but the liver supplies sufficient cholesterol to meet all of the body's own needs. *(#636)* Joseph Stokes of Boston University says that an average total cholesterol value of 190 milligrams per deciliter in adults more than 18 years old is a realistic goal for the year 2000. *(#627)*

Many studies have related dietary fat and cholesterol to blood cholesterol, and blood cholesterol to cardiovascular disease. Because of this, the AHA recommends monitoring personal consumption of cholesterol and keeping it less than 100 milligrams per 1,000 calories in the diet, not to exceed 300 milligrams per day.[3] *(#636)*

Stokes also favors incorporating the AHA dietary guidelines for fat into the Year 2000 Health Objectives. He says that the percentage of calories from fat should be less than 30 percent; the percentage of calories from saturated fat should be less than 10 percent; and the ratio between polyunsaturated and saturated fatty acids in the diet should be approximately 1:1. *(#627)*

Leslie VanDermeer, an occupational health nurse, says that screening of serum cholesterol levels should be available to all employees working at a company with a medical unit or a nursing department on the premises. *(#217)*

Other witnesses also emphasized the importance of follow-up of those with high cholesterol readings. The American Heart Association testimony calls for federal funds to help states develop and implement cholesterol screening programs. It emphasizes that such programs must involve not only screening but also appropriate referral and treatment activities. *(#636)*

Several witnesses referred to the need for individuals to reduce their fat and cholesterol intake. Several also favored additional research into the link between diet and cholesterol.

Witnesses also endorsed efforts to increase the

percentage of food products that are labeled according to their fat and cholesterol content. Dietitian Marilyn Guthrie says that the food industry should cooperate not only in labeling food, but also in lowering the amount of fat, saturated fat, and cholesterol in the products. She also recommends more support for businesses to offer cholesterol-lowering programs. Better data on the cost versus benefits of initiating dietary changes could provide the impetus for more structured programs. (#077) Chapter 12 contains a more detailed discussion of nutrition and cholesterol control.

TARGET POPULATIONS

Many witnesses emphasized the need to develop objectives to target high-risk groups and those who are especially hard to reach. These include Blacks, Hispanics, the elderly, males, and children, along with the medically or economically disadvantaged. Also, in many instances, individuals fall into two or more of these categories, multiplying many times the problems faced in changing their lifestyles or getting them into and maintaining treatment. For example, Kizer says that data from two statewide surveys in California demonstrate that priority must be given to ethnic minorities with a high prevalence of hypertension and to the medically or economically disadvantaged. He believes that adult males within these groups, in particular, should be targeted. (#591)

Blacks

Michael Jarrett of the South Carolina Department of Health and Environmental Control says the Year 2000 Health Objectives should specifically address awareness among high-risk groups such as Black males. (#108) John Thomas and William Neser of Meharry Medical College also emphasize the increased prevalence of hypertension among Blacks and note that although dramatic decreases in cardiovascular disease and hypertension have occurred in the overall population, the Black community has not seen that kind of decline. Possible risk factors for all groups, according to Thomas and Neser, are parental hypertension, weight gain, and smoking. Weight control, they emphasize, is an important nonpharmacological risk reduction measure. (#261)

Hispanics

Studies have shown that although Hispanics may have a better general knowledge about hypertension than Blacks, they still lag behind Whites in the percentage of known hypertensives who are taking medication and whose hypertension is under control.[4] Crawford speaks of the high cholesterol levels among Hispanics in San Antonio. The problem is more pronounced in Hispanics than in non-Hispanic Whites across socioeconomic groups. According to a local study among those with elevated cholesterol levels, fewer Hispanics are aware of it than non-Hispanic Whites, he testified. Of those in both groups who are aware, only one-fourth are under treatment and, of these, only about 40 percent have their levels controlled. Crawford believes that the problem with high cholesterol may be partially responsible for Hispanics not experiencing the kind of decline in ischemic heart disease seen in the general population in recent years. He called for an objective to reduce the prevalence of moderate-to high-risk cholesterol levels among young Hispanic men. (#743)

Elderly

The elderly are at special risk for CVD, according to Rosalie Young of Wayne State University: "As a major killer and disabler of the elderly, heart disease accounts for 45 percent of the mortality, 18 percent of the hospital days, another 18 percent of the bed days, and 10 percent of physician visits of the 65-plus cohort." Research she conducted for the National Institute of Aging indicates that it also "takes a major toll on the patient's general well being and mental health, and produces substantial physical and mental strain among family caregivers." (#478)

A special focus on the elderly is necessary, according to Rebecca Richards who conducts a wellness program for older adults in Wisconsin. She favors adding an objective to increase public and professional awareness about the risks and appropriate management of hypertension in older adults. Hypertension is the leading reason for doctor visits among older adults in Wisconsin, but many physicians still resist treating older people; she cited Cassel and Walsh on the subject: "The dogmas that hypertension is a benign disease in old age, that it is a natural result of aging, that old people need higher blood pressure to perfuse aging organ systems, and that antihypertensive therapy is of no value and too dangerous in persons over 65 years of age are all too frequently heard."[5] (#183)

Children

Although several witnesses discussed the apparent relationship between the existence of CVD risk factors in children or teens and later manifestation of the disease, agreement was not reached on how to identify and treat them.

Thomas and Neser discuss a study which found that hypertension and weight gain or smoking among Black parents are "significant independent predictors" of hypertension among their children; they suggest that "if such individuals were detected during early childhood (5–6 years), intervention could be instituted that could prevent or alter the course of later hypertension and thus morbidity and deaths due to hypertension and atherosclerotic cardiovascular disease." (#261)

However, Darwin Labarthe of the University of Texas Health Science Center at Houston warned that it may be difficult to identify those who will be at high risk in adulthood based on blood pressure or cholesterol levels in adolescence because patterns are not consistent. Cross-sectional survey data from around the world suggest that blood pressure rises during childhood and adolescence, and cholesterol level falls, he says. Therefore, it may not be possible to target individuals for prevention strategies at an early age. (#299)

Richard Niwinski, Terry Davis, and Rosemary Yancheck of Chapman College state that even if children at risk could be identified, some strategies, such as dietary interventions, might not be worthwhile because "not enough data has been collected to show the effect of diet in the age groups from two to twenty-five years." Rather, they suggest that educational programs for the parents of these children be considered. (#182)

Labarthe says the Southwest Center for Prevention Research is conducting research at the University of Texas that may help determine appropriate interventions for teenagers. (#299)

IMPLEMENTATION

The implementation issue that arose most often was lack of funding for research, evaluation, and surveillance.

The American Heart Association calls for objectives that reflect the need for the federal government to continue to dedicate "sufficient funding" to research in cardiovascular disease, "because it is only through continued research that disease prevention and health promotion activities will prosper." (#636) Similarly, the American College of Cardiology proposes objectives emphasizing research on cardiovascular disease prevention and application in practice, as well as more physician education in primary and secondary prevention. (#552)

Richards says that the ability to comply with antihypertensive medication is a special problem with older people and urges that surveillance and evaluation research include older subjects. (#183) Noting that his information collection and client tracking systems have been "deemphasized due to lack of funds and diminished resources," Stephen McDonough of the North Dakota State Department of Health and Consolidated Laboratories indicates that he is thus less able to assess categories of high blood pressure control. (#479)

REFERENCES

1. U.S. Department of Health and Human Services: Prevention '86/'87: Federal Programs and Progress. Washington, D.C.: U.S. Government Printing Office, 1987

2. American Heart Association: Position statement: Dietary guidelines for healthy American adults. A statement for physicians and health practitioners by the nutrition committee. Circulation 77(3):721A–724A, 1988

3. Ibid.

4. Barrios E, Iler E, Mulloy K, et al.: Hypertension in the Hispanic and Black population in New York City. J Nat Med Assoc 79(7):749-752, 1987

5. McDonald WJ: Medical, psychiatric and pharmacological topics. Geriatric Medicine, Vol. I. Edited by CK Cassel, JR Walsh. New York: Springer-Verlag, 1984

TESTIFIERS CITED IN CHAPTER 24

077 Guthrie, Marilyn; Virginia Mason Clinic (Seattle)
082 Hanneman, Richard; Salt Institute
108 Jarrett, Michael; South Carolina Department of Health and Environmental Control
182 Niwinski, Richard; Davis, Terry; Yancheck, Rosemary; Chapman College (San Diego)
183 Richards, Rebecca; North Woods Health Careers Consortium (Wausau, Wisconsin)
217 VanDermeer, Leslie; Hunter College (New York
261 Thomas, John and Neser, William; Meharry Medical College
299 Labarthe, Darwin; University of Texas Health Science Center at Houston
478 Young, Rosalie; Wayne State University
479 McDonough, Stephen; North Dakota State Department of Health and Consolidated Laboratories
552 Klocke, Francis; American College of Cardiology
558 Babbitz, Matilda; American Association of Occupational Health Nurses
591 Kizer, Kenneth; California Department of Health Services
627 Stokes, III, Joseph; Boston University
636 Ballin, Scott; American Heart Association
743 Crawford, Michael; University of Texas Health Science Center at San Antonio
800 Stoto, Michael; Institute of Medicine

25. Cancer

Cancer is the second leading cause of death in the United States, constituting approximately 20 percent of all deaths. The leading killers are lung, colorectal, and breast cancers. Over 30 percent of Americans now living eventually will develop some form of cancer. Many cancer deaths are preventable, however. The American Cancer Society estimates that about 178,000 people died in 1989 from cancer, who might have been saved by earlier diagnosis and treatment.[1] (#177)

"'Cancer' is not a single disease," according to Michael Skeels of the Oregon Department of Human Resources, "but rather a diverse set of clinical and epidemiological entities. Perhaps the only feature that cancers share in common is the underlying process, which involves a loss of control of normal cell growth." (#321)

Although many approaches to preventing cancer were mentioned in the hearings, this chapter focuses primarily on cancer screening and on secondary prevention issues. It highlights two forms of cancer that affect women—breast and cervical cancers—and a type of cancer that is increasing at a rapid pace, malignant melanoma. Many of the risk factors most often associated with prevention of cancer—smoking, dietary habits, exposure to toxic substances, and other environmental causes—are addressed at length in Chapters 10, 12, 17, and 18.

Witnesses make the point that the people stricken by cancer are just as diverse as the disease itself, and efforts must be made to target screenings, prevention programs, and treatments to the needs of each specific group. Many testifiers express grave concern about the cancer morbidity and mortality rates among Blacks. Robert Rutman of the University of Pennsylvania says, "The excess cancer risk facing the Black population is not only a major moral and ethical problem, it also is a costly financial one." Hispanics, too, are singled out for special attention, as are women who need to be brought into screening programs, especially mammography screening.

Harold Freeman of the American Cancer Society is concerned that the United States, as a nation, is not attending to the poor, minorities, and others who are not part of the mainstream. "We have directed most of our attention to those who can understand our language and pay our price. Unfortunately, many people are dying who are not in that category." (#443)

Although only 12 witnesses focused their testimony specifically on cancer, 52 addressed it in discussions of other topics.

SPECIFIC CANCERS

During the course of the seven hearings, lung cancer—the most common fatal cancer for both men and women—received considerable attention. However, other cancers were not overlooked. According to Skeels,

> In males, the second and third most common primary sites for fatal cancer are the prostate and the large intestine (colorectal cancer). In 1987, breast cancer was the second, and colorectal cancer the third leading type of fatal malignancy in females.[2] (#321)

Recognizing the importance of colorectal cancer, Linda Randolph of the New York State Department of Health suggests an objective of "increasing the proportion of adults who have occult blood testing, sigmoidoscopy, and digital rectal examinations performed at regular intervals." (#177) Oral cancer, discussed at some length especially by dentists and dental hygienists, is covered in Chapters 10 and 26.

Breast and Cervical Cancer

Although effective screening techniques exist to detect breast and cervical cancer, many women are not taking advantage of them. Witnesses testifying about these cancers emphasized the importance of increasing the percentage of women who are screened.

Until recently surpassed by lung cancer, breast cancer was the leading cause of mortality in women. According to American Cancer Society statistics cited by witnesses, approximately 142,000 cases of invasive breast cancer are diagnosed each year, and one third of the women who develop breast cancer in 1989 will die of it.[3] Morbidity and mortality from this disease could be reduced, several witnesses emphasize, if more women used the three screening techniques: breast self-examination, physical exam, and mammography.

Similarly, inadequate use of screening is resulting in needless deaths from cervical cancer. Witnesses call for increases in the number of women who undergo Pap smears to check for cervical cancer.

Ann Norman of the University of Washington focused on the need to get more older women screened: approximately one out of every ten women in this country will develop breast cancer, and 75 percent of those cancers will be detected among women 50 years of age or older.[4] She notes that although older women are at greater risk of dying from breast or cervical cancer than younger women, they are less likely to participate in cancer screening.[5] Norman also cites research showing that older women are about as likely as younger women to survive these cancers if they are detected early.[6] (#336)

Norman and others note that the National Cancer Institute (NCI) *Goals for the Year 2000: Cancer Control for the Nation*[7] addresses screening of older women, whereas the 1990 Objectives failed to target this group. She argues that NCI goals should be included in the Year 2000 Health Objectives. Those goals are (1) to increase the percentage of 50- to 70-year-old women who have an annual physical breast examination combined with mammography to 80 percent (it is now 45 percent for physical examination alone and 15 percent for mammography), and (2) to increase the percentage of women 40 to 70 years old who have a Pap smear every three years from 57 to 80 percent. (#336)

In addition to older women, witnesses suggest that low-income and non-White women be targeted in programs aimed at increasing screening utilization. (#020; #256; #452; #488; #615) Alvin Mauer and Mona Arreola of the University of Tennessee, Memphis, report that a year-long study of women admitted to a local hospital for treatment of breast or uterine cancer showed that poor women were coming in for breast cancer treatment at a later stage than others. Their study found that the reasons for the advanced stage at diagnosis could not be explained easily.

The results of the study indicated that, unfortunately, none of the simpler hypotheses were upheld. The women interviewed knew about cancer and its warning signs; they experienced no difficulties in gaining access to health care. The problem of delayed presentation appeared to be related to underlying psychosocial-behavioral factors that confounded the identification of a simple solution.[8] (#256)

Jose Lopez of the San Antonio Tumor and Blood Clinic made similar observations about Hispanics. He cites figures from one study in New York on knowledge and use of breast cancer detection among Hispanics: fewer Hispanic women did breast self-examination within the last year than non-Hispanic women; fewer Hispanic women have had a mammogram; and fewer have had a Pap smear. (#488)

An important impediment to the use of mammography is cost, according to witnesses. Even with the recent addition of mammography coverage to Medicare, gaps remain. Guy Newell and Charles LeMaistre of the University of Texas M.D. Anderson Hospital and Tumor Institute suggest a number of ways to reduce the cost of mammography screenings; for example, fewer films could be taken in routine screenings.[9] Newell and LeMaistre emphasize that cost and other barriers must be overcome so that more women can undergo mammograms.

Increased use of mammography depends on scientific consensus, policy making, marketing strategies, and cost reduction, among other factors. Endorsement of mammography screening by the medical profession coupled with availability at reasonable costs for the individual will be required for the widespread application of mammography screening. Until screening for breast cancer becomes a routine preventive practice, deaths from breast cancer will continue to be an increasing public health problem. (#484)

Addressing specifically the need to overcome barriers to testing among older women, Norman says that more research is needed on psychosocial factors, the role of physicians in assuring that older women are screened, and other areas. Innovative programs and approaches to the use of screening among older women should be tested as well. (#336)

Malignant Melanoma

Malignant melanoma was portrayed as an ideal candidate for an aggressive prevention program by William Robinson of the University of Colorado Health Sciences Center. He said that this type of skin cancer, which almost always affects Caucasians, has reached epidemic proportions. The incidence of malignant melanoma is increasing faster than any other cancer, yet the disease is largely preventable. (#708)

The rising incidence of the disease is due to increased exposure to sunshine and ultraviolet light, caused by changes in clothing habits and migration to the sunbelt, Robinson explained. It is a disease of the upper middle class. Those affected typically have brown, light brown, or light reddish hair and non-brown eyes. "We know what causes it, and we know who to target for the educational campaigns that need to be carried out," he says. This is an area in which a concerted prevention campaign could greatly reduce morbidity and mortality. (#708)

POOR AND MINORITIES

The inadequate utilization of breast and cervical screening techniques among Blacks and Hispanics is part of a broader-based gap in cancer prevention in those communities, witnesses reported.

Although limited national data on cancer rates among Hispanics indicate that they apparently have lower rates of some of the most common malignancies, several factors contribute to an increased risk of some types of cancer mortality, according to Lopez. He cites several factors to account for the increased risk, including later stage of cancer at diagnosis; lack of access to the health care delivery system; and certain knowledge, attitudes, and practices regarding cancer that are peculiar to Hispanics. (#488)

Lopez says that Hispanics are more fearful of getting cancer than other people, but they show, at best, a moderate awareness of the major risk factors for the disease. It is necessary to overcome psychological, cultural, and economic barriers to reach the Hispanic community with cancer programs, he added; "Hispanics tend to be fatalistic, feel there is a stigma attached to cancer, and have questions and concern about the treatment and the costs." (#488)

Hispanics in California follow the national pattern of "substantially lower" cancer incidence than non-Hispanic Whites, but Lester Breslow of the University of California, Los Angeles is concerned that as Hispanics "adopt the culture and way of life" of the area, there will be a "very sharp rise" in their cancer rates. He calls for Year 2000 Health Objectives to give "explicit attention to minority problems." (#026) John Bruhn of the University of Texas Medical Branch at Galveston points out that in some areas of Texas and for some types of cancer (stomach, liver, and gallbladder for males; uterine and cervical cancer for females), Mexican-Americans already are more

vulnerable than Whites. He says that "targeted education programs and readily available screening clinics should be of high priority." (#235)

The picture is even bleaker for Blacks, who "still have the highest overall age-adjusted cancer rate for both incidence and mortality of any U.S. population," according to Osman Ahmed of Meharry Medical College. (#269) Judith Glazner of the Denver Department of Health and Hospitals quotes several statistics for Black women illustrating the gap: "Nationally, the incidence rate for breast cancer has increased 1 percent per year; but while the mortality rate for White women has remained unchanged, for Black women it has increased 1 percent per year." For uterine cancer, the mortality rate among White women has declined 2.4 percent per year for the past five years, whereas for Black women, it has decreased by only 1.1 percent.[10] (#377)

Margaret Hargreaves, Osman Ahmed, and their coauthors from Meharry Medical College cite American Cancer Society figures indicating that in the last 30 years, cancer death rates for Blacks increased 40 percent, whereas the White rate increased only 10 percent; 30 years ago, Black and White rates were about the same. Data for 1967–1973 show that fewer Blacks than Whites had cancer diagnosed at an early stage when the chances of cure are greatest.[11] Blacks are less knowledgeable than Whites about warning signs and cancer tests, they noted. (#615)

The NCI recognizes the need to reach minority groups if its goal of reducing cancer mortality 50 percent by the year 2000 is to be met, according to testimony, and the NCI is beginning to address these issues. Minority representatives emphasized that culturally sensitive information about cancer and cancer detection tests is essential to any health education effort. Cancer in minority populations is discussed further in Chapter 6.

Testimony from the American Cancer Society (ACS) underscores the increased risk of cancer among poor people. Harold Freeman, ACS spokesman, reports that there is a 10–15 percent lower survival rate among poor people in America, regardless of race. At least half of the difference in survival is due to late diagnosis. He says that the increased prevalence of risk factors, such as smoking, poor nutrition, environmental exposures, and alcohol intake, also contribute to the variations.[12] (#443)

Primary prevention aimed at controlling risk factors could probably control two-thirds of the cancers, according to Freeman. However, efforts aimed at improving secondary prevention—primarily early diagnosis—are also important because the poor tend to seek care late. Instilling preventive habits is not easy,

Freeman acknowledges: "It is difficult to convince someone who is being shot at to have a rectal exam." *(#443)*

REFERENCES

1. American Cancer Society: Cancer Facts and Figures, 1989. Atlanta: 1989

2. National Center for Health Statistics: Health United States, 1989. (DHHS Publication No. [PHS] 90-1232), 1990

3. American Cancer Society: op. cit., reference 1

4. Seidman H, Mishinski M, Gelb S, et al.: Probabilities of eventually developing or dying of cancer—United States, 1985. CA Cancer J Clin 35(1):36–56, 1985

5. Gallup Organization: 1983 survey of public awareness and use of cancer detection tests for the American Cancer Society. New Jersey: The Gallup Organization, 1983

6. Baranovsky A, Myers MH: Cancer incidence and survival in patients 65 years of age and older. CA Cancer J Clin 36(1):26–41, 1986

7. Greenwald P, Sondik EJ (Eds.): Cancer Control Objectives for the Nation. 1985–2000. National Cancer Institute. NCI Monographs, No.2. (NCI Publication No. 86-2880), 1986

8. Mauer AM, Rosenthal T, Murphy J, et al.: Delayed Diagnosis in Breast and Uterine Cancer: A Study in Secondary Prevention. Unpublished study, Memphis: University of Tennessee, 1986–1987

9. American Cancer Society: Workshop on strategies to lower the cost of screening mammography, July 16–18, 1986. Executive Summary. Cancer 60:1700–1701, 1986

10. National Cancer Institute: Cancer Statistics Review, 1973–1986. (NIH Publication No. 89-2789), May 1989

11. American Cancer Society: Cancer Facts and Figures for Black Americans. New York: 1986

12. American Cancer Society: Cancer in the Economically Disadvantaged: A Special Report. Prepared by the Subcommittee on Cancer in the Economically Disadvantaged. June 1986

TESTIFIERS CITED IN CHAPTER 25

020 Bernstein, Robert; Texas Department of Health
026 Breslow, Lester; UCLA School of Public Health
177 Randolph, Linda; New York State Department of Health
235 Bruhn, John; University of Texas Medical Branch at Galveston
256 Mauer, Alvin and Arreola, Mona; University of Tennessee, Memphis
269 Ahmed, Osman; Meharry Medical College
321 Skeels, Michael; Oregon Department of Human Resources
336 Norman, Ann Deucy; University of Washington, School of Social Work
377 Glazner, Judith; Denver Department of Health and Hospitals
443 Freeman, Harold; State University of New York at Buffalo
452 Santee, Barbara and Alexander, Alpha; National Board of the YWCA of the United States

484   Newell, Guy and LeMaistre, Charles; University of Texas M.D. Anderson Hospital
488   Lopez, Jose; San Antonio Tumor and Blood Clinic
615   Hargreaves, Margaret; Meharry Medical College
708   Robinson, William; University of Colorado Health Sciences Center

26. Oral Health

Testimony on oral health covered the entire life span, from infancy to old age. The 53 witnesses who addressed oral health as a major part of their testimony discussed prevention of tooth decay and gum disease—the focus of the 1990 oral health objectives—as well as other areas such as access to dental health services, professional education, oral cancer, and the role of dental hygienists in achieving oral health goals.

Discussions of health priorities and preventive health strategies sometimes overlook oral health or treat it as an adjunct to other health goals. However, the witnesses who addressed oral health needs and objectives make it clear that this is a critical part of health—particularly preventive action taken to improve health in terms of personal well-being and to reduce lost work hours and costs. *(#163; #391)* Expenditures for dental care in 1987 reached $35 billion and have continued to increase.[1] *(#156)* According to Cyndi Newman, representing the American Dental Hygienists' Association:

> It has been obvious in the past that oral health has been considered separate from general total body health. I would like to suggest that it *should* be considered an integral part of total health. Oral health *must* be a basic component of all health education, treatment, and maintenance programs. Good oral health must no longer be considered optional for health status. *(#163)*

Witnesses also highlighted some new opportunities for making significant gains in oral health. For example, research in the last decade has made eradication of dental caries a realistic goal, according to Stephen Moss of New York University. *(#439)* New objectives were proposed to reflect that progress.

However, testimony also revealed areas in which progress is lagging. One such area is community water supply fluoridation. Fluoridation has been called the foundation of oral health, yet many communities are still without systemic fluoridation.

One issue that arose repeatedly is the vast disparity in oral health across various population subgroups; objectives should reflect or target the dental health needs of these groups, according to witnesses. Subgroups identified include the elderly, institutionalized, homeless, handicapped, minorities, migrant workers, and low-income people. Although specific objectives on oral health are proposed, witnesses feel that the process of setting objectives and measuring progress toward them is impeded by incomplete data on the oral health status and needs of many population subgroups. The Association of State and Territorial Dental Directors (ASTDD) says that an objective for 1990, that calls for a system to periodically assess oral health status, needs, and use of services is the single most important national dental health objective. *(#106)*

Another intervention discussed was professional education. Thomas Truhe of the Princeton Dental Resource Center says that the public receives most of its information on dental health from dentists, but fewer than 40 percent of practicing dentists consider their profession a primary source of information.[2] He believes that new research findings and other important information should be disseminated more effectively to dental professionals so that they can be better educators. *(#369)*

FLUORIDATION

"In the 1990 Objectives, water fluoridation was the foundation for the prevention of dental disease," says Myron Allukian representing the American Association of Public Health Dentistry. "That should continue in the year 2000." There was widespread consensus on that issue among those testifying. Witnesses urge that the 1990 target of having 95 percent of the population on community water systems receive the benefits of fluoridation, be carried over to the Year 2000 Health Objectives, although many think it an unrealistic goal. *(#435)*

According to Allukian, 60 percent of the population served by community water supplies had fluoridated water in 1975; by 1985, this had increased to only 61.4 percent.[3] *(#435)* John Brown of the University of Texas Health Science Center at San Antonio says that the promotion of water supply fluoridation is static: "Its benefits must be more effectively explained, so that those with this measure will defend it and those without it will acquire it." *(#029)*

The ASTDD calls for changes in a 1990 objective

that at least 50 percent of school children living in fluoride-deficient areas without community water systems should be served by an optimally fluoridated school water supply. He says that no real progress has been made toward this goal and there is no real prospect of attaining it. The ASTDD recommends replacing this objective with one that includes alternative ways to receive fluoride, such as mouth rinses, tablets, or both. *(#106)* The importance of using fluoride dentifrice twice daily is also underscored. *(#154)*

INFANTS AND CHILDREN

Many witnesses agree that a new objective aimed at preventing baby bottle tooth decay should be added; a public education campaign that alerts parents and other care givers to the problem could dramatically reduce its incidence. *(#154; #242; #353; #445; #705)*

Baby bottle tooth decay occurs when baby bottles filled with liquids containing natural or added sugars—such as milk, infant formula, fruit juice, or a soft drink—are used as pacifiers. When an infant who is awake takes in the liquid, the sugars are diluted with saliva and swallowed. However, if the infant falls asleep the sugars have time to react with bacteria and form acids that cause serious cavities. Discontinuing the use of liquids containing natural or added sugars in bedtime bottles would prevent this problem.

The national prevalence of baby bottle tooth decay is not known. In Head Start programs in San Antonio, 10–20 percent of preschoolers show the rampant form of this condition, according to Brown. *(#029)* David Johnsen of Case Western Reserve University estimates that 15 percent of urban and rural underserved children and over 50 percent of children in some Native American groups have the condition. He recommends that the prevalence be determined and high-risk groups identified. *(#109)*

Another new objective proposed by many witnesses involves the use of pit and fissure sealants to prevent dental caries in children. Sealants are a significant advance in caries prevention that were not addressed by the oral health objectives for the year 1990. Witnesses call for all children to have access to this procedure at public and private dental clinics. *(#242; #353; #445)* The eradication of caries in children is now a realistic goal, according to Stephen Moss of New York University, who notes that a survey of pediatric dentists' own children found that 90 percent of those less than 12 years old had no cavities. *(#439)*

The American Academy of Pediatric Dentistry emphasizes that sealants and two other proven preventive strategies—fluoride dentrifice and systemic fluoride—should be the focus of the Year 2000 Health Objectives on reduction of caries. Members of the academy and witnesses from other dental professional groups, as well as from the sugar industry, call for eliminating those of the 1990 objectives aimed at reducing the availability of cariogenic foods in schools. Those objectives are criticized for being untenable and unmeasurable, for failing to take into account uncertainties about which foods pose the most serious oral health threats, and for distracting attention from proven methods of reducing caries. *(#154; #197)*

ADULTS

For adults, witnesses focused on caries, periodontal disease, oral trauma, and oral cancers. Public education, personal dental hygiene, and regular dental care were identified as important prevention strategies for adults.

As the population ages, the number of adults with caries is increasing, according to Jane Weintraub of the University of Michigan, who explains that caries (not gum disease as was previously thought) are the major cause of tooth loss in adults.[4] The 1990 Objectives set targets for caries reduction in only one age group: nine year olds. Weintraub and others recommend that targets be expanded to include other ages, even adults, and that specific types of caries be included in some objectives. *(#391)*

Much of the adult population has periodontal disease, according to Dan Middaugh of the University of Washington.[5] To reduce the rates, new initiatives aimed at increasing public awareness of the importance of daily oral hygiene and regular professional care will be necessary, witnesses say. *(#353)* Although some testifiers note that the relationship between gingivitis and periodontal disease in adults is not clear *(#029; #106),* most witnesses favor continuing to include it in the objectives.

The American Cancer Society estimates that there are 30,600 new cases of oral cancer a year.[6] As Woodrow Myers of the Indiana State Board of Health says:

> Smokeless tobacco has been linked to cancer, specifically oral cancer. Use of oral snuff increases the risk of oral cancer several fold, and among long-term snuff dippers, the excess risk of cancers of the cheek and gum may reach

fiftyfold. Smokeless tobacco use is responsible for the development of a portion of oral leukoplakias in both teenage and adult users. *(#405)*

According to Percy Butcher of the American Dental Association, reductions in tobacco and alcohol use are important preventive strategies for oral cancers. *(#242)* Several witnesses expressed concern about the use of smokeless tobacco, particularly among youth and young adults. The testimony in this area is summarized in Chapter 10. Although smokeless tobacco use is a separate topic, a few witnesses recommended that it be included under oral health to emphasize its link to oral disease.

Increased public awareness of the risk factors and symptoms of oral cancer is necessary to decrease the morbidity and mortality from it; early detection and treatment of oral cancer result in higher cure rates. *(#249; #262)*

Another condition recommended for the new objectives is oral trauma. Although a 1990 objective concerned the use of mouthguards, there is some feeling that it must to be strengthened. Other strategies mentioned for preventing oral traumas include the use of seatbelts. *(#391)*

OLDER ADULTS

Some of the most compelling testimony about adult oral health needs concerned the elderly. None of the 1990 Objectives addressed this group specifically, although the elderly are the fastest growing segment of the population in this country and have serious dental health needs, according to witnesses. The American Society for Geriatric Dentistry (ASGD) notes that as more elderly keep their natural teeth, caries are an increasing problem. Also, as the numbers of elderly increase, so will the need for dental service, witnesses point out. The at-risk elderly must be identified so that prevention programs aimed at reducing caries can be introduced, according to the ASGD. *(#062)*

Oral mucosa disease is another problem for the elderly with dentures, the ASGD says, and a goal for the year 2000 should be to reduce the prevalence of oral mucosal lesions in the aging population by 50 percent. *(#062)*

Special attention also must be given to the oral health of the institutionalized elderly. The ASGD notes that they have a far greater need for dental care than those who are not institutionalized. *(#062)* Testimony reveals that in many institutions, elderly residents are not offered regular dental care. A new Texas law requiring that nursing home residents be offered dental services (at their own expense) on a regular basis is hailed as a model. *(#306)* The ASGD suggests that oral health programs be mandatory at all nursing homes by the year 2000. *(#062)*

UNDERSERVED POPULATIONS: PROBLEMS AND STRATEGIES

The theme sounded most often in the testimony on oral health is the disparity in oral health among population subgroups. In addition to the elderly, other subgroups identified include Blacks, Native Americans, Hispanics, residents of some rural areas, migrant workers, the handicapped, the homeless, the institutionalized or homebound, and low-income people. Objective setting should reflect the special needs of these groups, according to witnesses.

Allukian says that children in inner-city Boston have 55 percent more surfaces affected by tooth decay than the national average and that Black children in the United States have 2.5 times as many untreated cavities as White children. He also reports that a study of the homeless in Boston, in which the median age was 33, found that 97 percent needed treatment; 18 percent had pain or infection at the time of screening; 9 percent had suspicious soft tissue lesions; and 28 percent had not been to a dentist for an average of 14 years. *(#435)*

Newman says that although Native Americans on reservations have dental coverage through the Indian Health Service, oral health care is not always available locally. As a result, many Native Americans suffer from poor oral health. She describes the needs in rural Washington State where she works.

> The Indian Health Service in this area needs to refocus their attention on education, preventive therapies, and doing outreach to those Native Americans who are not receiving care. I see that a large number of Indian children are not receiving the oral health care that they need. I hear constant complaints of toothaches from school children. It is not uncommon to see rampant decay in these children. *(#163)*

The barriers to access faced by these groups typically involve the availability of providers, sociocultural issues, and cost. Brown describes the problem in San Antonio.

Effective oral disease prevention measures and oral health promotion activities are not reaching the community, especially those groups most at risk. Resources are disparate, often difficult to locate, duplicated, of poor quality in some instances and absent in others. Often ethnic, cultural, educational, and language diversity of communities is not sufficiently taken into account. Existing networks such as well baby clinics, WIC [Special Supplemental Food Program for Women, Infants and Children] programs, school systems, workplace health programs, health care facilities for the homeless, migrant health workers, community health centers, nutrition centers, retirement centers, and nursing homes need to be utilized to promote oral health and prevent oral disease by scientifically-based effective measures. *(#029)*

IMPLEMENTATION

The need for more and better data about oral health is intertwined throughout much of the testimony, especially as it relates to underserved populations. *(#062; #106; #109)* For example, Butcher states that because certain ethnic and socioeconomic groups have higher decayed, missing, or filled surfaces scores than the population as a whole, "such groups should be over-sampled to reflect more precisely the degree of difference." *(#242)* The American Association of Public Health Dentistry emphasizes the need to develop baseline data for each objective, so that progress can be measured throughout the decade. "Later data collection," it states, "can more comprehensively describe other aspects or dimensions of the objective" but is "no substitute for the understanding provided by baseline data." *(#156)*

Witnesses pointed out that health professionals, including dentists, hygienists, and even physicians, could play an expanded role in delivering preventive services to underserved populations. Hygienists can be especially useful in reaching the elderly, according to Betty Waedemon of the American Dental Hygienists' Association. *(#306)*

Waedemon says that hygienists could provide important preventive services in nursing homes. Many nursing homes cannot afford to have a dentist on staff, and the residents' dental needs are neglected, according to witnesses. Waedemon says that hygienists would be less expensive than dentists; therefore, institutions may be able to afford to have one on staff full- or part-time. *(#306)*

More dentists also should be trained in geriatric dentistry, according to the ASGD, which explains that dentists should have an understanding of normal and pathological aging, communication skills, and other specialized areas to treat the elderly effectively. Very few programs in the United States offer such training; thus, specific targets in this area are proposed for the year 2000. *(#062; #306)*

Several dental hygienists mentioned their role in bringing preventive services to groups such as the handicapped or those living in remote areas where dental services are unavailable, but said that restrictions on their practice can limit those opportunities. States may restrict them to working under either direct or general supervision of a dentist. In Washington State, for example, hygienists can work under the general supervision of a dentist in institutions, but they must have direct supervision in homes or private practice, according to testimony. Hygienists such as Newman say that these restrictions should be relaxed. *(#163)*

Physicians and other health providers also can play an important role in encouraging good dental health and identifying oral cancers or other conditions, according to testimony. They should be prepared for that role and encouraged to become involved in oral disease prevention. *(#154)*

Mobile dental units can help bring preventive services to those who are hard to reach. The ASGD reports that mobile units operating out of dental schools can be effective in long-term care institutions if they are designed properly. *(#062)* Other witnesses note their value in remote areas and for populations that are unable or unlikely to come to a clinic. *(#041)*

Several testifiers note that one approach to providing preventive dental services to underserved children is expanding school-based programs. Brown proposes that by the year 2000, at least 50 percent of school children be participating in school-based comprehensive health programs. He says that these should include fluoride and dental sealant programs, assessments and referral systems, comprehensive oral health education, and mouthguard programs. *(#029)*

Financial barriers to obtaining preventive dental services also were discussed. Many witnesses said that Medicare and Medicaid, as well as private insurers, should cover comprehensive preventive dental services. Several witnesses called for including dental services in more employee benefit packages. Weintraub proposes that by the year 2000, 75 percent of employed adults have dental insurance. In 1985, 58 percent of the employed population was covered to some extent, according to testimony.[7] *(#391)*

REFERENCES

1. National Center for Health Statistics: Health United States, 1989 (DHHS Publication No. [PHS] 90-1232), 1990

2. Opinion Research Corporation: Dental care: What people know. Surveying the "knowledge gap". A study on attitudes about dental health conducted by Opinion Research Corporation, 1983

3. U.S. Department of Health and Human Services: The 1990 Health Objectives for the Nation: A Midcourse Review. Washington, D.C.: U.S. Government Printing Office, 1987

4. Balit HL, Btaun R, Maryniuk GH, et al.: Is periodontal disease the primary cause of tooth extraction in adults? J Am Dent Assoc 114:40–45, 1987

5. Corbin SB, Kleinman DV, Lane JM: New opportunities for enhancing oral health: Moving toward the 1990 objectives for the nation. Public Health Rep 100(5):515–524, 1985

6. Silverberg E, Lubera JA: Cancer statistics, 1989. CA Cancer J Clin 39(1):3–20, 1989

7. National Institute for Dental Research: Oral Health of United States Adults. The National Survey of Oral Health in U.S. Employed Adults and Seniors: 1985–1986. National Findings. (NIH Publication No. 87-2868), August 1987

TESTIFIERS CITED IN CHAPTER 26

029 Brown, John; University of Texas Health Science Center at San Antonio
041 Swanson, Terri; Colorado Dental Hygienists' Association
062 Ettinger, Ronald; American Society for Geriatric Dentistry
106 Isman, Robert; The Association of State and Territorial Dental Directors
109 Johnsen, David; Case Western Reserve University
154 Moss, Stephen; American Academy of Pediatric Dentistry
156 Easley, Michael; American Association of Public Health Dentistry
163 Newman, Cyndi; Clallam County Department of Health (Washington)
197 Setton, Sarah; The Sugar Association
242 Butcher, Percy; American Dental Association
249 Davis, A. Conan; Alabama Department of Public Health
262 Fleming, Lisa; Alabama Dental Hygienists' Association
306 Waedemon, Betty; American Dental Hygienists' Association
353 Middaugh, Dan; University of Washington
369 Truhe, Thomas; Princeton Dental Resource Center
391 Weintraub, Jane; University of Michigan
405 Myers, Jr., Woodrow; Indiana State Board of Health
435 Allukian Jr., Myron; Boston Department of Health and Hospitals
439 Moss, Stephen; New York University
445 Greenfield, William; New York University
705 Johnson, Dana; Colorado Dental Association

27. Other Chronic Diseases and Disabling Conditions

The category "chronic disease" encompasses a vast and diverse collection of conditions and disabilities. One definition, developed by the Association of State and Territorial Chronic Disease Program Directors and adopted by some states, follows.

> Chronic disease is an impairment or deviation from normal, having any of the following characteristics: is related to avoidable behavioral risk factors; is permanent; leaves residual disability; is caused by irreversible pathological alterations; requires special training of the patient for rehabilitation; may require a long period of supervision, observation, or care. *(#470)*

Many such conditions were covered in the testimony, each involving specific prevention interventions. However, considerable testimony was concerned with general issues applying to chronic and disabling conditions as a whole. As Matthew Liang of Harvard Medical School observes, "Although each disease has its unique biology, the impact each has on the patients' energy, psychological and physical functioning, emotional state, and productivity is similarly pervasive and handicapping." *(#132)*

Patience Drake of the Michigan Department of Management and Budget and Robert Dolsen of the Statewide Health Coordinating Council emphasize that those with chronic diseases face special problems because the health care system is oriented toward acute disease and does not offer the necessary systematic response to all people with chronic needs for health services. *(#420)* Liang says there is a need to recast current approaches to chronic disease. Only by doing this can his proposed year 2000 objective of reducing its impact be met.

> A fundamental change in the paradigm which drives health care delivery and organization is needed. We will have to switch our view from cure to care; from preoccupation with the disease to the illness that results from the disease; from preoccupation with impairments to function; and from concerning ourselves with

death to life and the quality of existence with illness. *(#132)*

This chapter describes testimony from 52 witnesses about several chronic conditions and disabilities: diabetes, musculoskeletal conditions, hearing disorders, vision disorders, and developmental and chronic disabilities. Although chronic diseases strike people of all ages, witnesses stressed the particular toll they take on the elderly and the very young. Regardless of their age, however, all those disabled with chronic diseases deserve an opportunity to live full, productive lives, according to the American Foundation for the Blind: "It is not contradictory to pursue the objective of promoting the health and fitness of people with impairments, disabilities, and handicaps, along with the objective of reducing the incidence of impairments, disabilities, and handicaps." *(#116)*

The two most common chronic disease killers—heart disease and cancer—are discussed in Chapters 24 and 25. Many of the behavioral risk factors for chronic diseases are treated in Chapters 10 through 13.

DIABETES

Witnesses who addressed the topic of diabetes emphasized that it is a serious disease that should be included in the Year 2000 Health Objectives. Daniel Porte of the Seattle Veterans Administration Medical Center, representing the American Diabetes Association, provides some statistics. Diabetes is the seventh leading cause of death in the United States, with 130,000 deaths annually; it is the number one cause of new cases of adult blindness, responsible for 5,800 cases each year, many of which can be prevented. Further, it accounts for approximately one-fourth of new cases of end-stage renal disease in the United States. Diabetic nephropathy is the most common cause of renal failure in persons age 25–64 years, and 40–45 percent of nontraumatic leg or foot amputations are due to diabetes. In addition, individuals with diabetes are two to four times more likely to self-report a previous heart condition or report a heart attack or stroke, Porte says.[1] *(#699)* Most of the diabetes in the population is called Type II or "adult onset." This form of the disease, which offers the best opportunities for prevention, was the focus of most of the testimony.

Weight control is the most commonly mentioned form of primary prevention. According to Porte and others, controlling body weight can delay the onset of Type II diabetes by 10–20 years.[2] (#261; #699) However, much testimony about diabetes involves the importance of secondary and tertiary prevention—avoiding the complications of the disease. The American Diabetes Association (ADA) recommends that the prevention program developed in 1987 by the National Diabetes Advisory Board (NDAB) be incorporated into the Year 2000 Health Objectives. (#699) Reducing the incidence of diabetic complications is one of its goals.[3] (#457)

Several witnesses say that patient compliance with doctor-prescribed regimens and regular monitoring are important means of controlling the course of the disease. (#626) According to Victor Hawthorne of the University of Michigan, there is new evidence that screening for microalbuminuria could prevent kidney complications. (#410) In addition to preventing or delaying onset of the disease, measures such as treating diabetic retinopathy at an early stage and being more aggressive in testing hypertension in early diabetes nephropathy also can prevent diabetes morbidity. (#132)

Other parts of the NDAB agenda call for improved training of health professionals on topics such as the importance of assiduous skin and foot care (#132), as well as better patient and public education. Anne Esdale, representing the Michigan Society for Public Health Education, says that patient education about diabetes reduces hospitalization and health care costs. (#061) Alan Altschuler, an ADA spokesperson, notes that primary care doctors should be taught to use the most modern techniques for detection and treatment of diabetes. (#457) Several witnesses call special attention to the increased problem of diabetes among Hispanics and Blacks and the importance of making special efforts to reach these groups. (#457; #491; #496; #567) This issue is discussed in more detail in Chapter 6.

MUSCULOSKELETAL CONDITIONS

Witnesses who addressed musculoskeletal conditions focused their remarks on three particular preventable health problems: osteoporosis, osteoarthritis, and gout.

Osteoporosis

Osteoporosis is a reduction in bone mass that leads to easily fractured, fragile bones. The condition is most common in postmenopausal women, but individuals who take medications such as corticosteroids that alter bone mass are also at increased risk. Witnesses characterized osteoporosis as a common and costly condition. Figures cited from the 1984 and 1987 consensus development conferences of the National Institutes of Health and the Food and Drug Administration indicate that 24 million Americans have osteoporotic fractures. Even more have serious bone mass reductions (osteopenia) that are likely to result in fractures in the future. The annual cost for acute hospital care alone approaches $10 billion. Hip fractures cause most of the mortality and morbidity. Other common sites include the spine, wrist, and pelvis. The fracture rates, mortality, and cost are expected to double by the year 2000, according to testimony from Paul Miller of the University of Colorado Health Sciences Center.[4] (#367)

Witnesses reported that primary reductions in bone mass (i.e., reductions not associated with another condition or medication) are a result of aging and decreased estrogen levels due to menopause. Genetic disposition also plays a role: women with small frames, Caucasians, and Asians are more susceptible to the condition. (#367)

Prevention can play a critical role in reducing the morbidity and mortality from osteoporosis, witnesses agreed. Maria Greenwald, representing the National Osteoporosis Foundation (NOF), identifies several measures required to reduce osteoporotic fractures: build greater bone density when young; prevent bone loss that begins in the middle years; rebuild bone density among the elderly; and prevent falls. (#281)

Although studies suggest that attaining peak bone mass is highly dependent on calcium intake and activity during adolescence and the twenties, when bone mass reaches its peak. (#367) Although reaching teens with information about preventing osteoporosis is not easy, it is vitally important, according to Charles Chestnut of NOF: "It is obviously extremely difficult for young women aged 15 to be concerned about a disease that may occur 40 years later; however, it has been noted that osteoporosis may be a pediatric disease, and that the ultimate prophylaxis for osteoporosis may exist in the teenage female." (#332) Several witnesses propose objectives aimed at increasing exercise and calcium intake. These include expanding public and professional education about the importance of bone mass and ways to prevent osteoporosis. Other witnesses set specific targets for calcium intake or exercise levels. Dietitians Barbara Bruemmer and Darlene Fontana of the Pacific Medical Center in Seattle, for example, suggest that virtually all contacts with health professionals for girls age 8 to 20 assess calcium intake and that health curriculum textbooks provide information on the link between calcium and osteoporosis. *(#030)*

For older individuals, preventive strategies are aimed at increasing bone mass or reducing further deterioration. The NOF calls for increasing the number of postmenopausal women on estrogen replacement therapy (ERT) by the year 2000. According to testifiers, this is one of the few interventions known to reduce hip fractures. They also note that because of side effects, the appropriateness of ERT must be determined on an individual basis. Two testifiers report positive results in studies using drugs to increase bone density. However, it is still unclear whether these increases will lead to a reduction in fractures. *(#281; #367)*

Several witnesses note the potential value of monitoring bone mass to identify quantitatively those at risk for osteoporosis. New radiological tests can detect a 2−3 percent bone loss, according to Miller; used properly—not as a mass screening technique—these tests can assist physicians in determining whether ERT is appropriate for postmenopausal women. As an objective for the year 2000, Miller and others recommend educating health professionals and the public about the indications for bone mass measurement and favorable third-party reimbursement for the procedure. *(#214; #332; #367)*

As with many topic areas, success in reaching the proposed objectives will depend on effective public and professional education, witnesses agreed. Other needs identified include additional research into the cause and prevention of osteoporosis; better prevalence and incidence figures about spinal osteoporosis; improved techniques for detecting bone mass loss; and better coordination among government, private, professional, and public groups involved in the field.

Arthritis

According to testimony, arthritis afflicts more than 37 million Americans and exacts an enormous toll in lost workdays and reduction in the quality of life.[5] *(#373)*

Wayne Tsuji of the Washington State Arthritis Foundation emphasizes primary prevention approaches to osteoarthritis. He notes that risk factors for the condition include advancing age, obesity, injuries, adverse workplace environment, and hip dysplasia. Preventive strategies should be directed toward reducing these risk factors, where possible. Tsuji proposes a prevention agenda that emphasizes weight control, ergonomic measures in the workplace, prevention and appropriate treatment of athletic injuries, and early diagnosis of children with hip dysplasia. *(#339)*

Other witnesses also address some of these factors. According to Liang, congenital hip dislocation in newborns is a preventable cause of osteoarthritis, but screening for the condition is lapsing. He urges better education of pediatricians and medical students about its importance. *(#132)* The Arthritis Foundation emphasizes the importance of weight reduction for prevention of osteoarthritis of the knee. *(#134)*

The importance of secondary prevention also is underscored in testimony. Debra Lappin, a representative of the National Arthritis Foundation, says that it could make "an astounding difference" in preventing complications such as deformity and limitations in mobility. Lappin says that drug treatment, physical and occupational therapy, and physical medicine (e.g., joint replacement) are the most effective ways of controlling the disease, but that these techniques are not reaching all who could benefit from them. *(#373)* Liang notes that patients with polyarthritis, particularly those with rheumatoid arthritis and children with arthritis, are not being treated with agents that could lead to remission or better control of the disease. He says patients are not being referred for appropriate physical or occupational therapy and are being overtreated with steroids. *(#132)*

Michael Condit, also representing the Arthritis Foundation, makes a compelling case for the tragedy associated with rheumatoid arthritis, which often strikes younger people.

Of moderately severe or mildly severe patients, about half are not able to work anymore. It is not so much that they cannot do any work, as they find themselves in the unfortunate position of falling in the cracks of our systems. They are too disabled to work, but not disabled enough to have some help. *(#685)*

Gout

Testimony about gout also emphasizes the inadequate dissemination of effective interventions. Although gout is called "one of the few forms of arthritis that is almost completely controllable," it still causes considerable morbidity. The Arthritis Foundation says that "no effective primary preventive measures exist" for gout, making the application of secondary measures to reduce disability "an attractive alternative." Overall, the prevalence of gout based on doctor diagnoses is 1 million cases, but self-reports are double that, according to the foundation.[6] Fully 80 percent of those suffering from gout are men; the first attack usually occurs between ages 40 and 50. (#134) According to Liang, many patients are being misdiagnosed and put on potentially dangerous drugs because synovial fluid analysis—the diagnostic tool—is not being interpreted correctly by laboratories. (#132) Lappin notes that low-income and minority groups are not receiving available treatment and says that an objective for the year 2000 should be to increase access to available treatment. She says that disability from gout among Blacks is three times that in Whites. (#373)

HEARING DISORDERS

About 22 million people in the United States suffer from a hearing impairment.[7] (#396) Although several of the 1990 Objectives, particularly those involving prenatal care and newborn screening, could have an impact on reducing hearing disorders, none of them specifically targeted the prevention of hearing loss. Several witnesses propose such objectives for the year 2000.

Testimony highlights the point that risk factors for hearing loss are known and largely preventable, but interventions must begin early in life. (#361) Much of the testimony falls into two general categories: (1) prenatal care and screening newborns and children, and (2) reduction in damage-causing noise.

Many witnesses emphasize the importance of newborn screening. Marion Downs of the University of Colorado Health Sciences Center proposes that by the year 2000, 80 percent of all newborns be screened for hearing disorders by electrophysiological screening. In 1986, only 5 percent of newborns were screened, she says, and only at major hospitals in larger cities.[8] (#361) Shirley Sparks of Western Michigan University, representing the American Speech-Language-Hearing Association, calls for screening of high-risk

infants. (#396)

Witnesses agree about the importance of proper diagnosis and treatment of otitis media in children as a means of preventing hearing loss. Glenna Jojola-Ellison of the All Indian Pueblo Council calls for a 50 percent reduction in the incidence of diagnosed otitis media by the year 2000. Her strategy for reducing the incidence and severity of the condition includes improved prenatal care, development of high-risk registries, encouragement of breast-feeding or discouragement of bottle propping, isolation of sick children in day-care/group baby-sitting environments, and eliminating exposure to cigarette smoke. She and others also emphasize the importance of public education about the dangers and signs of early ear disease. (#113) Hearing loss in young children is especially dangerous because it can interfere with language development. Jojola-Ellison emphasizes the importance of addressing problems related to hearing loss, such as learning disabilities. (#113) Downs suggests as a target for the year 2000 that 80 percent of primary care physicians screen all children age 1 to 3 for language delays from recurrent otitis media. Professional medical organizations should provide training materials for physicians and develop ways to make the screening cost-effective and routine. (#361) Sparks emphasizes the need to educate care givers about conditions that put language development at risk. (#396)

Testimony on hearing loss also emphasizes noise reduction. Witnesses cite several sources of potentially dangerous noise. According to one witness, musicians suffer hearing loss and research is needed into ways to control noise damage. (#152) Sally Lusk of the University of Michigan says that 14 million workers are exposed to hazardous noise,[9] and because the noise is not always controllable, protective devices are needed. However, she describes the difficulty in convincing workers to use these devices and urges research into ways to achieve better compliance. (#424)

Others speak of controlling community noise from sources as diverse as rock music and rifles. Michael Marge of Syracuse University proposes that by the year 2000, 80 percent of states and their communities have ordinances prohibiting hazardous noise levels. (#433) Downs suggests that by the year 2000, 50 percent of the population should be able to identify noxious noise that may endanger their hearing and should possess or know how to obtain adequate ear protection for unavoidable harmful noise levels. (#361)

In addition to prevention of hearing loss, some testifiers call for reducing secondary disability from hearing loss that has been sustained. Sparks says that by the year 2000, disability from communication disorders among the elderly should be reduced by increasing the use of assistive devices and other support measures. She suggests as an objective that there be no increase in the incidence of communication disorders, despite the projected increase in the number of elderly. *(#396)*

VISION DISORDERS

Vision impairments are a common problem in the United States. According to testifiers, more than 11.4 million Americans are visually impaired, and about 500,000 are legally blind. More than 100 million Americans wear corrective lenses.[10] *(#758)* Testifiers link vision impairment to a large number of problems, including unintentional injury, poor school performance, reduced work productivity, and decreased alertness or independence among the elderly because of sensory deprivation. *(#213)* Good vision also is related to the safe operation of motor vehicles, and Robert Kleinstein of the University of Alabama at Birmingham recommends that by the year 2000, all drivers be tested for vision when renewing their driver's licenses. *(#720)*

Testimony from the American Public Health Association (APHA) Vision Care Section identifies several areas for increased public awareness, including the importance of early detection and treatment of eye problems and the role of environmental factors, such as posture, nutrition, and luminance, in vision problems.

About one out of every 20 Americans has low vision. Many are unable to read ordinary print or watch television, even with correctional glasses or contact lenses. Low vision problems range from legal blindness to any vision impairment that, even with conventional glasses, prevents participating in or enjoying a desired visual activity.

The APHA notes that individuals with low vision should be alerted that they probably can be helped. *(#758)* According to John Tumblin of the American Optometric Association (AOA), most people with low vision can achieve vision improvement with professional help. *(#213)*

Several witnesses emphasize the importance of regular eye exams for everyone from preschoolers to older people. Robert Reinecke of the American Academy of Ophthalmology emphasizes that traditional school vision-testing programs are not enough. "Unfortunately, these exams usually are done for children over six years of age, thus missing the children at the time that they are most susceptible to treatment of the visual loss." *(#455)* He and others call for vision screening in schools and preschools to reach the very young. *(#455; #720)*

To increase the number of eye exams among the elderly, the AOA proposes that routine vision services be available under Medicare Part B for all older patients, especially those who are in institutions or homebound. *(#455)* In an effort to help the disadvantaged elderly gain access to quality eye care, the American Academy of Ophthalmology has a toll-free number through which those 65 and older can be assigned to a nearby volunteer ophthalmologist who will either accept insurance or give them free care, if needed, and who will provide follow-up. *(#068; #455)*

The APHA says that by the year 2000, employers should be fully informed about the importance of establishing an occupational vision program. *(#198)* The AOA proposes on-the-job vision assessment and calls for a 50 percent reduction in eye injuries in industry from 1990 levels. It also emphasizes the need of eye protection for athletes and those regularly exposed to ultraviolet radiation. *(#213)*

Saunders Hupp of the University of South Alabama discusses the ocular complications of diabetes: diabetes is the leading cause of new blindness among adults age 20 to 74, but it can be prevented with early intervention.[11] Hupp calls for a 60 percent reduction in the incidence of legal blindness due to diabetes by the year 2000; this can be achieved if all segments of the population receive eye exams early enough to detect problems when they are treatable. Hupp notes that large numbers of diabetics— especially indigent people—are not receiving regular eye exams and says that physicians should be educated about new eye treatments for diabetes patients. *(#265)*

DEVELOPMENTAL AND CHRONIC DISABILITIES

Although disabilities originate from a variety of sources and at various times, testimony often focused on problems common to all disabled people. One issue raised several times is lack of access to health services, especially preventive services, which is discussed in detail in Chapters 7 and 8.

Another approach is to reduce secondary disabilities in disabled people. For example, several witnesses mention the problem of decubitus ulcers, both in the context of the disabled and in relation to the elderly and acute care hospital patients. *(#087; #139; #568; #639; #732)*

In addition to these general goals for the disabled, several specific disabilities were discussed in testimony. Mental retardation received the most comments. However, the point also was made that the most common conditions often get the most attention whereas many other conditions—often classified as "other"—get short shrift from planners despite the extensive morbidity associated with them. *(#420)* Drake and Dolsen mention postpolio sequelae, lupus, myasthenia gravis, multiple sclerosis, chronic viral diseases, and other examples. *(#420)*

Dementia and Alzheimer's disease also are identified by witnesses as important chronic illnesses, especially in the elderly. According to a survey conducted by reviewer Robert Katzman, University of California, San Diego, the incidence of new cases of dementia in those age 80 in New York is as great or greater than that of myocardial infarction, and exceeds that of stroke.[12] These conditions are not preventable, and individuals with them are likely to have additional disabilities, he notes. *(#794)*

Mental Retardation

Approximately 2–3 percent of babies born each year will be diagnosed at some point in their lives as mentally retarded.[13] *(#048)* Witnesses from organizations representing the mentally retarded emphasize that many of these cases are preventable.

Mary De Riso of the American Association on Mental Retardation (AAMR) says that both psychosocial and biomedical prevention activities are necessary. Poverty; lack of economic opportunity; and inadequate jobs, nutrition, or housing all contribute to mental retardation and should be addressed, according to De Riso. On the biomedical side, the AAMR seeks increased support for immunization programs, prenatal care, mandatory lead screening, and other interventions aimed at reducing the incidence of mental retardation. *(#045)*

Several 1990 Objectives are aimed at preventing mental retardation, and Sharon Davis, representing the Association for Retarded Citizens of the United States, urges that these be updated and retained in the Year 2000 Health Objectives. She says that by the year 2000, the prevalence of mental retardation from known causes should be cut in half. *(#048)*

Robert Guthrie of the State University of New York at Buffalo recalls President Nixon saying in 1971 that half of all mental retardation could be prevented with what was known then. This underscores the point he and other witnesses make that knowledge about how to prevent mental retardation has outpaced concerted efforts to achieve these gains. Guthrie notes in particular the need for leadership and coordination at both the national and the state levels. *(#529)* Several witnesses also emphasize the goal of caring for more of the mentally retarded through community health services rather than in institutions by the year 2000. *(#012; #048)* However, Milton Baker of the National Council on the Handicapped recognizes that "such a community direction toward integration requires a disciplined plan of action and cannot take place without multiple supports and built-in monitoring." *(#012)*

REFERENCES

1. National Diabetes Data Group (Ed.): Diabetes in America. (NIH Publication No. 85-1468), August 1985

2. Ibid.

3. National Diabetes Advisory Board: The National Long Range Plan to Combat Diabetes, 1987 (NIH Publication No. 87-1587), 1987

4. NIH Conference proceedings: Consensus Conference: Osteoporosis. J Am Med Assoc 252:799, 1984

5. Lawrence RC, Hochberg MC, Kelsey JL, et al.: Workgroup report: Estimates of the prevalence of selected arthritic and musculoskeletal diseases in the United States. J Rheumatol 16(4):427–441, 1989

6. Ibid.

7. National Center for Health Statistics: Vital and Health Statistics: Current Estimates from the National Health Interview Survey, 1988. Series 10, No. 173 (DHHS Publication No. [PHS] 89-1501), October, 1989

8. Swigart ET (Ed.): Neonatal Hearing Screening. San Diego: College-Hill Press, 1986

9. Occupational Safety and Health Administration: Noise Control. A Guide for Workers and Employers. OSHA 3048, Washington, D.C.: U.S. Department of Labor, 1980

10. American Academy of Ophthalmology: Eye Care for the American People. San Francisco, 1987

11. National Diabetes Data Group: op. cit., reference 1

12. Katzman R, Aronson M, Fuld P, et al.: Development of dementing illnesses in an 80-year-old volunteer cohort. Ann Neurol 25(4):317-324, 1989

13. Oliphant PS, Geiger-Parker B, Gundell GW: Programs for Preventing the Causes of Mental Retardation. Presented to the Governor's Council on the Prevention of Mental Retardation by the Association for Retarded Citizens, New Jersey. New Brunswick: New Jersey Governor's Council on the Prevention of Mental Retardation, 1985

TESTIFIERS CITED IN CHAPTER 27

012 Baker, Milton; Syracuse Developmental Services Office
030 Bruemmer, Barbara; Pacific Medical Center and Fontana, Darlene; University Hospital (Seattle)
045 De Riso, Mary; American Association on Mental Retardation
048 Davis, Sharon; Association for Retarded Citizens of the United States
061 Esdale, Anne; Michigan Chapter, Society for Public Health Education
068 Garber, Norma; American Association of Certified Allied Health Personnel in Ophthalmology
087 Haus, Therese; Columbia University
113 Jojola-Ellison, Glenna; The All Indian Pueblo Council (Albuquerque)
116 Kirchner, Corinne; American Foundation for the Blind
132 Liang, Matthew; Harvard University
134 Long, Mary; Arthritis Foundation
139 Maklebust, JoAnn; Harper Hospital (Detroit)
152 Monaghan, Susan; Hunter Bellevue School of Nursing
198 Sheps, Cecil; American Public Health Association
213 Tumblin, John; American Optometric Association
214 Turner, Suzanna; National Osteoporosis Foundation
261 Thomas, John and Neser, William; Meharry Medical College
265 Hupp, Saunders; University of South Alabama
281 Greenwald, Maria; University of California, Los Angeles
332 Chestnut, III, Charles; University of Washington
339 Tsuji, Wayne; Washington State Arthritis Foundation
361 Downs, Marion; University of Colorado Health Sciences Center
367 Miller, Paul; University of Colorado Health Sciences Center
373 Lappin, Debra; National Arthritis Foundation
396 Sparks, Shirley; Western Michigan University
410 Hawthorne, Victor; University of Michigan
420 Drake, Patience; Michigan Department of Management and Budget and Dolsen, Robert; Statewide Health Coordinating Council
424 Lusk, Sally; University of Michigan
433 Marge, Michael; Syracuse University

455 Reinecke, Robert; Wills Eye Hospital
457 Altschuler, Alan; Prudential-Bache Securities, Inc.
470 Bright, Frank; Ohio Department of Health
491 Haffner, Steven; University of Texas Health Science Center at San Antonio
496 Young, Eleanor; University of Texas Health Science Center at San Antonio
529 Guthrie, Robert; State University of New York at Buffalo
567 Diehl, Andrew and Stern, Michael; University of Texas Health Science Center at San Antonio
568 Brandon, Jeffrey; University of New Orleans
626 Hiss, Roland; University of Michigan
639 Parrino, Sandra; National Council on the Handicapped
685 Condit, J. Michael; Kelsey-Seybold Clinic
699 Porte, Jr., Daniel; Seattle Veterans Administration Medical Center
720 Kleinstein, Robert; University of Alabama at Birmingham
732 Hill, Nina; International Center for the Disabled
758 Whitener, John; American Public Health Association, Vision Care Section
794 Katzman, Robert; University of California, San Diego

APPENDIX A: TESTIFIERS FOR THE YEAR 2000 HEALTH OBJECTIVES

Acampora, Gabrielle; Greater New York Association of Occupational Health Nurses
Ackerly, Mary Jane, et al.; Southern Arizona Lactation Association
Adams, Frederick; Connecticut Department of Health Services*
Adams, Gordon, Moses, Dennis and Baubman, Janne; Chapman College (San Diego)
Addiss, Susan; Quinnipiack Valley Health District (Connecticut)
Aguirre-Molina, Marilyn and Lubinski, Christine; National Council on Alcoholism*
Ahmed, Ismael; Arab Community Center (ACCESS) (Detroit)
Ahmed, Osman; Meharry Medical College
Ahn, Jung; New York University
Alden, John; American College of Preventive Medicine*
Alderman, E. Joseph; Georgia Department of Human Resources*
Aldrich, Robert; University of Washington
Alexander, K., Pebenito, C. and Meskill, G.; Chapman College (San Diego)
Allen, Nancy; University of California, Los Angeles
Allensworth, Diane; American School Health Association*
Allensworth, Diane; American School Health Association* and Baldi, Susan; Santa Rosa College (San Francisco)
Allukian, Jr., Myron; Boston Department of Health and Hospitals
Altschuler, Alan; Prudential-Bache Securities, Inc.
Ames, Margaret; ASPO/Lamaze Association*
Anderson, Dave; American Automobile Association
Anderson, Jennifer; Colorado State University
Andrew, Sylvia; Our Lady of the Lake University of San Antonio
Angelo, Dolores; University of Colorado Health Sciences Center
Anthony, Virginia; American Association of Child and Adolescent Psychiatry*
Antisdel, Suzanne; Michigan Public Health Association
Archer, Mary; National Wellness Society
Armitage, Karen; New Mexico Health and Environment Department
Arnold, Charles; Metropolitan Life Insurance Company
Arnold, Milton; American Academy of Pediatrics
Arrell, Vernon; Texas Rehabilitation Commission
Artz, Lynn; University of Alabama at Birmingham
Auerbach, Kathleen; University of Chicago, Wyler Children's Hospital
Aust, Carolyn; University of Colorado Health Sciences Center
Austin, Richard; Michigan Department of State Police
Babbitz, Matilda; American Association of Occupational Health Nurses*
Bahr, Raymond; St. Agnes Hospital (Baltimore)
Baker, Marian; Rivertown, Wyoming
Baker, Milton; Syracuse Developmental Services Office
Balassone, Mary Lou; University of Washington
Ballin, Scott; American Heart Association*
Banyay, Beverly; Community College of Beaver County (Pennsylvania)
Banzhaf, III, John; Action on Smoking and Health (Washington, D.C.)
Barkauskas, Violet; University of Michigan
Barnes, Marlene; Taylor, Michigan
Barreras, Rita; Colorado Department of Social Services
Barrett, Tom; Center for Psychological Growth (Denver)
Bastien, Deborah; Galveston, Texas

* Testimony received in writing from a consortium organization, statement attributed to organization.

Batiste, Edna; Detroit Department of Health
Beckerman, Anita; College of New Rochelle (New York)
Beckham, Bradley; Colorado Department of Health*
Beinke, Allen; Texas Water Commission
Bell, Allen; Texas Air Control Board
Bell, Carl; Community Mental Health Council (Chicago)
Bell, Thomas; University of Washington
Benjamin, George; National Safety Council*
Bennett, Ruth; Columbia University
Berg, Alfred; University of Washington
Berliner, Howard; New Jersey Department of Health*
Bermingham, Paula; Clearlake, California
Bernard, Louis; Meharry Medical College
Bernshaw, Nicole; Salt Lake City, Utah
Bernstein, Robert; Texas Department of Health*
Bertin, Joan and Taras, Ana; American Civil Liberties Union Foundation, and Stellman, Jeanne; Columbia University
Besaw, David; Wisconsin Tribal Health Directors
Biery, Richard; Kansas City Health Department
Black, James; Oregon Department of Agriculture
Black, Robert; Monterey, California
Blackburn, George; Harvard University
Blaine, James; American Public Health Association, Laboratory Section*
Blair, Steven; Institute for Aerobics Research (Dallas)
Blayney, Keith; University of Alabama at Birmingham
Blockstein, William; University of Wisconsin-Madison
Blum, Steven; American College Health Association*
Blumenthal, Daniel; American Public Health Association, Medical Care Section*
Blumenthal, Daniel; Morehouse School of Medicine
Bolan, Robert; American Diabetes Association
Boll, Thomas; University of Alabama at Birmingham
Bond, Dorothy; Grose Ile, Michigan
Bonnett, Joyce; Woodhaven, Michigan
Bonta, Diana; Los Angeles Regional Family Planning Council
Bortz, II, Walter; Palo Alto Medical Foundation
Bouldin, Agnes and Ricci, Edmund; University of Pittsburgh
Boylan, Jean; Professional Respite Care (Denver)
Bradley, Chet; Wisconsin Department of Public Instruction
Brand, E. Cabell; Recovery Systems Inc. (Virginia)
Brandon, Jeffrey; University of New Orleans
Bray, George; University of Southern California
Breault, George; U.S. Public Health Service
Breen, James; George Washington University (Washington, D.C.)
Breslow, Lester; University of California, Los Angeles
Brewer, Thomas; Nutrition Action Group (San Francisco)
Bright, Frank; Ohio Department of Health*
Brindis, Claire and Lee, Phillip; University of California, San Francisco
Brinkley, Jr., Fred; Texas State Board of Pharmacy
Brooks, Chet; Texas State Senate
Brooks, Christine; University of Michigan

* Testimony received in writing from a consortium organization, statement attributed to organization.

Brown, John; University of Texas Health Science Center at San Antonio
Brown, Les; Washington Governor's Council on Physical Fitness, Health and Sport
Bruemmer, Barbara; Pacific Medical Center and Fontana, Darlene; University Hospital (Seattle)
Bruhn, John; University of Texas Medical Branch at Galveston
Bruhn, Kathleen; Birmingham Area Council of Camp Fire
Brunswick, Ann and Rier, David; Columbia University
Brunwasser, Albert; Allegheny County Health Department (Pennsylvania)
Bublitz, Deborah; University of Colorado Health Sciences Center
Bukoff, Allen; Wayne State University
Buller, Ann; Texas Department of Human Services
Butcher, Percy; American Dental Association
Buttery, C. M. G.; Virginia Department of Health*
Calderone, Fernando; Lincoln Park, Michigan
Calonge, Ned; University of Colorado Health Sciences Center
Campbell, Jacquelyn; Wayne State University
Campbell, Kay; The Phoenix Project (Kirkland, Washington)
Campbell, Paul; Health Industry Manufacturers Association*
Campos, Beverly; University of Colorado Health Sciences Center
Cardona, Gilbert; Los Angeles Human Relations Commission
Carpenter, Charles C. J.; Brown University
Carr, Katherine; American College of Nurse-Midwives
Carter, William; Seattle Veterans Administration Medical Center
Cave, Ginger; San Antonio Branch, Texas Society to Prevent Blindness
Champion, G. Suzanne; La Leche League International
Chand, Aima; Southwest Detroit Community Mental Health Services
Chang, Francis; South Cove Community Health Center (Boston)
Chater, Shirley; Texas Woman's University
Checkoway, Harvey; University of Washington
Chen, Jr., Moon; Ohio State University
Chestnut, III, Charles; University of Washington
Chiu, Sunny; Michigan Department of Public Health*
Cisneros, Henry; City of San Antonio
Clancy, Nancy, Flood, Jeannette and Witherspoon, Ann; Chapman College (San Diego)
Clark, James; American Optometric Association
Clever, Linda Hawes; Pacific Presbyterian Medical Center (San Francisco)
Clydesdale, F. M.; University of Massachusetts at Amherst
Cohen, Sharon; The University of Rochester
Collen, Morris; The Permanente Medical Group
Collins, Harvey; California Department of Health Services
Condit, J. Michael; Kelsey-Seybold Clinic (Houston)
Conway, Dorothy; California Conference of Local Health Department Nutritionists
Cook, Anne; Seattle, Washington
Cornman, John; The Gerontological Society of America
Corry, Maureen; March of Dimes Birth Defects Foundation*
Crawford, Michael; University of Texas Health Science Center at San Antonio
Crocker, Allen; Children's Hospital (Boston)
Cunningham, Allan; Columbia University
Curtis, Joseph; City of New Rochelle Department of Human Services (New York)
Dahl, Ernest; American River College (Sacramento)

* Testimony received in writing from a consortium organization, statement attributed to organization.

Darity, William; University of Massachusetts at Amherst
Davidson, Ezra; King-Drew Medical Center (Los Angeles)
Davis, A. Conan; Alabama Department of Public Health*
Davis, Sharon; Association for Retarded Citizens of the United States*
De Riso, Mary; American Association on Mental Retardation*
Delgado, Jane; The National Coalition of Hispanic Health and Human Services Organizations (COSSMHO)*
Demmin, Tish; Midwives' Alliance of North America*
Denno, Donna; University of Michigan
Desmarais, Linda; International Lactation Consultant Association*
Dickinson, Dena; California Public Health Association
Dickson, Bob; Texas Commission on Alcohol and Drug Abuse
DiClemente, Ralph; University of California, San Francisco
Diehl, Andrew and Stern, Michael; University of Texas Health Science Center at San Antonio
Dietzen, Karen; International Lactation Consultant Association
Dilloway, Rose; Alliance for the Mentally Ill—Wayne County Coalition
Dodds, Janice; Society for Nutrition Education*
Dohrenwend, Bruce; Columbia University
Dorf, Alexis; Education for Childbirth (Ridgefield, Connecticut)
Dorfman, Sharon; Focus Technologies Corporation (Greenbelt, Maryland)
Dotterer, Betty; American Academy of Ophthalmology*
Dowling, Teri; San Francisco Department of Public Health
Downs, Marion; University of Colorado
Doyle, Radora; Associated Milk Producers
Drake, Patience; Michigan Department of Management and Budget, and Dolsen, Robert; Statewide Health Coordinating Council
Duffy, Kathy; Harborview Medical Center, and Wilkins, Jennifer; Pullman, Washington
Duffy, Sonia; University of Michigan; Michigan Cancer Foundation
Dunn, Marion; Livonia, Michigan
duPont, Terry; American Association for Respiratory Care*
Dwyer, Kevin; National Association of School Psychologists
Easley, Michael; American Association of Public Health Dentistry*
Eberst, Richard; Adelphi University (Long Island)
Edington, D. W.; University of Michigan
Egan, M. Jean; Michigan Dietetic Association
Eichelberger, Martin; Children's Hospital National Medical Center (Washington, D.C.)
Eisenberg, Leon; Harvard University
Ellis, Mary; Iowa Department of Public Health*
Entmacher, Paul; Metropolitan Life Insurance Company
Eriksen, Michael; University of Texas Health Science Center at Houston
Ernst, Eunice K. M.; National Association of Childbearing Centers
Escobedo, Marilyn; Bexar County Hospital, San Antonio
Esdale, Anne; Michigan Chapter, Society for Public Health Education
Ettinger, Ronald; American Society for Geriatric Dentistry
Evans, Caswell; Los Angeles County Department of Health Services
Fainsinger, Ann; Alliance for Aging Research*
Fales, Martha; University of Washington
Farabee, Helen; Benedictine Health Promotion Center (Austin)
Feinstein, Ronald; University of Alabama at Birmingham
Fennelly, Kathy and Cabezas, Dagmaris; Columbia University

* Testimony received in writing from a consortium organization, statement attributed to organization.

Ferguson, Wilda; Virginia Department for the Aging
Fields, M. Joan; Detroit Department of Health
Firman, James; United Seniors Health Cooperative (Washington, D.C.)
Fleming, Lisa; Alabama Dental Hygienists' Association
Fletcher, Carol; Grocery Manufacturers of America*
Floberg, Jill; Olympia Physical Therapy Service
Flores, George; Metropolitan Health District, San Antonio
Flores, Juan; Center for Health Policy Development (San Antonio)
Fosco, Angelo; Laborers' International Union of North America
Foster, Carol; Children's Hospital of Los Angeles
Foster, Sylvia; Best Beginnings (Hillsboro, Oregon)
Fowler, Helene; La Leche League International
Fox, Claude Earl; Alabama Department of Public Health*
Frederick, Jacqueline; New Jersey Department of Education
Free, Alfred; Miles Inc. (Elkhart, Indiana)
Freedman, Mary Anne; Association for Vital Records and Health Statistics*
Freeland, Thomas and Del Polito, Carolyn; American Society of Allied Health Professions*
Freeman, Harold; State University of New York at Buffalo
Freeman, Howard; University of California, Los Angeles
Freeman, S. David, et al.; Lower Colorado River Authority
Frissell, Nelson; City-County Health Department, Casper, Wyoming
Fuhrer, Robert; Lincoln Park, Michigan
Gaffney, Donna; Columbia University
Gaines, George; Detroit Department of Health
Garber, Norma; American Association of Certified Allied Health Personnel in Ophthalmology*
Gardner, Rebecca; National Association of State NET Program Coordinators*
Gargas, Donald; Yakima Valley Farm Workers Clinic (Toppenish, Washington)
Garrison, Preston; National Mental Health Association*
Gartner, Audrey; National Self-Help Clearinghouse
Geyman, John; University of Washington
Gilchrist, Lew; University of Washington
Ginley, Thomas; American Dental Association*
Givens, Austin; American Occupational Medical Association*
Glasscock, Betty; University of Alabama at Birmingham
Glazner, Judith; Denver Department of Health and Hospitals
Gleason, Mary Ann; Denver Health Care for the Homeless Project
Goldberg, Sheldon; American Association of Homes for the Aging*
Goldstein, Bernard; University of Medicine and Dentistry of New Jersey, Robert Wood Johnson Medical School
Goldston, Stephen; University of California, Los Angeles
Gorchow, Margo; Botsford General Hospital (Farmington Hills, Michigan)
Gossett, Leo; Texas Department of Public Safety
Gossman, Marilyn and Walter, Jane; American Physical Therapy Association*
Gossman, Marilyn, et al.; University of Alabama at Birmingham
Gottman, Roberta; Wayne State University
Gragg, Donald; Southern California Permanente Medical Group
Graham, Robert; American Academy of Family Physicians*
Grant, Christine; New Jersey Department of Health*
Grant, Linda; Washington State Association of Alcoholism and Addictions Programs
Gray, Isabel; Texas Woman's University

* Testimony received in writing from a consortium organization, statement attributed to organization.

Grayston, J. Thomas; University of Washington
Greenberg, Michael; Rutgers University
Greenfield, William; New York University
Greenwald, Maria; University of California, Los Angeles
Grieder, Karen; Texas Association of Community Health Centers
Griffith, M. Linden; Washington Seniors Wellness Center
Griffith, Patrick; Morehouse School of Medicine
Grigsby, Sharon; The Visiting Nurse Foundation
Grimord, Mary; Texas Woman's University
Groschel, Dieter; American Society for Microbiology*
Groves, David; Comerica Incorporated (Detroit)
Guerra, Fernando; San Antonio Metropolitan Health District
Gurian, Gary; City of Allentown Bureau of Health (Pennsylvania)
Guthrie, Marilyn; Virginia Mason Clinic (Seattle)
Guthrie, Robert; State University of New York at Buffalo
Hacker, Sylvia; University of Michigan
Haffner, Steven; University of Texas Health Science Center at San Antonio
Hagar, Phyllis; Sacramento/Placer Mental Health Association
Hagens, William; Washington State House of Representatives
Hager, Carl; Citizens Commission on Human Rights, Seattle Chapter
Haggerty, Robert; William T. Grant Foundation (New York)
Hagopian, Agnes; Dearborn, Michigan
Halamandaris, Val; National Association for Home Care*
Hall, Cynthia; Potomac, Maryland
Hall, Euphemia; New York State Hospital Review and Planning Council
Halpin, Thomas and Evans, Karen; Ohio Department of Health*
Han, Eugene E.S.; Korean Health Education, Information and Referral Center (Los Angeles)
Handsfield, H. Hunter; Seattle-King County Department of Public Health
Hanneman, Richard; Salt Institute*
Hanson, Donnie and Vennewitz, Peter; Washington State Department of Social and Health Services*
Hanson, Penelope; Rapid City Regional Hospital (South Dakota)
Hanson, Shirley; The Oregon Health Sciences University
Hargreaves, Margaret, et al.; Meharry Medical College
Harkavy, Lorraine; LMH Health Associates (Potomac, Maryland)
Harmon, Robert; Missouri Department of Health*
Harris, Kathy; Detroit Department of Health
Hartigan, Robert; Michigan State Alliance for the Mentally Ill
Hartwell, Jr., Shattuck; The Cleveland Clinic Foundation
Haus, Therese; Columbia University
Havel, Jim; The National Alliance for the Mentally Ill*
Haviland, James; Seattle, Washington
Hawken, Patty; University of Texas Health Science Center at San Antonio
Hawks, Debra; American Academy of Pediatrics* and American Public Health Association*
Hawthorne, Victor; University of Michigan
Hay, Betty Jo; Mental Health Association in Texas
Hayes-Bautista, David; University of California, Los Angeles
Hayes, Donald; Sara Lee Corporation
Hayes, Ellen; Alliance for the Mentally Ill, Oakland County Michigan
Haynes, Alfred; Charles R. Drew Postgraduate Medical School

* Testimony received in writing from a consortium organization, statement attributed to organization.

Hays, Kathy; Crofton, Maryland
Head, Albert; Detroit Department of Health
Heckmann, Glenn; Texas Board of Pardons and Paroles
Hedrick, Hannah; American Medical Association
Helton, Anne; Bellaire, Texas
Hendee, William; American Medical Association*
Henderson, Claudine; Houston Council on Alcoholism and Drug Abuse
Henderson, Flavia; Mile High Council on Alcoholism and Drug Abuse
Henderson, James; Pacific Bell
Henry, Linda; The Children's Hospital (Denver)
Hernandez, C.; Kentucky Cabinet for Human Resources
Hertel, Victoria; Colorado Department of Health
Heston, Thomas; University of Washington
Heximer-Nelson, Daleen; Lact-Natch Breastfeeding Clinic (Albuquerque)
Heydinger, David; West Virginia Department of Health*
Hickey, Mary Jeanne; Weymouth, Massachusetts
Hill, Elaine and Clark, Casey; University of Colorado Health Sciences Center
Hill, Joseph; Detroit Department of Health
Hill, L. Leighton; University of Texas Health Science Center at Houston
Hill, Nina; National Council on the Handicapped
Hirsch, Pamela; Humana Hospital (Hoffman Estates, Illinois)
Hiss, Roland; University of Michigan
Hoerr, Sharon; Michigan State University
Hollers, Kay; National Association for Home Care*
Holmes, Marge; San Antonio Alliance for the Mentally Ill
Holtan, Neal; St. Paul Department of Community Services
Honer, Vicki; Roanoke Childbirth Educators
Hoover, Stephanie; American Occupational Therapy Association*
Horrigan, Robert; Trenton, New Jersey
Hovell, Mel; San Diego State University
Howe, III, John; University of Texas Health Science Center at San Antonio
Howell, Delores; Royal Oak, Michigan
Hughes, Vergie, et al.; Georgetown University
Hullet, Sandral; West Alabama Health Services
Hunter, Katherine; Baptist Medical Center, Montclair (Alabama)
Hunter, Paul; American Medical Student Association/Foundation*
Hupp, Saunders; University of South Alabama
Hurst, Victor; American Association of Retired Persons*
Hutchins, Earl; National Stroke Association*
Hwalek, Melanie; SPEC Associates (Detroit)
Hyslop, Thomas; Harris County Health Department (Texas)
Igoe, Judith; University of Colorado Health Sciences Center
Isenberg, Henry; Long Island Jewish Medical Center
Isman, Robert; The Association of State and Territorial Dental Directors*
Jackson, Rudolph; Morehouse School of Medicine
Jacobs, Louise; Salt Lake City, Utah
Jacobson, Miriam; Washington Business Group on Health*
Jamieson, Marjorie; The Block Nurse Program (Minneapolis)
Jarrett, Michael; South Carolina Department of Health and Environmental Control*

* Testimony received in writing from a consortium organization, statement attributed to organization.

Jasso, Ricardo; Nosotros Human Services Development (San Antonio)
Jelliffe, Derrick; University of California, Los Angeles
Johnsen, David; Case Western Reserve University
Johnson, Carl; South Dakota Department of Health
Johnson, Dale; University of Houston
Johnson, Dana; Colorado Dental Association
Johnson, Dorothea; AT&T
Johnston, Carden; American Academy of Pediatrics
Johnston, Marlin; Texas Department of Human Services
Jojola-Ellison, Glenna; The All Indian Pueblo Council (Albuquerque)
Jones, Elizabeth; International Lactation Consultant Association
Jones, Jean; Ohio Department of Education
Jones, Tom; Northwest Portland Area Indian Health Board
Jordan, Harold; Meharry Medical College
Joseph, Pat; United States Air Force, Lowry Air Force Base, Denver
Joseph, Stephen; New York City Department of Health
Jubb, Wanda; Michigan Department of Education
Judson, Franklyn; Denver Public Health Department
Jukes, Thomas; University of California, Berkeley
Justice, Blair; University of Texas Health Science Center at Houston
Kahler, Jr., Harold; Wellness Councils of America (WELCOA)
Kamberg, Larry; Washington State Environmental Health Association
Kaminsky, Kenneth; Wayne County Intermediate School District (Michigan)
Karlin, Steve; National Recreation and Park Association*
Katz, Alfred; University of California, Los Angeles
Katz, Jane; Bronx Community College
Katz, Michael; University of Texas Health Science Center at San Antonio
Katzman, Robert; University of California, San Diego
Kauffman, JoAnn; Seattle Indian Health Board
Kay, Clyde; Louisiana Primary Care Association
Kelly, Edna; La Leche League International
Kennedy, Kathleen; Dental Hygienists' Association of the State of New York
Kenney, Lawrence; Washington State Labor Council, AFL-CIO
Kerrigan, Margo; Phoenix Area Indian Health Service
Khoury, Radwan; Arab-American and Chaldean Communities Social Services Council (Detroit)
King, Carole; American Academy of Pediatrics*
King, William; Kohaut, Edward C.; Johnston, F. Carden, et al.; The Children's Hospital of Alabama
Kinsman, Katherine; South Dakota Department of Health*
Kirby, William; Texas Commission on Education
Kirchner, Corinne; American Foundation for the Blind
Kizer, Kenneth; California Department of Health Services*
Klatt, Linda; Minnesota Lactation Consultants
Kleinstein, Robert; University of Alabama at Birmingham
Kligman, Evan; Society of Teachers of Family Medicine
Klingbeil, Karil; University of Washington
Klocke, Francis; American College of Cardiology*
Knight, Sharon, et al.; Tacoma-Pierce County Health Department (Washington)
Kopelman, J. Joshua; The OB-GYN Associates (Denver)
Kopple, Joel; University of California, Los Angeles

* Testimony received in writing from a consortium organization, statement attributed to organization.

Kovar, Richard; Country Doctor Community Clinic (Seattle)
Kramer, Morton; The Johns Hopkins University
Kreyer, Virginia; United Church of Christ
Kullman, Mary Ellen; Arthritis Foundation*
Kunst, Robert; Cure AIDS Now (Miami)
Kuntzleman, Charles; Fitness Finders (Spring Arbor, Michigan)
Kupfer, George; Milwaukee Health Department
Kutner, Linda; Mooresville, North Carolina
Labarthe, Darwin; University of Texas Health Science Center at Houston
Lacayo, Carmela; National Association for Hispanic Elderly*
LaCerva, Victor; New Mexico Health Services Division
Lafferty, William; Washington State Department of Public Health*
Lanese, Mary Grace; St. Luke's Hospital of Kansas City
Lange, Charles; Loyola University (Chicago)
Lappin, Debra; National Arthritis Foundation
Large, Lou; La Porte Independent School District (Texas)
Larsen, Michael; Mississippi State Department of Health*
Lassek, William; Department of Health and Human Services, Region III
Lauwers, Judith; International Lactation Consultants Association
Lawrence, David; Kaiser Foundation Health Plan of Colorado
Lawrence, Marlene; Community Hospital (Battle Creek, Michigan)
Lawrence, Ruth; University of Rochester Medical Center
Leaper, Jeannine; South Coast American Society for Psychoprophylaxis in Obstetrics
Lechowich, Karen, et al.; The American Dietetic Association*
Leininger, Madeleine; Wayne State University
Lester, Betty; Michigan
Leuchter, Henry; Mental Health Association of Franklin County (Ohio)
Leventhal, Marcia; New York University, and BrooksSchmitz, Nancy; Columbia University
Levine, Steven; University of Michigan
Lewis, Charles; Better Breast Health Society (San Antonio)
Liang, Matthew; Harvard University
Lima, Bruno; The Johns Hopkins University
Lipsher, Julian; Hawaii State Department of Health*
Livingston, Charles; Highway Users Federation*
Logan, Thomas; Alliance for Health*
Logsdon, Donald; INSURE Project (New York)
Long, Beverly; World Federation for Mental Health
Long, Mary; Arthritis Foundation*
Longworth, Judith; Detroit Receiving Hospital
Lopez, Alfredo; National Migrant Referral Project
Lopez, Jose; San Antonio Tumor and Blood Clinic
Lorincz, Andrew; University of Alabama at Birmingham
Lourie, Eileen; Phoenix Area Indian Health Service
Love, Melinda; Detroit Department of Health
Lovell, James; National Hearing Aid Society*
Low, Lisa Kane; American College of Nurse-Midwives*
Lucas, Adetokunbo; Carnegie Corporation of New York
Lurie, David; Minneapolis Health Department
Lurie, Sue; Texas College of Osteopathic Medicine

* Testimony received in writing from a consortium organization, statement attributed to organization.

Lusk, Sally; University of Michigan
Lyons, Vern; National Association of Social Workers*
Macdonald, Steven; University of Washington
Mack, Douglas; Kent County Health Department (Michigan)
Mackniesh, Joan; Life Balance Company (Novi, Michigan)
Mahan, Charles; Florida Department of Health and Rehabilitative Services*
Maklebust, JoAnn; Harper Hospital (Detroit)
Maloney, Carol Ann; Rockwood, Michigan
Mangione, Ellen; Colorado Department of Health
Mann, George; Meharry International Health Center
Mann, Margot; Forest Hills Lactation Center (New York)
Manson, Spero; University of Colorado Health Sciences Center
Marge, Michael; Syracuse University
Marine, Susan; Boulder, Colorado
Marine, William; University of Colorado Health Sciences Center
Markstrom, Mae; Lake Superior State University and Baker, Mary and Stanley Light, Dixie; Wellness C.A.R.E.
    Center (Sault Sainte Marie, Michigan)
Marmet, Chele; Lactation Institute and Breastfeeding Clinic (Encino, California)
Marsh, Frank; University of Colorado Health Sciences Center
Martin, A. Damien; Hetrick-Martin Institute (New York)
Martin, Robert; Society of Teachers of Family Medicine
Masheter, Carol; University of Connecticut
Mauer, Alvin and Arreola, Mona; University of Tennessee, Memphis
Maynard, Olivia; Michigan Office of Services to the Aging
Mazur, Ronald; University of Massachusetts at Amherst
McCallum, Charles; University of Alabama at Birmingham
McCardwell, Betty; Dearborn, Michigan
McCarron, David, et al.; The Oregon Health Sciences University
McCarthy, Diane; Health Policy Agenda for the American People (Chicago)
McCreight, Lillian; Association of State and Territorial Directors of Nursing*
McCubbin, Hamilton; National Council on Family Relations
McDonough, Stephen; North Dakota State Department of Health and Consolidated Laboratories*
McEvoy, Marianne; New Born Nursing Concepts (Pequannock, New Jersey)
McFarlane, Judith; Texas Woman's University
McGregor, Deborah; Virgin Islands Department of Health
McGuire, Judi and Crowder, Aletha; The National PTA*
McHugh, Catherine; Cleveland Metropolitan General Hospital
McKinney, Charles; Gay Men's Health Crisis (New York)
McNeely, Simon, Vincent, Edith and Stalvey, J. Rendal; Society of State Directors of Health, Physical Education
    and Recreation*
McNeil, Jo; South Puget Sound Community College
Mecklenburg, Robert; Potomac, Maryland
Medrano, Martha; University of Texas Health Science Center at San Antonio
Meeks, Robert; University of Alabama at Birmingham
Mellinger, Amanda; California State Department of Education
Mendelsohn, Sally; Midwives' Alliance of North America
Mental Health Association in California
Merijanian, Jeanette; The University of Montevallo (Montevallo, Alabama)
Messenger, Tom; Association of Food and Drug Officials*

* Testimony received in writing from a consortium organization, statement attributed to organization.

Metzger, Cheryl and Easley, Michael; American Public Health Association, Dental Health Section*
Michael, Jerrold; University of Hawaii School of Public Health
Michaels, Nancy; La Leche League International
Middaugh, Dan; University of Washington
Miller, Paul; University of Colorado Health Sciences Center
Miller, Sanford; University of Texas Health Science Center at San Antonio
Milne, Thomas; Southwest Washington Health District
Miner, John; Massachusetts Mental Health Center
Misener, Terry; University of South Carolina
Missirlian, Arthur and Missirlian, Penny Ann; Sports Courts (Omaha)
Moldeven, Meyer; Del Mar, California
Monaghan, Susan; Hunter Bellevue School of Nursing
Monahan, Paul; Yakima Valley Farm Workers Clinic (Toppenish, Washington)
Montgomery, William; Mount Carmel Mercy Hospital (Detroit)
Moore, D. L.; Texas Cancer Council
Morrison, Jacqueline; Wayne State University
Morse, Roy; Institute of Food Technologists
Morton, Max; Adolph Coors Company
Moss, Stephen; American Academy of Pediatric Dentistry*
Moss, Stephen; New York University
Mossinghoff, Gerald; Pharmaceutical Manufacturers Association*
Mostow, Steven; Rose Medical Center (Denver)
Motta, Glenda; International Association for Enterostomal Therapy*
Mulford, Christine; International Lactation Consultant Association of Eastern Pennsylvania
Mullan, Ronald; Dearborn, Michigan
Mullen, Patricia; University of Texas Health Science Center at Houston
Mullins, Stella; Mental Health Association in Texas
Mundinger, Mary; Columbia University
Munoz, Eric; Long Island Jewish Medical Center
Murphy, Sheldon; University of Washington
Murtaugh, Alice; New York
Myers, Hurley; Southern Illinois University
Myers, Toby; The Pivot Group (Houston)
Myers, Jr., Woodrow; Indiana State Board of Health*
Nakamura, Peter; Portland Area Indian Health Service
Neifert, Marianne; St. Luke's Hospital (Denver)
Neill, Carol; Alum Rock Union Elementary School District (California)
Newall, Guy and LeMaistre, Charles; University of Texas Health Science Center at Houston
Newbrun, Ernest; The Dental Health Foundation (San Rafael, California)
Newcomer, Robert and Pasick, Rena; University of California, San Francisco
Newman, Cyndi; Clallam County Department of Health (Washington)
Nicola, Bud; Seattle-King County Department of Public Health
Nitzkin, Joel; Monroe County Health Department (New York)
Niwinski, Richard, Davis, Terry and Yanchek, Rosemary; Chapman College (San Diego)
Norman, Ann Duecy; University of Washington
Norris, Emilie; Westland, Michigan
Novack, Thomas and Stover, Samuel; University of Alabama at Birmingham
O'Brien, Patricia; Royal Oak, Michigan
O'Gorman, Leo; Brazoria County Health Department (Texas)

* Testimony received in writing from a consortium organization, statement attributed to organization.

O'Malley, Patrick and Johnston, Lloyd; University of Michigan
O'Reilly, Maureen; Dearborn, Michigan
O'Rourke, Thomas; University of Illinois
Oberle, Mark; University of Washington
Oderkirk, Donald; Berrien County Health Department (Michigan)
Oliva, Michael; Aurora, Colorado
Olsen, Larry and St. Pierre, Richard; Pennsylvania State University
Orlandi, Mario; American Health Foundation
Orleans, Miriam; University of Colorado Health Sciences Center
Ortega, Herbert; Pan American Health Organization
Osterbusch, Suzanne; National Council for the Education of Health Professionals in Health Promotion*
Ostergren, Walter; Life Planning/Health Services, Inc. (Dallas)
Ostfeld, Adrian; Yale University
Ostrowski, John; Michigan
Owen, Jack; American Hospital Association*
Papenfuss, Richard; Association for the Advancement of Health Education*
Parcel, Guy; University of Texas Health Science Center at Houston
Parker, John; Detroit Department of Health
Paronich, Elizabeth; Plymouth, Massachusetts
Parrino, Sandra; National Council on the Handicapped*
Pate, Russell; University of South Carolina
Patrick, Donald; University of Washington
Perry, Jean; American Alliance for Health, Physical Education, Recreation and Dance*
Pessl, Molly; Evergreen Hospital Medical Center (Kirkland, Washington)
Philipps, Carol; Wisconsin Department of Public Instruction
Phillips, Karen; Birmingham, Alabama
Pinckney, Edward; Beverly Hills, California
Piper, Lynne; Carol County Health Department (Maryland) and Van Doren, Sandy; Westminster, Maryland
Pitkin, Ila; Richland, Washington
Player, Ernestine; Association of State and Territorial Public Health Social Work*
Porte, Jr., Daniel; Seattle Veterans Administration Medical Center
Powell, Shirley; Southeastern Michigan Food Coalition
Pratt, David; Mary Imogene Bassett Hospital (Cooperstown, New York)
Prothrow-Stith, Deborah; Massachusetts Department of Public Health*
Pulrang, Peter; Washington State Bureau of Parent and Child Health Services
Quick, James; University of Texas at Arlington
Rader, Herbert; The Salvation Army in the United States
Ramos, Leonor; San Antonio District Dental Hygienist Society
Randolph, Linda; New York State Department of Health*
Ranney, Helen; University of California, San Diego
Raven, Peter and Drinkwater, Barbara; American College of Sports Medicine*
Reault, Hilda; Livonia, Michigan
Reeves, Philip; American Public Health Association, Community Health Planning Section*
Reger, Roy; Colorado Department of Health
Reid, Elaine; Sacred Heart Medical Center (Spokane, Washington)
Reinecke, Robert; Wills Eye Hospital (Philadelphia)
Reiss, Joan; Mental Health Association, Sacramento-Placer
Reveal, Marge; American Dental Hygienists' Association*
Rice, Dorothy; University of California

* Testimony received in writing from a consortium organization, statement attributed to organization.

Rice, Ilene; Heartstart Publications (St. Paul)
Rice, Katharine; Carleton, Michigan
Richards, N. Mark; Pennsylvania Department of Health*
Richards, Rebecca; North Woods Health Careers Consortium (Wausau, Wisconsin)
Richards, Ruth; University of California, Los Angeles
Richardson, Donald; Los Angeles, California
Richland, Jud; Association of State and Territorial Health Officials*
Riordan, Hugh; Oliva W. Garvey Center for the Improvement of Human Functioning (Wichita)
Ripple, Florence; Alliance for Mentally Ill, Downriver (Romulus, Michigan)
Rivara, Frederick; Harborview Injury Prevention and Research Center (Seattle)
Robinson, Joseph; Lonza Inc. (Fairlawn, New Jersey)
Robinson, William; University of Colorado Health Sciences Center
Rockwell, Bruce; The Colorado Trust
Rodriguez, Gloria; Sea-Mar Home Health Services (Seattle)
Roemer, Milton; University of California, Los Angeles
Roemer, Ruth; University of California, Los Angeles
Rogers, Paul; Hogan and Hartson (Washington, D.C.)
Roland, Deborah; Seattle-King County Department of Public Health
Romero, Emilio; University of Texas Health Science Center at San Antonio
Romney, Seymour; Albert Einstein College of Medicine of Yeshiva University
Rose, Annette; Mount Vernon Neighborhood Health Center (Yonkers, New York)
Rose, Jackie; Clackamas County Department of Human Services (Oregon)
Rosenblatt, Roger; University of Washington
Rosenfield, Allan; Columbia University
Rosner, Robert; Smoking Policy Institute (Seattle)
Ross, James; Maryland
Roth, Jeff; National Research Council
Rothert, Marilyn; Michigan State University
Russ, Blanche; Parent-Child, Inc. (San Antonio)
Rutman, Robert; University of Pennsylvania
Ruzek, Sheryl; Temple University
Saalberg, James; CUNA Mutual Insurance Group
Salas, Nancy and McCurdy, Robert; Colorado Department of Health*
Salive, Marcel and Parkinson, Michael; Association of Preventive Medicine Residents
Salive, Marcel and Wolfe, Sidney; Public Citizen Health Research Group (Washington, D.C.)
Sall, James; Detroit Department of Health
Samuelson, Carole; Jefferson County Department of Health (Alabama)
Sanders, Louise; Board of Nurse Examiners (Texas)
Santee, Barbara; Women and AIDS Resource Network
Santee, Barbara and Alexander, Alpha; National Board of the YWCA of the U.S.A.
Sapp, Mary; Benedictine Health Resource Center (San Antonio)
Schadegg, Kira, et al.; Huntingdon Valley Nursing Mothers (Pennsylvania)
Scheckler, William; University of Wisconsin
Schiff, Donald; American Academy of Pediatrics
Schlegel, John; American Pharmaceutical Association*
Schlotfeldt, Rozella; Cleveland Heights, Ohio
Schmidt, William; Wisconsin Division of Health
Schoewe, Hazel; Dearborn Heights, Michigan
Schopp, Rae; La Leche League International

* Testimony received in writing from a consortium organization, statement attributed to organization.

Schramm, Carl; Health Insurance Association of America*
Schumacher, Karin; National Stroke Association
Schwartz, Randy; Society for Public Health Education*
Schwarz, Lewis; Morristown Memorial Hospital (New Jersey)
Schwarz, Richard; State University of New York Health Science Center at Brooklyn
Schweers, Nancy; Travis Park Infant Nutrition Program (San Antonio)
Scitovsky, Anne; Palo Alto Medical Foundation
Scott, H. Denman; Rhode Island Department of Health
Scott, Roseann; University of Colorado Health Sciences Center
Seffrin, John, et al.; American School Health Association*
Segal, Tobelle; California Dental Hygienists Association
Setton, Sarah; The Sugar Association
Sharkey, Brian; University of Northern Colorado
Sheehan, George; The Second Wind, Inc. (Red Bank, New Jersey)
Sheps, Cecil; American Public Health Association*
Shoults, Harold; The Salvation Army*
Showstead, Philip; Seattle-King County Department of Public Health
Siefert, Kristine; University of Michigan
Silver, George; Yale University
Singer, Raymond; Mount Sinai School of Medicine
Siscovick, David; University of Washington
Skeels, Michael; Oregon Department of Human Resources
Skrip, Louise; Dearborn, Michigan
Sleet, David; San Diego State University
Sloan, Daniel; Parkview Episcopal Medical Center (Pueblo, Colorado)
Smith, Elizabeth; Miami, Florida
Smith, George; Tennessee Department of Health and Environment*
Smith, Linda; Mary Immaculate Hospital (Yorktown, Virginia)
Smith, Marie; American Society of Hospital Pharmacists*
Smith, Peggy B.; Baylor College of Medicine
Smith, Richard; Henry Ford Hospital (Detroit)
Sneegas, Karla; South Carolina Department of Education
Sobel, David; The Permanente Medical Group
Society for Prospective Medicine
Somers, Anne; University of Medicine and Dentistry of New Jersey, and Weisfeld, Victoria; Robert Wood Johnson
    Foundation
Sowinski, Joan; Colorado Department of Health
Spain, Carol; Health Officers Association of California
Spannraft, Elizabeth; Libertyville, Illinois
Sparks, Shirley; Western Michigan University
Spear, Robert; University of California, Berkeley
Speckmann, Elwood; National Dairy Council*
Speert, Ellen; American Art Therapy Association
Spencer, William; Baylor University
Spengler, Robert; Vermont Department of Health*
Stevens, Michelle; Severn, Maryland
Stevens, Nancy; Kaiser Permanente, Northwest Region
Stewart, Frances; Michael Reese Hospital and Medical Center (Chicago)
Stock, J. S.; Livonia, Michigan

* Testimony received in writing from a consortium organization, statement attributed to organization.

Stokes, III, Joseph; Boston University
Stoto, Michael; Institute of Medicine
Stout, Chuck; Colorado Department of Health
Stover, Samuel; University of Alabama at Birmingham
Strantz, Irma; Los Angeles County Department of Health Services
Strauther, John; Detroit Department of Health
Strembel, Shirley; Arizona Healthy Mothers, Healthy Babies
Sugarman, James; National Association of Retired Senior Volunteer Program Directors*
Sugarman, Jule; Washington State Department of Social and Health Services*
Sullivan, Daniel; Hawaii Department of Education
Sumaya, Ciro; University of Texas Health Science Center at San Antonio
Surgeon General's Workshop on Health Promotion and Aging
Swanson, Terri; Colorado Dental Hygienists' Association
Sweezy, Sandra; Beth Israel Hospital (Boston)
Sykes, James; The National Council on the Aging*
Tableman, Betty; Michigan Department of Mental Health
Tallia, Alfred, Spitalnik, Debbie and Like, Robert; University of Medicine and Dentistry of New Jersey
Tarrant, Karen; Michigan Department of State Police
Teague, Wayne; Alabama Department of Education
Thomas, John and Neser, William; Meharry Medical College
Thompson, Alvin; University of Washington
Thompson, Ellen; American Public Health Association, Food and Nutrition Section*
Tice, R. Dean; National Recreation and Park Association*
Tiedje, Linda; Michigan State University
Toler, Fred; Texas Commission on Law Enforcement Officer Standards and Education
Tomaino, Louis; Our Lady of the Lake University of San Antonio
Tonsberg, Robert; Indian Health Service/Wind River Indian Reservation (Fort Washakie, Wyoming)
Trager, Frances; Alliance for the Mentally Ill of Michigan
Treser, Charles; University of Washington
Trietsch, Gary; Texas State Department of Highways and Public Transportation
Trinca, Carl; American Association of Colleges of Pharmacy*
Trostmann, Cathy; Houston, Texas
Truhe, Thomas; Princeton Dental Resource Center
Tsuji, Wayne; Washington State Arthritis Foundation
Tucker, Gary; University of Washington
Tumblin, John; American Optometric Association*
Turner, Ronald; Community Health Awareness Group (Detroit)
Turner, Suzanna; National Osteoporosis Foundation*
Turnock, Bernard; Illinois Department of Public Health*
Utah Nutrition Council
Van Citters, Robert; University of Washington
VanDermeer, Leslie; Hunter College (New York)
Varkaly, Elizabeth; Garden City, Michigan
Vash, Carolyn; Altadena, California
Vida, George; Flat Rock, Michigan
Vigil, Everett; The Jicarilla Apache Tribe (Dulce, New Mexico)
Volle, Robert; National Board of Medical Examiners*
Waddill, Louise; Board of Nurse Examiners for the State of Texas
Waedemon, Betty; American Dental Hygienists' Association

* Testimony received in writing from a consortium organization, statement attributed to organization.

Wagner, Betty; La Leche League International*
Wagner, Edward; Group Health Cooperative of Puget Sound
Waldrep, Kent; Kent Waldrep National Paralysis Foundation (Dallas)
Wallace, Jr., William; New Hampshire Division of Public Health Services
Waller, John; Wayne State University
Wandberg, Robert; Minnesota Department of Education, and Geer, Lois; University of Minnesota
Wardrop, Richard; Aluminum Company of America
Warner, Kenneth; University of Michigan
Warshaw, Leon; New York Business Group on Health
Washam, W. Thomas; Aluminum Company of America
Watanabe, Michael; Asian Pacific Planning Council (Los Angeles)
Watkins, Jr., Thomas; Michigan Department of Mental Health
Watts, Malcolm S. M.; University of California, San Francisco
Weiner, Lyn and Morse, Barbara; Boston University
Weinstein, I. Bernard; Columbia University
Weintraub, Jane; University of Michigan
Welch, Dick; Minnesota Department of Health*
Welch, Robert and Sokol, Robert; Wayne State University/Hutzel Hospital (Detroit)
Weller, Thomas; Harvard University
Wente, Susan; Jefferson Davis Hospital (Houston)
Wentworth, Berttina; American Public Health Association, Laboratory Section*
West, Jack; Puro Corporation of America (Maspeth, New York)
West, Jerome; Five Sandoval Indian Pueblos, Inc. (Bernillo, New Mexico)
West, M. Patricia; Colorado Department of Health
West, Margaret; University of Washington
White, Francine; National Association of Community Health Centers*
Whitener, John; American Public Health Association, Vision Care Section*
Wieland, Holly; Silver Spring, Maryland
Wiener, Raj; Michigan Department of Public Health*
Wilburn, Susan; Pacific Medical Center (Seattle)
Wilhoit, Gene; National Association of State Boards of Education*
Wilkinson, William; University of Washington
Williams, Corinne; California Dietetic Association
Williams, Diane; Hospice Home Health (San Antonio)
Williams, James; National Education Association, Health Information Network*
Williams, Robert; Baylor College of Medicine
Williamson, Donald; Alabama Department of Public Health
Wilson, Marjorie; Olympia, Washington
Winawer, H.; Utah State Office of Education
Windle, Anne; American Public Health Association, Public Health Education Section*
Windsor, Richard; University of Alabama at Birmingham
Winfree, Jeanette; Physical Therapy Services (Galveston, Texas)
Wirtschafter, David; Southern California Kaiser Permanente
Wood, Loring; NYNEX Corporation
Woodrum, James; Wellness and Prevention Program, Inc. (Houston)
Wooldridge, Nancy; Alabama Dietetic Association
Work, Rebecca; University of Alabama at Birmingham
Wright, Al; County of Los Angeles Department of Health Services
Wright, Terri; Detroit/Wayne County Infant Health Promotion Coalition

* Testimony received in writing from a consortium organization, statement attributed to organization.

Yaffe, Bertram; New England Conference for Disease Prevention, Health Protection and Health Promotion (NECON)

Young, Alma; Mount Sinai School of Medicine

Young, Eleanor; University of Texas Health Science Center at San Antonio

Young, James; University of Texas Health Science Center at San Antonio

Young, Rosalie; Wayne State University

Young, "Snip" Walter; Colorado Department of Health*

Zal, Harriette; Southern California Association of Occupational Health Nurses

Zerger, Ardis; Dearborn, Michigan

Zielinski, Linda; Boise, Idaho

Zito, Dominick S.; Preventive*PLUS (Paramus, New Jersey)

Zola, Irving; Brandeis University

Zuzich, Ann; Wayne State University

---

* Testimony received in writing from a consortium organization, statement attributed to organization.

APPENDIX B: YEAR 2000 HEALTH OBJECTIVES CONSORTIUM

National Organizations

Academy of General Dentistry
Aerobics and Fitness Association of America
Alcohol and Drug Problems Association of North America
Alliance for Aging Research
Alliance for Health
Amateur Athletic Union
American Academy of Child and Adolescent Psychiatry
American Academy of Family Physicians
American Academy of Ophthalmology
American Academy of Orthopaedic Surgeons
American Academy of Pediatric Dentistry
American Academy of Pediatrics
American Alliance for Health, Physical Education, Recreation and Dance
American Art Therapy Association
American Association for Clinical Chemistry
American Association for Dental Research
American Association for Marriage and Family Therapy
American Association for Respiratory Care
American Association for the Advancement of Science
American Association of Certified Orthoptists
American Association of Colleges of Pharmacy
American Association of Dental Schools
American Association of Homes for the Aging
American Association of Occupational Health Nurses
American Association of Pathologists' Assistants
American Association of Public Health Dentistry
American Association of Public Health Physicians
American Association of Retired Persons
American Association of School Administrators
American Association of Suicidology
American Association of University Affiliated Programs for Persons with Developmental Disabilities
American Association on Mental Retardation
American Cancer Society
American College Health Association
American College of Cardiology
American College of Clinical Pharmacy
American College of Health Care Administrators
American College of Healthcare Executives
American College of Nurse-Midwives
American College of Nutrition
American College of Obstetricians and Gynecologists
American College of Occupational Medicine
American College of Physicians
American College of Preventive Medicine
American College of Radiology
American College of Sports Medicine
American Council on Alcholism
American Dental Association

American Dental Hygienists' Association
American Diabetes Association
American Dietetic Association
American Federation of Teachers
American Geriatrics Society
American Heart Association
American Home Economics Association
American Hospital Association
American Indian Health Care Association
American Institute for Preventive Medicine
American Institute of Nutrition
American Kinesiotherapy Association
American Lung Association
American Meat Institute
American Medical Association
American Medical Student Association
American Nurses' Association
American Nutritionists Association
American Occupational Therapy Association
American Optometric Association
American Orthopaedic Society for Sports Medicine
American Osteopathic Academy of Sports Medicine
American Osteopathic Association
American Osteopathic Hospital Association
American Pharmaceutical Association
American Physical Therapy Association
American Physiological Society
American Podiatric Medical Association
American Psychiatric Association
American Psychiatric Nurses' Association
American Psychological Association
American Public Health Association
American Red Cross
American Rehabilitation Counseling Association
American School Food Service Association
American School Health Association
American Social Health Association
American Society for Clinical Nutrition
American Society for Microbiology
American Society for Parenteral and Enteral Nutrition
American Society of Acupuncture
American Society of Addiction Medicine
American Society of Allied Health Professions
American Society of Hospital Pharmacists
American Society of Human Genetics
American Society of Ocularists
American Speech-Language-Hearing Association
American Spinal Injury Association
American Statistical Association
American Thoracic Society
Arthritis Foundation
Asian American Health Forum

ASPO/Lamaze Association
Association for Applied Psychophysiology and Biofeedback
Association for Fitness in Business
Association for Hospital Medical Education
Association for Practitioners in Infection Control
Association for Retarded Citizens of the United States
Association for the Advancement of Automotive Medicine
Association for the Advancement of Health Education
Association for Vital Records and Health Statistics
Association of Academic Health Centers
Association of American Indian Physicians
Association of American Medical Colleges
Association of Clinical Scientists
Association of Community Health Nursing Educators
Association of Food and Drug Officials
Association of Maternal and Child Health Programs
Association of Pediatric Oncology Nurses
Association of Rehabilitation Nurses
Association of Schools of Public Health
Association of State and Territorial Dental Directors
Association of State and Territorial Directors of Nursing
Association of State and Territorial Directors of Public Health Education
Association of State and Territorial Health Officials
Association of State and Territorial Public Health Laboratory Directors
Association of State and Territorial Public Health Nutrition Directors
Association of State and Territorial Public Health Social Work
Association of Teachers of Preventive Medicine
Association of Technical Personnel in Ophthalmology
Black Congress on Health, Law and Economics
Blue Cross and Blue Shield Association
Boys Scouts of America
Business Roundtable
Camp Fire
Cardiovascular Credentialling International
Catholic Health Association of the United States
Chamber of Commerce of the United States
Children's National Medical Center
College of American Pathologists
Council for Responsible Nutrition
Council of Medical Specialty Societies
Dairy and Food Nutrition Council of the Southeast
Emergency Nurses Association
Eye Bank Association of America
Federation of American Societies for Experimental Biology
Federation of Nurses and Health Professionals (AFT)
Food Marketing Institute
Future Homemakers of America
Gerontological Society of America
Girl Scouts of the United States of America
Great Lakes Association of Clinical Medicine
Grocery Manufacturers of America
Group Health Association of America

Health Industry Manufacturers Association
Health Insurance Association of America
Highway Users Federation for Safety and Mobility
Institute of Food Technologists
International Association for Enterostomal Therapy
International Lactation Consultant Association
International Life Sciences Institute
International Patient Education Council
La Leche League International
Learning Disabilities Association of America
March of Dimes Birth Defects Foundation
Maternal and Child Health Network
Maternity Center Association
Midwives' Alliance of North America
Migrant Clinicians Network
Mothers Against Drunk Driving
National AIDS Network
National Alliance for the Mentally Ill
National Alliance of Black School Educators
National Alliance of Nurse Practitioners
National Association for Hispanic Elderly
National Association for Home Care
National Association for Human Development
National Association for Music Therapy
National Association for Sport and Physical Education
National Association of Biology Teachers
National Association of Childbearing Centers
National Association of Community Health Centers
National Association of Counties
National Association of County Health Officials
National Association of Elementary School Principals
National Association of Governors Council on Physical Fitness and Sports
National Association of Neonatal Nurses
National Association of Optometrists and Opticians
National Association of Pediatric Nurse Associates and Practitioners
National Association of Retail Druggists
National Association of RSVP Directors
National Association of School Nurses
National Association of Secondary School Principals
National Association of Social Workers
National Association of State Alcohol and Drug Abuse Directors
National Association of State Boards of Education
National Association of State NET Program Coordinators
National Black Nurses' Association
National Board of Medical Examiners
National Center for Health Education
National Coalition of Hispanic Health and Human Services Organizations (COSSMHO)
National Commission Against Drunk Driving
National Committee for Adoption
National Committee for Prevention of Child Abuse
National Conference of State Legislatures
National Consumers League

National Council for International Health
National Council for the Education of Health Professionals in Health Promotion
National Council on Alcoholism and Drug Dependence
National Council on Disability
National Council on Health Laboratory Services
National Council on Patient Information and Education
National Council on Self-Help and Public Health
National Council on the Aging
National Dairy Council
National Environmental Health Association
National Extension Homemakers Council
National Family Planning and Reproductive Health Association
National Federation of State High School Associations
National Food Processors Association
National Head Injury Foundation
National Health Council
National Health Lawyers Association
National Hearing Aid Society
National Institute for Fitness and Sport
National Kidney Foundation
National League for Nursing
National Lesbian and Gay Health Foundation
National Medical Association
National Mental Health Association
National Museum of Health and Medicine
National Nurses Society on Addictions
National Organization for Women
National Organization on Adolescent Pregnancy and Parenting
National Osteoporosis Foundation
National Pest Control Association
National Pressure Ulcer Advisory Panel
National PTA
National Recreation and Park Association
National Safety Council
National School Boards Association
National Society of Allied Health
National Society to Prevent Blindness
National Strength and Conditioning Association
National Stroke Association
National Wellness Institute
National Women's Health Network
NEA Health Information Network
Nursing Network on Violence Against Women
Oncology Nursing Society
Organization for Obstetric, Gynecologic, and Neonatal Nurses (NAACOG)
Paralyzed Veterans of America
People's Medical Society
Pharmaceutical Manufacturers Association
Planned Parenthood Federation of America
Population Association of America
Produce Marketing Association
Salt Institute

Salvation Army
Society for Nutrition Education
Society for Public Health Education
Society of Behavioral Medicine
Society of Hospital Epidemiologists of America
Society of Prospective Medicine
Society of State Directors of Health, Physical Education and Recreation
South Cove Community Health Center
State Family Planning Administrators
United States Conference of Mayors
United Way of America
Visiting Nurse Associations of America
Voluntary Hospitals of America
Washington Business Group on Health
Wellness Councils of America (WELCOA)
Western Consortium for Public Health
Women's Sports Foundation

State Organizations

Alabama
Alaska
American Samoa
Arizona
Arkansas
California
Colorado
Connecticut
Delaware
District of Columbia
Florida
Georgia
Guam
Hawaii
Idaho
Illinois
Indiana
Iowa
Kansas
Kentucky
Louisana
Maine
Maryland
Massachusetts
Michigan
Minnesota
Mississippi
Missouri
Montana
Nebraska
Nevada
New Hampshire

New Jersey
New Mexico
New York
North Dakota
Ohio
Oklahoma
Oregon
Pennsylvania
Puerto Rico
Rhode Island
South Carolina
South Dakota
Tennessee
Texas
Utah
Vermont
Virginia
Washington
West Virginia
Wisconsin
Wyoming

APPENDIX C: LOCAL COSPONSORS FOR YEAR 2000 REGIONAL HEARINGS

Birmingham

University of Alabama at Birmingham, School of Public Health
Alabama Medicaid Agency
Cooperative Health Manpower Education Program
Alabama Department of Public Health
Meharry Medical College
Morehouse School of Medicine
University of Alabama at Birmingham, Geriatric Education Center
Veterans Administration Medical Center

Los Angeles

University of California, Los Angeles, School of Public Health
California Department of Health Services
The Henry J. Kaiser Family Foundation
Charles R. Drew University of Medicine and Science

Houston

Texas Department of Health
University of Texas Health Science Center, School of Public Health
University of Texas Health Science Center, Prevention Center

Seattle

University of Washington, School of Public Health and Community Medicine
Alaska Native Medical Center
American Lung Association of Washington
Center for Health Research, Kaiser Permanente
Coalition for Rural Health
Columbia River Association of Occupational Health Nurses
Department of Health and Human Services, Public Health Service, Region X
Division of Health, Washington State Department of Social and Health Services
Group Health Cooperative of Puget Sound
The Henry J. Kaiser Family Foundation
National Environmental Health Association
Northwest Association of Occupational Medicine
Oregon State Health Division
Oregon State Public Health Association

Washington Association of Occupational Health Nurses
Washington State Association of Local Public Health Officials
Washington State Board of Health
Washington State Environmental Health Association
Washington State Labor Council
Washington State Medical Association
Washington State Nurses Association
Washington State Public Health Association

Denver

University of Colorado Health Sciences Center
Colorado State Health Department
Colorado Action for Healthy People
Colorado Public Health Association

Detroit

Wayne State University
General Motors Corporation
The University of Michigan, School of Public Health
W. K. Kellogg Foundation

New York

Host: Metropolitan Life Insurance Company

Cosponsors:

Columbia University School of Nursing
Columbia University School of Public Health
National Center for Health Education
The New York Business Group on Health